CICELY SAUNDERS

A LIFE AND LEGACY

CICELY SAUNDERS

A LIFE AND LEGACY

BY **DAVID CLARK,** PhD, FAcSS, OBE

School of Interdisciplinary Studies
University of Glasgow
Scotland, UK

Oxford University Press is a department of the University of Oxford. It furthers
the University's objective of excellence in research, scholarship, and education
by publishing worldwide. Oxford is a registered trade mark of Oxford University
Press in the UK and certain other countries.

Published in the United States of America by Oxford University Press
198 Madison Avenue, New York, NY 10016, United States of America.

Library of Congress Cataloging-in-Publication Data
Names: Clark, David, 1953– author.
Title: Cicely Saunders : a life and legacy / by David Clark.
Description: Oxford ; New York : Oxford University Press, [2018]
Identifiers: LCCN 2017052990 | ISBN 9780190637934 (hardback : alk. paper)
Subjects: | MESH: Saunders, Cicely M., Dame. | St. Christopher's Hospice. |
Hospice Care—history | Palliative Care—history | Physicians | History, 20th Century |
England | Biography
Classification: LCC R726.8 | NLM WZ 100 | DDC 616.02/9—dc23
LC record available at https://lccn.loc.gov/2017052990

9 8 7 6 5 4 3

Printed by Sheridan Books, Inc., United States of America

*In memory of my parents – Joseph Henry Winn Clark
and Ethel Clark (née Spavin)*

CONTENTS

ACKNOWLEDGEMENTS

A work so long in gestation as this accumulates many debts of gratitude. I am thankful to all those people who, in varying ways, have assisted me in my endeavour over the years.

To those of you whose interviews have contributed to this book, I am deeply grateful. I am also indebted to those who joined me in conducting some of the interviews. Neil Small deserves a special mention, for his collegiality over many years and for the fascinating material he collected from Cicely Saunders that proved so helpful here. Among other academic colleagues, Jane Seymour, Michelle Winslow, Yasmin Gunaratnum, Carlos Centeno, Lisbeth Thoresen, Michael Wright, Sam Ahmedzai, and Martina Holder have each, at different times, illuminated my understanding of my subject. The several translators of *Watch with Me* have also given encouragement and insight.

At Oxford University Press in New York I had wonderful support. My editor, Andrea Knobloch, showed faith in the project throughout; Rebecca Suzan read and commented helpfully on my early draft chapters; Tiffany Lu gave detailed support in the later stages; Emily Perry was an astute and efficient production editor; and Cat Ohala copy-edited the manuscript with thoroughness and sensitivity.

Additional help on specific matters was given by various people at different points and I thank them for that: Rosemary Burch, Christine Kearney, Aleksander Jedrosz, Robert Twycross, Mary Baines, Gillian Ford, Denise Brady, Balfour Mount, David Allport, Ruth Ashcroft, Anthony Greenwood, Isobel Fitzgerald O'Connor, Avril Jackson, Andrew Goodhead, and Denise Brady.

At the Archives and Special Collections of King's College London, Chris Olver and Lianne Smith helped me enormously, showing great enthusiasm for the work, and, together with their colleagues, made for efficient and very enjoyable archival visits, during which their assistance and attention to detail were exemplary. At Roedean School, Jackie Sullivan, Archivist and Assistant Librarian, and at Dauntsey's School, Julie Romijn, Foundation Office Secretary, were likewise generous and attentive in responding to my requests and preoccupations.

As the holder of a Wellcome Trust Investigator Award during the crucial period of writing this book, I must acknowledge the ongoing support of the Trust. It has given me freedom to work on the biography in detail. In earlier years it supported the oral history work that laid some of the foundation for the current volume, along with two specific Wellcome Witness Seminars which also proved very helpful. Not least, it funded the cataloguing of the Cicely Saunders Archive at King's, that is now such a resource for anyone interested in her life and work.

Whilst writing this book, I have been fortunate to enjoy the support and interest of many colleagues at the University of Glasgow. In addition to those actively involved in the Glasgow End of Life Studies Group, I pay special thanks to Anne Anderson, who has done so much over several years to encourage me in my endeavours and to guide me through the delicate balancing act between personal scholarship and wider academic duties.

My dear friend and fellow sociologist Anne Grinyer read the entire first draft of the manuscript, gave helpful and encouraging feedback, and, through her engagement in the unfolding story, bolstered my confidence and determination to keep going.

Christopher Saunders, Cicely's brother, was tireless in supporting my efforts on numerous occasions, keeping in touch throughout the years, but always with an admirable 'hands off' approach to my writing. His unwavering trust has meant a great deal to me.

Finally, my wife, Fiona Graham, has accepted the distracted presence of life with a biographer. She has tolerated and enjoyed endless anecdotes from me about the life and work of Cicely Saunders, and has cast an eagle eye over passages of my more purple prose. She has been the perfect foil to writing this book and I thank her from the bottom of my heart.

LIST OF FIGURES

CICELY SAUNDERS

A LIFE AND LEGACY

Prologue: Whys and Wherefores

I FIRST GOT TO KNOW Cicely Saunders in 1994 and, throughout the years until her death in 2005, we collaborated on a number of projects, initially focussed around my wish to capture the emerging history of the modern hospice and palliative care movement, and also to preserve its oral testimony and documentary record. She was enthusiastic in her support for my first and rather tentative application to the Wellcome Trust to initiate this work and, like me, was surprised by the broad avenues that later opened up in what at first seemed a rather narrow course of academic endeavour. As this proceeded, I began to understand the colossal contribution that Cicely herself had made to this history and I looked for ways to recognise it in a manner which would be available to others in the future. She had devoted her professional life to a marginal and often undervalued activity — the care of those with advanced and terminal disease. She had forged a clinical model for this work which took account of physical, social, psychological, and spiritual dimensions. She then devised an organisational vehicle which could not only deliver such care, but also could generate and disseminate new knowledge in the field and serve to support those who wished to serve in it. The effects were global in proportion and the reverberations are continuing.

I started my efforts by writing a number of specific and rather focussed articles on her work as well as trying to edit and collate some of her contributions. It was about five years into this process that I realised how important it would be to embark upon a new biography of Cicely, one which would build on and extend the foundational work of Shirley du Boulay, first published in 1984. I wanted to understand better the complex relationship between the personal and the professional aspects of Cicely's life and attempt to see her in a more rounded context. This book is the result.

The wider project began with a series of 'on the record' interviews at St Christopher's Hospice conducted by my colleague Neil Small. I then became actively involved in supporting the initial cataloguing of a large portion of Cicely's papers, mainly those from the 1950s to the 1980s. This was some of the groundwork that led to the eventual full consolidation of her archive at King's College London, where it is now housed as a remarkable resource for research and teaching. Over the years I have enjoyed unfettered access to all of her papers. Through the interviews and particularly the cataloguing, it was possible to get a sense of the tremendous range of Cicely's activities and the depth of influences that had shaped her beliefs, philosophy, and practice. Some of the material was remarkably personal. Close work on the papers also flushed out a vast body of her published writing, some of it hard to access or forgotten, and much of it undocumented in her rather under-stated curriculum vitae. In time, it was possible to assemble a full bibliography of her publications and also to start annotating each one.

Her correspondence was legion. From 1958, when she acquired a secretary and a dictating machine, she wrote often lengthy and rich letters to friends, colleagues, and associates all around the world. I was able to select about seven hundred of these for inclusion in a volume of her letters which was published in 2002 and which, she considered, gave a fairly unvarnished account of her activities up to the late 1990s[1]. In addition, in 2003 we produced a much shorter but immensely popular book of her more reflective writings and spiritual preoccupations, that has gone on to be translated into several languages[2]. The success of this spurred me on to suggest a larger volume of her selected papers, particularly those focussing on clinical work, service development, and the emerging research base within hospice and palliative care. This selection was published just a few months after she died[3]. The *Letters* and *Selected Writings* together make a useful reference source for anyone wanting to understand Cicely Saunders better and they should be read as companion volumes to this biography — making up, I hope, an enduring trilogy. *Watch with Me* has, in turn, been described as Cicely's 'autobiography'[4].

After hearing her speak at a conference in Sheffield in 1999, I suggested to Cicely that there were elements of her story that needed to be captured in more depth, more candidly, and in ways that went beyond the rhetorical repetitions of her public interviews. Paraphrasing an advertisement for beer at that time, I said I 'want to reach the parts that other interviewers haven't reached'. She didn't recognise the marketing reference, but immediately sensed my purpose: 'come to the house and we will do the interviews there'. I felt I had gained access to a more private setting. For the next five years I visited her periodically at 50 Lawrie Park Gardens, where she lived on the ground floor. We always sat in the same place, at right angles to one another, she in her favourite chair and me at the end of the sofa in a sitting room full of homely clutter, books, CDs and records, newspapers, magazines, and letters. The first interview there took place on 23 August 1999 and the last one on 5 October 2004. The final interview I conducted with her was recorded, sitting next to her bed in Nuffield Ward at St Christopher's Hospice on 8 March 2005. I last saw her there on 11 June 2005, but this time without my sound recorder. I was visiting simply to pay my respects and to say goodbye.

Cicely proved a daunting person with whom to work, but at the same time a rather relaxed collaborator. Her mind was sharp and she even thought it was getting sharper with advanced age. She didn't have much of an appetite for small talk, but was prone to fire questions at me about the current state of palliative care, often focussing on some very specific detail about which I often felt unprepared. Her orientation to my increasingly in-depth preoccupation with her life and work started with mild bemusement, then edged into enthusiastic support, but never strayed into editorial control or manipulation.

Orientations

The commitment to writing this biography, first made in 1999, has at times weighed heavily upon me in the interim. Following Cicely's death in 2005, there were many tributes, obituaries, and personal reflections, both spoken and written. At her memorial service in Westminster Abbey the following year, there were eloquent accounts from those who had known her much longer and far better than me. It seemed too early to be starting a new full-length assessment of her life. There were also my own pressures of work, deadlines, and commitments, and generally the things that happen, as John Lennon put it, 'while you're busy making other plans'. In 2009, I moved away from the coalface of palliative care research to take up a new set of academic responsibilities. With a degree of sadness, I sent to King's College Archives more than sixty boxes of Cicely's papers, that had been with me for several years. But the task of the biography and my commitment to it remained, sitting on my shoulder, maturing in my mind, and I reassured myself that in due course the time would be right to make a start. When, in 2015, I received a Wellcome Trust Investigator Award, space opened up for new ideas and priorities. I also realised that time was fairly short if my book was to be published in 2018 — to mark the centenary of Cicely's birth. I began writing in May 2016 and concluded the first full draft one year later.

As I got going, I faced some immediate challenges common to many biographers. Two among these predominated. First, what 'tense' should the book adopt? I decided (mainly) to eschew the historical present favoured by some historians and to tell the story in the past tense. Second, and more worrisome, was how to refer to my subject. Initially I felt uneasy with 'Cicely'. It seemed too cosy, lacking in distance, respect even. But 'Saunders' seemed too formal, remote, and looked ridiculous when applied to the early years. I decided to adopt no fixed pattern. It would be 'Cicely' in childhood, 'Miss Saunders' at Roedean and Oxford, 'Nurse Saunders' in the war years, back to Miss Saunders for her time as an almoner, 'Dr Saunders' in due course, and eventually 'Dame Cicely'. It proved tortuous and more irritating the further I proceeded. In the end, I abandoned it all as a bad lot and simply went for 'Cicely'.

In much of my work on hospice and palliative care I have referred to my orientation as that of the 'critical friend' — supportive of the wider enterprise, but bringing to its analysis a searching approach rooted in social science thinking and an historical perspective. I have adopted the same principles here. No one could fail to admire Cicely's contribution to the development of modern hospice and palliative care. It is important to salute this. At the same time, her methods, character, and beliefs all shaped that work and were consequential for it, as well as for Cicely herself and those around her. Likewise, this work and her experience were influenced by wider forces as she lived through monumental changes in national life and global society spanning nine decades. These dimensions all bear careful scrutiny and require a balanced analysis. I have tried to walk this line — avoiding both hagiography and opprobrium. Others can judge the degree to which I have been successful. I am not a professional biographer, but I have used my skills and knowledge as a sociologist and historian to underpin my approach. C. Wright Mills[5] famously described sociology as the encounter between 'biography' and 'history', and that is the orientation I have adopted here.

Technical Matters

Without interrupting the flow of the story, I have tried to be quite full in referencing my sources. Significant among these are the twenty-two personal interviews with Cicely, conducted by me after the idea of a posthumous biography had been agreed, and carried out with that in mind. Before that I did two 'on the record' interviews in 1997, to add to the five which Neil Small had conducted in 1995 – 1996. So for this book, I draw in depth on a total of twenty-nine recorded conversations. I quote from or allude to these in many places, giving details in the notes. In the subset of twenty-two interviews, there was much oral history material on past times and experiences, but in the later years in particular, the sessions often began or were concluded with some observations on recent events. These covered happenings at St Christopher's as well as significant detail on Cicely's health problems and physical decline. They make up a powerful set of recordings and transcriptions which have been invaluable to me in preparing this work. Occasionally, I also make use of interviews with Cicely, conducted by others and mainly available in the public domain, and these are referenced accordingly. I also draw on interviews carried out with others who knew Cicely — in her personal, family, and working life — and these too are referenced in full.

In places I have relied heavily on Cicely's correspondence. Wherever letters are used I give the date of writing and the name of the recipient. I do the same with letters written to Cicely. In the relevant examples, I reference material that can be found in more detail in my volume of her *Selected Letters*. Where I use letters that are not included in that volume, they can be found in the Cicely Saunders's Archive at King's College London, as indeed can all the published letters. I make use of the Shirley du Boulay biography, giving citations from the paperback second edition, which appeared in 1994[6], ten years after it had first been published. It contains a new preface by the author and an 'afterword' on euthanasia by Cicely herself. For the later period of Cicely's life, I also make occasional use of the updated du Boulay and Rankin[7] version of the biography, that was published in 2007. Several other references are to material in the King's College Archives. This material has an online finding aid. Some of it is also 'closed' until specific dates, though because I had agreed the work with Cicely in her lifetime and, until she died, had access to all areas of her papers, there have been no restrictions on my access for the purposes of writing this biography. My references to this material give sufficient detail to allow it to be located in the King's College Archives.

Cicely was a prolific writer. Starting with her first article in the *St Thomas's Hospital Gazette* in 1958, she went on to produce some three hundred published works. These ranged from clinical case studies to literature reviews and commentaries, reflective pieces, reworked lectures, edited books, research reports, and biographical reflections as well as, in later life, a substantial number of forewords and introductions to the work of others. I have collated all these works and hold copies of the full set. They are referenced throughout this book and all of them would repay ongoing scrutiny. A selection of them can be found in the *Selected Writings* collection.

There is a huge photographic record of Cicely's life and a very small selection from this is used here. I also draw on some sound and video recordings of Cicely, prepared for teaching purposes, or for wider broadcasting.

Reflections

The entire 'archive' of the life and works of Cicely Saunders is vast and varied. Only a part of it is formally catalogued and available at King's College London. Elsewhere lie many other documents, objects, recorded material, images, and artefacts that also add to our understanding of Cicely. I have treated all of this as source material. It makes up a complex and inviting assemblage of objects which have their own agency. To turn over her letters, carefully preserved in the early days as carbon copies of the original, or to read her annotated manuscripts, richly worked on with marginalia and corrections, is to get alongside their creator in a remarkably privileged way. To listen to her voice, with its changing modulations and pitch over time, is to be reminded of her passion, tenacity, and intellect. To read her well-ordered prose, itself carefully supported by her own extensive reading, is to discover a clinician who went far beyond the limits of day-to-day practice. These and many more dimensions I have tried to capture here.

The chapters cover chronological periods of up to twenty years at a time. During periods of maximum activity, these chapters are necessarily lengthy. I have structured the content of each chapter thematically rather than chronologically. The themes are clearly designated in subheadings. I discovered early in the process that I could not write a 'diary' of Cicely's life, nor would this be desirable or useful. Rather, I chose to divide her life into distinct time periods and within those I have attended thematically to the issues I consider most important. I have also faced the challenges of the sheer volume of source material. If I have been comprehensive in examining it, I may not have been in reporting it.

I have found writing this book has been the most compelling and enjoyable task in my entire professional life. I hope it will be read with pleasure and interest by the many people who knew Cicely personally, as well as by those who have been subsequently inspired by her. It is also a book for those with no prior knowledge of the Hospice Movement, palliative care, and the twists and turns of their shared evolution. It records a life of remarkable facets, achievements, and contradictions, and it is inspired by the belief of Cicely Saunders herself, that ultimately, as life ends, 'all will be well'.

Notes

1. Clark D. *Cicely Saunders. Founder of the Hospice Movement: Selected Letters 1959–1999.* Oxford: Oxford University Press; 2002 (hereafter *Letters*).

2. Saunders C. *Watch with Me: Inspiration for a Life in Hospice Care.* Sheffield: Mortal Press; 2003.

3. Saunders C. *Selected Writings 1958–2004.* Oxford: Oxford University Press; 2006.

4. Twycross R. Eulogy at the memorial service for Dame Cicely Saunders, Westminster Abbey, 7 March 2006, http://www.stchristophers.org.uk/about/damecicelysaunders/tributes, accessed 1 September 2017.

5. Wright Mills C. *The Sociological Imagination.* New York: Oxford University Press; 1959.

6. du Boulay S. *Cicely Saunders: The Founder of the Modern Hospice Movement,* 2nd ed. London: Hodder and Stoughton; 1994.

7. du Boulay S, with Rankin M. *Cicely Saunders: The Founder of the Modern Hospice Movement,* 3rd ed. London: SPCK; 2007.

1 | The Saunders of Hadley Hurst (1918 – 1938)

I think we were nouveau riche, if you ask me. So we had expensive holidays and schools and universities and things like that — all the things that he hadn't had.

I thought, 'Gosh, I look exactly like my father, absolutely *ready to pounce*' [1].

Beginnings

Cicely Mary Strode Saunders was born to Chrissie and Gordon Saunders on Saturday, 22 June 1918. Her parents' home, Linden Lodge, at 45 Bedford Avenue in Barnet, was situated in the English county of Hertfordshire. Despite its rural associations and market-town history however, 'Chipping' Barnet was an expanding suburban area in the emerging London commuter belt. A train service left frequently for the city and, as the crow flew, it was less than eight miles to Westminster Bridge, in the heart of the capital. It was in London that Gordon Saunders had his business and, from there, was making his fortune as a land agent. His only daughter would also be cleaved to the city, never living elsewhere, apart from her years at boarding school and then University. In July 2005, at age eighty-seven, she would die in Sydenham, south London, in the hospice she had created. A life circumscribed by the boundaries and aspects of a great metropolis would prove consequential all around the world.

The 1918 summer was cool and wet. The red pantiles of Linden Lodge shone damp in the north London rain. The detached suburban house, built at the turn of the century in the Edwardian style, was a desirable place for a couple expecting their first child. It was on the same road as Chrissie's parents' home. Chrissie had married an energetic man whose career was taking off and who was exempt from service in the Great War due to a schoolboy sporting injury. Unlike the young women all around her, she had no anxious waiting for news from the front. Safe from military duties, her relationship with Gordon developed as the war ground into a bloody stalemate and, in the process, claimed thirty-eight alumni from his old school — more than half the number on the school roll at the time he attended[2]. Married in June 1916, two years later the Saunders's first baby, a girl, had arrived.

They named their daughter Cicely. It might seem at once attractive, frilly, and Victorian, a variant of Cecily and Cecilia. But if they had reflected on meanings, it might seem a strange choice. Derived from Caecilius, an old Roman family name, that has its root in the Latin *caecus*, it means blind, or poorly sighted. It was also the name of a third-century Christian who founded a church in the Trastevere section of Rome, who was later venerated as a martyr and became the patron saint of musicians. More mundanely, it is the name of an aromatic white-flowered plant of the parsley family, with fern-like leaves. Perhaps it was simply the sound that appealed to her parents, something that fitted snugly with the social world to which they aspired. Later, among her family and friends, she would often be known affectionately as 'Cicel', whilst her American associates referred to her as 'Cecily'. As to her other names, 'Mary' was after her mother and 'Strode' had important family significance, also on the maternal side and about which we shall learn more in due course.

When Cicely was born, the war of 1914 – 1918 was moving into its final stages. Germany was throwing a last-ditch effort into the Western Front. In July, French troops launched a surprise counter-offensive, and the 'one hundred days' of effort from the Allies began which would end four years of conflict. In August, the battle of Amiens was a crucial victory and a black day for the German Army. The summer also saw the murder of the tsar and his family at Yekaterinburg, as the Bolsheviks took control of Russia. War and the consequences of war were everywhere to be seen. In London, the injured and mutilated casualties were ubiquitous on the streets and in the stations, returning home to what Lloyd George would soon call a 'country fit for heroes'. The fighting had also taken a terrible toll on those left behind. As historian Joanna Bourke observes: 'Three hundred thousand never saw their fathers again; 160,000 wives received the dreaded telegram informing them that their husbands had been killed. Countless others discovered the meaning of suffering'[3].

Emotional Landscape

Against this terrible backdrop, the new Saunders family, by contrast, appeared safe and secure. They had a comfortable home, with money coming in, and a pleasant neighbourhood in which to live. The material prospects looked promising and were well matched to Gordon's ambition and energy. But the courtship of Gordon and Chrissie had sounded some warning bells[4]. Chrissie's mother was keen to make the match, but Gordon proposed three times before

Chrissie agreed to marriage. An engagement of four years followed and, by the spring of 1916, Gordon Saunders seems to have married more out of pity than passion for his bride. The accounts we have of Chrissie at that time point to a woman of great beauty and style, but also one who was fragile, a perfectionist, and prone to recuse herself from those around her. Certainly Chrissie and Gordon made a handsome pair. One photograph of them (Figure 1.1) taken early in their life together shows a couple of remarkable bearing and elegance, but whilst Gordon's alert eyes sparkle, Chrissie looks questioning, even challenging, and there is a less-than-happy quality in her countenance. They seem poised on the brink of change and yet, at the same time, look elegiac for an order that is coming to an end, with all the uncertainties of what that might mean.

The tone was set in the first year of Cicely's life. Her godmother was Daisy, Gordon's sister, who worked as a governess and was later a school matron. Ten years older than Gordon and unmarried, Daisy took a keen interest in the new baby. Within months and struggling to cope, Chrissie 'gave over' the care of Cicely to her sister-in-law; but then, seeing the growing bond developing between them, she sent Daisy away in a fit of jealous confusion. A photograph taken about this time (Figure 1.2) shows Chrissie looking downcast and rather detached from the bright-eyed young daughter, now able to lift her head, who is laid across her mother's lap. The incident with Daisy and the associations of the photograph of mother and child portend other issues, and these would surface quite soon in the family life of the Saunders.

Two years after Cicely, came the birth of her brother John Frederick Stacy Saunders, in September 1920. The children bonded with their father, but during their childhood years were remote from their mother, and she from them. If

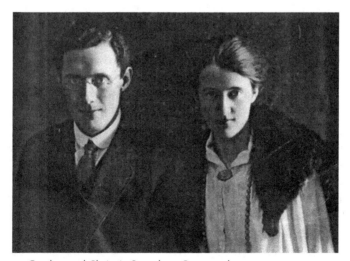

FIGURE 1.1 Gordon and Chrissie Saunders. *Source unknown.*

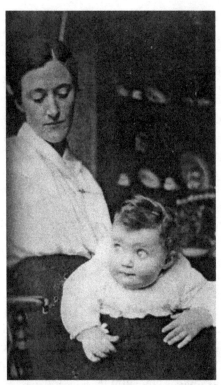

FIGURE 1.2 Chrissie Saunders and baby Cicely. *Source unknown.*

unhappy, perhaps depressed, Chrissie was self-contained, as long as she had a female companion to support her through the routines of the day. A steady stream of governesses, 'mother's helps', and nannies, and eventually a retinue of household staff took on the practical burden of raising the children, but this did not unlock space for happier or meaningful pursuits or for a deepening relationship between Chrissie and her husband. As the complement of household staff increased, it brought its own pressures to bear on Chrissie, who was unskilled in hiring, firing, and managing them, and who eventually abrogated all these responsibilities to someone else.

Though the emotional landscape was becoming inauspicious, the tensions did not prevent the Saunders from prospering materially. In 1922, they moved to Monkenholt, a large, white, Georgian house situated a short distance away on Hadley Green Road. Hadley is a Saxon word meaning 'high place'. Standing at 440 feet above sea level, its air is said to be the freshest in London. It was a place where, for centuries, wealthy families took holidays from the city, and its tranquillity was protected by adjacent common land which could not be developed. The grandfather of William Makepeace Thackeray, Anthony Trollope's sister, and medical missionary David Livingstone had all lived nearby.

With the knowledge of his profession as a land agent, Gordon had chosen well. The step up in accommodation was striking. Built around 1767, Monkenholt was distinguished by graceful bow windows and exquisite painted panelling[5]. The one-acre garden included a sunken pond, extensive rose beds, and an orchard, along with two magnificent cedars of Lebanon as old as the house. Servants, such as Mr. and Mrs. Read, the cook and butler, were employed, and companions for Chrissie became a regular feature of family life — 'Emily', Miss Morrison, and 'Stocky', in turn[6]. In her later years, Cicely could recall ' "the brilliant garden, full of secret places" where her father taught her tennis and cricket, and the "quiet, rather dim area at the bottom where my brothers and I built bonfires and toasted leaves" '[7]. It was at Monkenholt that her second brother, Christopher Gordon Strode Saunders, was born in March 1926. The family was now complete, but eventually Cicely would look back to this time and suggest that the breakup of her parent's marriage was already becoming inevitable.

Schooldays

Age four at the time of the move to Monkenholt, Cicely's formal education was getting underway. First she went to kindergarten in a house run by two unmarried sisters called Smythe, in Barnet. From there, she went on to a local private school to which she was taken each day by horse and carriage. This seemed to be the beginning of some unhappiness at school as well as tensions with her classmates. Next, and marking a break with home, was Southlands, a boarding school at Seaford, sandwiched between Newhaven and Eastbourne, on the Sussex coast of southern England. There, the matron was Aunt Daisy, who was now reconciled with Chrissie and beginning to spend holidays with the family. This may well have been behind the choice of school: Cicely was already tall for a girl of ten, and she was gauche and awkward with others, so whenever troubles blew up, her godmother was on hand to soothe and give solace, discreetly calling in on occasions when Cicely felt happier staying in bed for a day[8]. Her Aunt Daisy may well have been the primary reason for Cicely's contentment during her four years at Seaford.

For an intelligent and articulate girl, by age fourteen, Cicely's academic progress was not commensurate with her father's expectations. Whether this was a result of her motivation and application, or the quality of the pedagogy at Southlands, is hard to tell. Nevertheless, in 1932, without discussion, and to his daughter's enduring annoyance, her father sent her to Roedean, situated to the west of Seaford on the outskirts of the elegant resort of Brighton. Founded in 1885 as Wimbledon House, and relocated nearby with a new name in 1889, the school was created to prepare young women for entrance into the newly formed women's colleges at Cambridge — Girton and Newnham. When an art studio was built around 1910, Edward Burne Jones and George Watts and others of the pre-Raphaelite Movement contributed to the design. By the early 1920s, the school was thriving and had around 450 students and staff members combined, still under the leadership of the founding 'firm' of the three Lawrence sisters — Penelope, Dorothy, and Millicent[9]. The school's handsome Flemish–style main building, designed by Sir John Simpson, sat on forty acres, with playing fields, a swimming pool, and even a secret tunnel through the chalk and under the road to the flint shingle beach and rock pools below. Its cliff-top location was spectacular, facing directly out to sea. Roedean's pupils dressed in a distinctive short-sleeve tunic, known as a *djibbah*[10], that was worn over the top of a white long-sleeve blouse (Figure 1.3). There was a thick woollen djibbah for the morning and, for the afternoon, something made of silk or velvet, that the girls were encouraged to individualise. Roedean oozed an

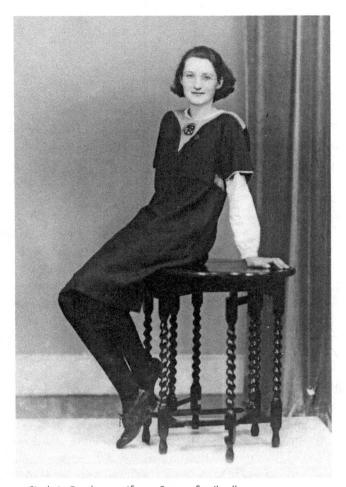

FIGURE 1.3 Cicely in Roedean uniform. *Source: family album.*

atmosphere of seriousness, privilege, and the preparation of girls for a life of achievement, in which they were encouraged to follow the biblically inspired school motto and 'honour the worthy'.

At Roedean

Despite its prestige, reputation, and extensive facilities, for a while things did not go well for Cicely at Roedean. She hated leaving home for Sussex. She refused to travel by train and had to be chauffeured to school, one might say as a spoiled and privileged teenager. At the root of this was stomach-turning loneliness and feeling like an outsider at Roedean. She was too shy to sit with others at the mid-morning cocoa, self-conscious, and without friends. Her father's throwaway but insensitive teasing rang in her ears: She was 'lanky, tall, and spotty'[11] and found it hard to like herself or to be liked by others. But, when a parcel containing a gold bangle sent to her from home was intercepted and stolen by another girl, Cicely was discreet about the misdemeanour, told no one, and then befriended the thief, who turned out to be 'another lost lonely girl who didn't know what to do with herself'[12]. It was the kind of circumspect behaviour that gained respect in the Roedean context, especially with Miss Mellanby, her housemistress, who was able to give a detailed report to the girl's parents[13]. Cicely later claimed she had no friend to tell about what had happened, but perhaps this sensitive and individual act of human kindness also foreshadowed the Cicely which was to come. Another augury was the onset of back problems. Like her mother, Cicely suffered from a slight curvature of the spine and it was becoming painful. Her Roedean routine started to include a daily session of laying on her back on the floor, watched over by her housemistress, who allowed no distractions, and hoped the problem could somehow be straightened out.

Whatever the discomforts, her orientation toward Roedean did begin to change. School magazines suggest an active and engaged pupil involved in several activities beyond the classroom. The girls played cricket, but not to a high standard, it seems. In the summer of 1935, Cicely's house team apparently showed a disgraceful lack of concentration when batting and, in one match, 'the fielding was wild at times and the fielders were slow on their feet'. Nevertheless, along with an able team captain, C.M.S. Saunders was singled out for praise and played well in the final of the inter-house competition[14]. She became a house prefect in the Michaelmas term of 1935 and a school prefect (one of seven) in the Lent term of 1936[15]. Cicely also went on to play in the house first twelve at lacrosse for the next couple of years, but cricket in 1936 seemed little improved on the previous season. In a picture taken with fellow prefects at that time, she stands tall at the back, looking quietly assured, and there are hints of the mature woman of strength and determination who would eventually emerge. She was by now head of number two house, a role she had taken on reluctantly but seems to have enjoyed.

In 1929, Roedean had purchased a property in nearby Rottingdean which it used as the base for a school mission — providing support to impoverished local children. Pupils were encouraged to get involved in a range of practical and social activities, and, on leaving, to donate money to the work on an ongoing basis. In 1936, Cicely was elected secretary of the school mission, foreshadowing the charitable interests she would take up in later life[16]. Likewise around this time, she attended Anglican confirmation classes and began to take more of an interest in religion. After that, she embraced a period of adolescent atheism. These combined interests and preoccupations would remain with her, transforming and changing as her later vocational and spiritual paths opened up and led her forward.

Cicely looked back on this time as a period when she gained a feeling for the underdog, something perhaps previously unknown to her given the nature of her upbringing. She worked hard at music, playing the violin, and in turn became more focussed on her other studies. She was inspired by the political and economic teaching of Aline Augusta Lion, who taught at the school from 1930 to 1951 and who had taken a D.Phil at Oxford and published a work of political philosophy on fascism[17]. Lion met Cicely's parents and encouraged an application from their daughter to read History at Oxford. Her father was delighted. His ambitions for Cicely, backed by the financial resources denied to him at the same age, would ensure she got the university education he had missed.

In her last year at Roedean, 1937, she donated two volumes on medieval political theory to the reference library and, on 19 June, one day after her nineteenth birthday, Oliver Sherwell Franks, Professor of Moral Philosophy at the University of Glasgow, presented her with a Speech Day sixth-form prize for history[18]. Her late run of academic effort met with disappointment, however. She was rejected by Lady Margaret Hall and Somerville College, Oxford, and only made the waiting list for Newnham College, Cambridge. Her final report, of March 1937, states rather mutedly: 'Good. She has done very well and deserves success . . . . Trying again Nov. 1937'[19]. Cicely then had to resort to a private 'crammer' and rote learning[20] before she was eventually accepted in 1938 into the Society for Homes Students at Oxford — her last choice.

For one whose subsequent achievements were so considerable, it might seem harsh to judge her early academic record negatively. As we shall see, once embarked at Oxford, Cicely was not initially singled out for high praise. She quickly left her studies when other more practical priorities emerged, although her eventual 'war degree', in which allowances were made for the period of conflict, was more distinguished. Her later postgraduate studies likewise failed to realise the medical doctorate to which they were oriented. That said, she developed an early passion for reading that stayed with her throughout her life. She seemed to have had a lifelong enthusiasm for learning, but not for the workman-like application that sometimes brings academic success even to those less talented than she. From childhood, there was something of the auto-didact about her. Aunt Daisy fed her religious texts, that she devoured with enthusiasm at an early age. She was the bookish child who found calm in the process of reading, in worlds which transcended her own and in the possibilities of other things beyond the material comfort in which she lived and the strains which were growing between her parents. It was a habit which sustained her throughout later life, when other travails and sorrow broke in.

In the later 1930s, tensions were also mounting in the world beyond southern England, and soon life there would be dramatically affected. Events in Germany were again setting Europe on the path to war. In the year when Cicely became a school prefect at Roedean, Adolf Hitler presided over a triumphalist Nazi Olympics in Munich. Months earlier, the German Army had re-entered the Rhineland, military conscription was beginning, and, by the winter of 1936, Hitler had formed a military alliance with Mussolini and an anti-Comintern pact had been signed with Japan. Situated right on the English Channel, only a short crossing to where enemy troops would eventually come to a halt in France, Roedean School was commandeered by the British Navy and evacuated in 1940[21]. Staff and pupils were relocated to northwest England, to the town of Keswick, in the Lake District. Some even went to Nova Scotia. If the second half of the 1930s saw growing political foment in Europe, however, it seemed oddly untroubling to life in the increasingly affluent Saunders family. Yet, it is hard to imagine that Gordon Saunders would not be thinking about the implications of war on his thriving business interests, and the material and reputational benefits that might be affected.

Hadley Hurst

In 1934, the family moved to the edge of Hadley Green, to the extensive property called Hadley Hurst. Its acquisition was a defining moment for Gordon Saunders and an astonishing statement about his business success. It also set the seal on his failing marriage; for, when the time came, he chose Hadley Hurst before his wife. Meanwhile, the Saunders's comfortable and increasingly upper-middle-class life moved to a new level of opulence and style that marked them out — placed them in a set of people at home in town and country — and shaped their manners, politics, and orientation to the world around them. Thought to have been designed by Christopher Wren and built in the years before 1707[22], Hadley Hurst's three-storey brick construction included eight bay windows, a hipped roof, and a wooden eaves cornice. Above the main doorway inside the house stood a 'broken' curved pediment in the Baroque style which led on to numerous panelled rooms, with fireplaces of Palladian design. When the Saunders moved in, the property had stable buildings which had been converted to staff accommodations and garages. It was rural opulence, a stone's throw from the city:

> We moved to Hadley when I was sixteen. And it was a great big Queen Anne . . . had an enormous garden . . . enough to have three tennis courts, two grass and one hard, and plenty of lawn and herbaceous border and lovely trees — two great big cedars at the front and two great big cedars at the back. And it was comfortable and with plenty of servants and a chauffeur and a Rolls, and stable yard, and cottages for the gardeners and a cottage for the butler and his wife. So it was fairly palatial and on Hadley Common, so outside was common and woods and so on . . . [23].

Philip Gordon Saunders

How had Gordon Saunders been able to bring off this triumph of material acquisition? At one level it was an achievement against the odds. His starting point had been unpromising, if not conspicuously disadvantaged. Born in Eton, near Windsor, to the west of London, in September 1889, Philip Gordon Saunders was the last of his twice-married father's seventeen children, five from the first marriage. His father, John Henry Saunders, born in 1836, died when Gordon was one year old. He had been court photographer to Queen Victoria and lived comfortably in Gerrards Cross. Yet after his death, the proceeds of a string of photography businesses — Hills and Saunders, that he had jointly owned in towns across the south of England — seem quickly to have been dissipated. Nevertheless, Gordon's mother, Elizabeth Saunders, who had been born in Oxford and widowed at forty-three, did a sterling job in keeping the family going and 'living on her own means'. Quite how that was done is unclear. She was a water colourist of some talent and often left the youngest children in the care of their elder siblings to pursue her painting.

For two decades, the British Census shows the changing composition of Gordon's family and household. In 1891, as a toddler, he was living in Iver, in Buckinghamshire. His sisters Daisy (age eleven) and Mabel (age eight) were also there, along with his brothers John (age eight) and Bernard (age five). The household was likewise home to half-sisters Mary (age thirty-three) and Catherine (age twenty-seven), along with his mother's nephew and niece Frederick Hills (age seven) and Charlotte Hills (age five). Ten years later, the household had moved to Ealing and still comprised seven people. Daisy, the half-sisters, and the niece and nephew had gone, but now Gordon's older half-brothers Frank (age twenty-three), a photographer's assistant, and Arthur (age twenty), an auctioneer's clerk, make an appearance, though they had been absent ten years earlier. By 1911, and still in Ealing, there were just three at home. Daisy, at thirty-one, had returned and was living there with her mother, now age sixty-four, along with twenty-one-year-old Gordon, who by this time was working as a surveyor.

Dauntsey's School

Against this background and whatever the extent of his mother's private means, it is puzzling to know how Gordon had been sent in his early teens to the fee-paying Dauntsey's Agricultural School in West Lavington, Wiltshire, in south-west England. Established in 1542 in accordance with the will of William Dauntsey, a master of the Worshipful Company of Mercers, the school had been re-named and moved to new premises in 1895. In 1904, there were sixty-one pupils on the school roll, comprising forty-nine boarders and twelve day boys[24]. This was the limit of the school's dormitory and classroom capacity. The headmaster from 1900 was Mr F.O. Solomon and the core activities were farming and agriculture. The school taught the boys various aspects of land and livestock management, with a strong practical orientation, and there was considerable interest in experimental methods and trials to compare the merits of different regimes on crop production and yields.

Sports also figured strongly. Gordon Saunders started in the autumn of 1904 and left in the summer of 1906. At Dauntsey's, he showed himself to be a keen cricketer and athlete, receiving a silver cricket shield at the Speech Day presentations in his first year, when he also came in third in the senior boys' one hundred-yard race[25]. Chiefly a batsman at cricket, he was not prolific. The 1905 season saw a string of low scores, until finally, on 17 July, he made twenty-three runs — his best performance for the school — against a team from nearby Urchfont. That year he played twenty innings for a total of 101 runs and a meagre innings average of 5.94[26]. He also played for the football team and his efforts in the 1904 – 1905 season, when twenty-six matches were played, were summarised thus in the school magazine: 'Vigorous and speedy; would make a useful outside left if he centred more accurately and showed more control over the ball'[27]. Although not recorded in the school record, it was here whilst playing football that he sustained an ankle injury. Although he was still playing sports at nineteen, the injury later ruled him out of army service. His subsequent vigour and energy, however, were unimpaired.

On leaving school out of the fourth form, at age sixteen, Gordon began to develop an ambition to restore the family fortune. He would rise above the hard-earned but soon-lost successes of the photography business and look to an occupation capable of realising major returns for flair, confidence, and a measure of risk taking. But, to begin, and in the absence of any capital of his own, he needed some kind of work to get him started. He had learned rudimentary surveying skills at Dauntsey's and quickly found work as a trainee surveyor with a firm called Giddy and Giddy on Packhorse Road in Gerrards Cross, not far from home. Later, he worked in Shrewsbury. But surveying was not a match for the scale of his ambition.

John D. Wood and Co.

By the account of his son Christopher, he began to look for a firm in London in which the senior partner was nearing retirement and the other partners were capable but not overly so — and where, in short, he might progress quickly[28]. His choice of firm was the estate agents John D. Wood and Company. Established in 1872, it specialised in property in London and the south of England. Based in Mount Street, Mayfair, opposite the Connaught Hotel, John Daniel Wood had founded the company at the age of twenty-three. When Gordon Saunders joined the business around 1912, Wood was in his sixties and contemplating retirement. This was just a few years after the 'people's budget' of 1909, in which Asquith's liberal government had introduced a charge of twenty percent on unearned appreciation in land values to be levied whenever estates were sold, inherited, or transferred. It also brought in increases in death duties and income tax with a surtax of 6d in the pound on incomes greater than £5,000. In such a context there was money to be made from the breakup of large land holdings and the sale of expensive properties. John D. Wood and Co. was able to benefit as the rich and landed classes squirmed at the imposition of financial penalties and sought to mitigate their exposure to taxation.

The firm was undoubtedly doing well when Gordon Saunders arrived, but his impact was immediate and positive. By 1916, with the founder now retired, Gordon was senior partner at the age of just twenty-eight. After the First World War, the company regularly took instructions on major houses and country estates. Such was its profile that the properties on its list were advertised over the entire back page of *The Times* newspaper and in expansive style in *Country Life* magazine. Notable sales included Dorchester House, Park Lane (later the Dorchester Hotel), Leeds Castle in Kent, and Parham Park in Sussex[29]. Signalling the company's expanding fortunes under Saunders's leadership, in 1930 it moved headquarters around the corner to Berkeley Square, where it remained for another fifty years. Gordon Saunders brought this about, as much as anything, by force of personality and sheer hard work. He was buccaneering, extroverted, tireless — a dynamo. Having started with nothing but his own native wit, no education beyond the age of sixteen, and no capital to get him going, Gordon had now become exceptionally wealthy. He set about enjoying his good fortune and giving to his family all the luxuries which had been denied to him as a child.

Mary Christian Knight

Little is known about Cicely's maternal lineage[30]. That side of the family had connections with the west of England, but in the later nineteenth century also had associations with South Africa. Cicely's maternal great-grandmother was Sarah Christian Ford, born in 1828 and married to John Ford, a grocer. At the age of sixty-nine, Sarah seems to have died on a ship, the *Dunvegan Castle*, whilst travelling to the Western Cape in June 1897. Her body was brought to Cape Town and her place of burial (and a photograph of the headstone) is recorded as Burgersdorp, Drakensberg District, Eastern Cape — a community far inland and about 160 miles south of Bloemfontein. We must assume that she was travelling there to visit her daughter Susan, who was living in Burgersdorp at that time. Susan Ford had been born in Newton Abbot, Devon, in 1857. In 1861, Susan, age four, and her six-year-old brother, George, were living with their mother and father in St Martin's, Leicester. By 1871 they were in Uxbridge, Middlesex, with Susan only. Susan married one Frederick (Fred) Knight, who was born in Gloster, Bristol, in 1852 and may have been a schoolmaster in England. His parents were Thomas Knight and Elizabeth Emma Knight. The wedding of Fred and Susan took place in her hometown of Newton Abbot in early 1885. It is not clear when they went to the Cape, perhaps in the early 1890s. It seems that Fred's brother, Edward Jukes Knight, had moved there too, and died in Burgersdorp around 1913.

The Burgersdorp settlement had been first established in 1846. The Afrikaaner Bond political party had been formed there in 1881 and, four years later, the town's isolation was reduced by a railway connection. Between 1869 and 1905 it had a theological seminary, run by the Dutch Reformed Church. In Burgersdorp, Fred Knight ran a somewhat unsuccessful local store. Cicely's mother, Mary Christian Knight, was born there in 1889. Chrissie, as she was soon known, had two brothers, George and Charles, with whom she remembered playing cricket under the hot sun. Their life appears to have been unhappy. Fred Knight's warmth and charm affected those around him, but it wasn't sufficient to make life bearable in Burgersdorp. His kindness got in the way of his business sense. His wife was said to be a dominating figure who eventually had some kind of breakdown. This may well have been precipitated by the tragic circumstances of her mother's death, leading in turn to the decision to return to England. Defeated by a lack of business acumen and the ravages of the South African conflict, experienced first-hand in 1900 when the Boers occupied Burgersdorp, the Knights moved back to Britain when Chrissie was in her mid teens and were recorded in the 1911 Census as living in a house called Bongola, in Bedford Avenue, Chipping Barnet, with Chrissie (age twenty-one) and George (age eighteen, a provisions trader); Charles seems to have moved on and was no longer at home. Fred was now employed as a shipping agent in the drapery business. There in Barnet, Susan could perhaps rekindle memories of better times in her own family history. She claimed descent from Sir John Strode (1624 – 1679) of the English west country (Susan's home area), who gained notoriety for enraging Charles I to the point where the King burst into Parliament seeking vengeance against

Strode. Thereafter, it was determined that no reigning monarch could enter the parliamentary chamber unannounced. The name of Strode carried historical weight to Cicely's grandmother, and this was transmitted to Chrissie, who eagerly added it to her first child's string of names as well as to those of her second son, Christopher[31], but it does not appear in the names of earlier generations of the family. Susan died in 1925, taking with her the original relevance of the Strode name.

Life with the Saunders

By any standards, the lives of Chrissie and Gordon Saunders were transformed in the years after their marriage. They were moving out of the indifferent circumstances of their families of origin and quickly making their way into the upper echelons of English middle-class society. But, if Gordon relished this with an ebullience that went from strength to strength, Chrissie was more diffident, enjoying the material luxuries it afforded, but, in her private spaces, troubled, ill at ease and, it was said, hard to please. It made for unhappiness in the marriage, that in the child-rearing years could be covered up by a measure of bourgeois propriety, but was to become increasingly visible as their offspring flew the coop.

Family Dynamics

By the time of the move to Hadley Hurst, the family's pattern of relationships was consolidating. Chrissie seems to have been closer to John, who was quieter in temperament than her other two children. Perhaps she found his easy-going, non-critical ways simpler to tolerate. Christopher was known as the mechanically minded boy, fascinated with trains, cars, and aeroplanes — a budding scientist in the making. Christopher had a serious and enquiring air, not unlike the picture of Gerald Durrell that emerges in his memoir *My Family and Other Animals*[32]. As a young child, he had struggled to say his full name, Christopher Gordon Saunders, that came out as 'Gobber', a nickname that stayed with him all through the later years. He and Cicely were more energetic in personality and had inherited their father's drive and intelligence. Except when the children were ill and she could go into nursing mode, Chrissie dispensed little demonstrable affection to any of her offspring. Even late in his life, Christopher continued to remember the complete absence of hugs or cuddles. But, if she was detached from her children, she was conscious of her place in society. Du Boulay recounts the story of a warm day, when Cicely asked her mother why she was wearing a hat. The reply was stern and aloof: 'You seem to forget, Cicely, that I am Mrs Saunders of Hadley Hurst'[33]. Chrissie was conscious of her status, terrified of losing it, and determined to hold on to her marriage and family, however unhappy they were in consequence.

After spells at kindergarten, John and Christopher were both sent to preparatory schools. At one of these, run by an Austrian family called Engelhardt, Christopher became friendly with the grandson of H.G. Wells. Later, at Highfield Boarding Preparatory School, near Liphook in Hampshire, and despite a term lost through ill health, Christopher performed exceptionally well academically. In contrast to his sister, he was small, but — like her — he was shy and one who found it difficult to fit in with his classmates[34]. John appears reserved and less talented, though he was to excel at sports and, with his sister, became an expert ballroom dancer.

In their teenage years, John and Christopher both attended Haileybury School, near Hertford. It was less than twenty miles from Hadley Hurst and within easy cycling range. John, if rather short-sighted, was brilliant at ball games. He was a sprinter, a fast wing three quarter at rugby, playing for the school first fifteen. He also made the second eleven at cricket. If not a spectacular scholar, John nevertheless went on to read Estate Management at Cambridge University, taking a two-year wartime degree. At a higher level, there were echoes of his father's time at Dauntsey's, gaining knowledge of agriculture and the practical business of land management, and mixing with those who would be returning home to take up such duties. But with war raging, by 1942, John Saunders was a soldier in the Queen's Own Royal West Kent Regiment and was soon to see a considerable measure of military action and foreign engagement. He married Barbara Wood before the war ended and served abroad for a time. They went on to have three children. He worked for a spell with the Duke of Westminster, and lived with his family in Chester. Then it was on to J. D. Wood itself, where in 1967 he found the plot of land on which St Christopher's Hospice would be built. But in these years, John did not enjoy good health. He had been a commander of flame-throwing tanks in the war and had seen some terrible sights. Typical of the era, he received no therapeutic help afterwards. He may well have suffered what was later termed post-traumatic stress disorder. His wife inherited money and, by age fifty-five, he was to retire, living quietly in Moreton in Marsh, Gloucestershire, in the English Cotswolds. Nevertheless, well into his seventies, John kept up his business interests as a company director with Rawlinson Wood Investments Ltd[35]. He died on 11 October 2015[36].

Christopher Saunders enjoyed notable academic success, rising up through the house and prefect system at school like his sister; but, unlike Cicely, he emerged with an outstanding academic record which pointed him straight towards Oxford and a four-year undergraduate degree in Chemistry, with which he graduated in 1948. In the interim, he laid the basis of a lifelong passion for rowing; at last, he had found a sport at which he could excel. From there it was on to an M.B.A. at Harvard Business School. He married Shirley Warren, and they too had three children. He spent around eleven years working with an agro-chemicals company, based in Cambridgeshire, and then five years with management consultants McKinsey and Company. When Gordon Saunders died, Christopher inherited money to invest in an engineering business of his own, selling up in 1985 to focus on investments and consultancy work of various kinds, and continuing to live, and to row, in Cambridge, where he was much enthused by the city's potential for growth through partnership between its University and business innovation.

Material Living

But back in the years before the Second World War, the Saunders children lived a life governed by the routines of boarding school and punctuated with holidays, organised on a lavish scale. Though the emotional life of the family was meagre, the material one was not. The Saunders were living high on the hog. The Channel island of Jersey was initially a favoured holiday location. There was a cruise to Gibraltar and Madeira, and a visit to Egypt. Beginning in about 1933, the picaresque artist colony of St Ives, on the north coast of Cornwall, became their regular destination (Figure 1.4). Beginning in the 1880s, artists and bohemians had taken up residence at St Ives in some of the disused warehouses that accompanied the decline in the fishing industry. It became a magnet for painters, sculptors, and others of an outré disposition. By the 1930s, it was becoming strongly associated with English modernism. It may have been here that Cicely gradually acquired something of her later love of painting and sculpture. Eventually, she was to marry an artist who loved colour and expression. In St Ives, she could have seen abstract work by the likes of Ben Nicholson or 'primitive' pieces by local painter Alfred Wallis. Perhaps Cicely slipped away at times from the family games and bathing parties or the conversational *longeurs* to explore the backstreets and alleyways that were the locus of the artistic energy that pervaded the town and brought with it a sense of danger that lay beyond her conventional upbringing.

This might have been difficult, however. Gordon Saunders preferred a crowd around him and liked to be the centre and instigator of organised activities. Disinclined to spend too much time with his wife, he invited friends to come on holiday. He could be over-bearing with them, but was also generous. They would often be a large group, of a dozen or more, staying at the Treloyhan Manor or Tregenna Castle, a Great Western Railway Hotel. 'Surf bathing' was the order of the day, practiced on wooden boards while lying flat in the shallow water. Cicely was good at it and admired by others for her skill[37]. Lilian Gardner, a young woman in her early twenties, was Chrissie Saunders's regular companion during Cicely's teenage years. She had joined the household in 1927 and gradually took on more and more responsibility for managing its day-to-day affairs. She was attractive and full of energy. One holiday photograph shows her with Cicely, arms linked and emerging from the sea in bathing caps and costumes along with Gordon, John, and Christopher.

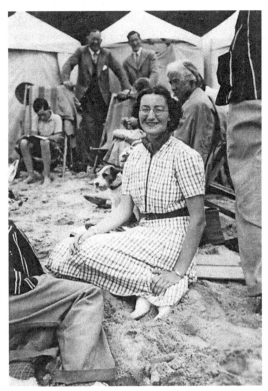

FIGURE 1.4 Cicely on holiday; Christopher reading, Gordon and John looking on. *Source: family album.*

Chrissie is nowhere to be seen. Herman and Doris (Dee) Diamant were often in the party. He was a Polish doctor and something of a property entrepreneur — based in Mayfair. Following Herman's death, Dee would later be Gordon's companion as, separated and at first disenchanted, he rattled around Hadley Hurst, and Chrissie lived in London. Looking back, Cicely captured the mood of those vacations:

> We went on holiday with friends. I remember going on holiday once and we had to split tables and I was sitting at a table with just my parents and suddenly saying, 'Goodness! Wouldn't it be awful if it was just us' — and realising that I'd dropped a real clanger[38]!

Scotland

Another popular holiday venue was the Scottish Highlands. The family would go to Glengarry, in Invernesshire, often accompanied by some of Gordon's clients, timber merchants from Yorkshire or industrialists from the Midlands[39]. This made it a more grown-up environment, where business as well as pleasure was on the agenda. Christopher wasn't allowed to be there until he was age ten.

They stayed in Glenquoich Lodge in the western reaches of Invergarry. The house had been built by Edward Ellie, who had made a fortune in the Hudson's Bay Company. The painter Edward Landseer was entertained there, albeit in a somewhat spartan environment. Then, in 1873, the brewing magnate and later Lord Burton took a thirty-one-year lease on the property, transforming it into a place of Highland sporting luxury. The King himself, Edward VII, stayed there on two occasions in 1904 and 1905. It sat right on the water's edge. High up in the glen, Loch Quoich with its shallow bays was the favoured fishing spot. An accomplished fly fisherman, Gordon worked his split-cane rod from a boat rowed by Cicely. The boys caught fingerlings in the burns, that they sometimes ate with tea and toast. It was a bastion of Highland tradition, as lived out by visitors and landowners whose native homes were in England.

Though well appointed, the lodge was massive and brooding. The air was pervaded by wood smoke and the smell of tobacco; the loch waters were dark with peat. No doubt whisky was the favoured drink. It was a place where businessmen could meet and make commercial alliances, and where fishing could dominate the days. The Saunders continued to visit even in wartime and on into the later 1940s, when Gordon would sometimes suggest eligible men for Cicely who might be invited along[40]. Even into the early 1950s, visits to Glenquoich Lodge were still part of Cicely's annual routine. But by 1955, the level of the loch was raised by one hundred feet when hydro-electric dams were installed, and Glenquoich Lodge was no more[41].

Emerging to Womanhood

We see in these experiences and illustrations the strong, defining influence of the Saunders family culture on Cicely. In turn, it is clear that culture was largely the creation of one person — Gordon Saunders. To understand Cicely at this time, we need to look closer at her relationship with her father. She reflected back warmly in later life on the time he spent with her, his endless patience with ball games in the garden, his bonhomie, and his generosity. Yet, her years at Roedean were undermined by his jibes about how she looked and, though she sided with him, she could see he was not kind to her mother either. It was at this time that she started to question his view of the world, posing challenges based on her education, her wide reading, but still rather limited life experience. Gordon was busy making profits, clinching deals, speculating, and having fun in the process. His leisure time was spent with a crowd of cronies. There is no evidence that he read anything much, either for pleasure or enlightenment. Aligned with the landed classes and sympathetic to them as, first, liberal and, later, socialist governments ate away at their privilege, we can only speculate that his politics were conservative and these suffused the household. Chrissie seems to have been a straw which bent in the wind. She was largely devoid of views and beliefs beyond the domestic circle. Meanwhile, at school,

Cicely was drinking deeply from the political teachings of Mlle Lion and exploring the polemical and atheistic world of George Bernard Shaw. When at home, she would clash with her father on matters of principle, and mealtimes were dominated by heated debate between them, with the others sitting passively on the side-lines. When this happened at breakfast, he would arrive late and flustered at the office, to the ongoing amusement of his colleagues[42].

These emerging principles and values were not yet clearly articulated by Cicely. Nor did she revolt against the life of privilege and comfort she was living. She could enjoy the indulgences of Hadley Hurst, the motor cars, the parties, and the dances, and remain content behind the cedar trees, as yet ignorant of the world beyond. Aspiring to Oxford or Cambridge was still unusual for her gender, but normative for her class. She struggled to gain entrance, but for her two younger brothers, Oxford and Cambridge followed as naturally as the night from the day.

Within this 'Oxbridge' ambience, an exploration of religion and atheism was not unusual. When she was a child, her parents led secular lives. They neither attended church nor appeared interested in matters of faith. Cicely's 'holy godmother' Daisy was the one point of contact with the tenets of Christianity. She had given Cicely a copy of *Pilgrim's Progress*[43] as a young girl. This Christian allegory from the seventeenth century had been written by a son of Bedfordshire, a county close to where Cicely had grown up. She was fascinated by its characters, topography, and narrative twists, concluding at the Land of Beaulah, where the pilgrims crossed the river of death and their words were recorded. It is not hard to see in Bunyan's story some of the elements of Cicely's life to come. Later, as her religious belief strengthened, she was able to populate her journey with meanings derived from the connection between 'faith and works'. Yet, if anything, this was despite, rather than because of, her upbringing: 'I had really no religious background at all other than Scripture lessons and a good godmother who was very quiet, never said anything very much, but gave me *Lives of the Celtic Saints* and things like that every now and again'[44].

Occasionally, there were distractions involving the opposite sex. There was Tony Holland, who helped her mother and worked in the office at Hadley Hurst. Cicely thought he was 'gorgeous' and they spent quite a bit of time together. Her father liked the match and told her she needed a man. But, when war came in 1939, Holland joined the Royal Air Force and, apart from a photograph she had of him in uniform, he 'sank without trace', only cropping up with a letter of congratulations years later when she became a Dame of the British Empire. Kingsley Gray was taken under Gordon's wing when his parents were in Malaysia. He attended school with Cicely's brother John and was a couple of years younger than her. Going up to Balliol College Oxford in 1939, he was soon in the army, in reconnaissance, where he was awarded the Military Cross. He called his armoured car after Cicely and wrote lots of letters, even after D Day in 1944, 'and then he fell in love with a blonde, so that was the end of that one'[45]. In each case, Cicely felt she had been keener on these men than they had been on her. This was not the case with the son of one of her mother's friends, who was often around the parties and social scene of Hadley Hurst. He had wanted to marry Cicely, something she thought would have been disastrous. As she put it decades later, looking back on her relationships at the time: 'it wasn't a man-less life, but none of it was particularly constructive'[46].

As Cicely approached the age of nineteen, she had no identifiable career path or vocation in mind. Romance was not filling her time. A life of faith was still to come. What was her motivation to aspire to Oxford? She had an obvious alternative in the prospect of joining her father's firm, but quickly rejected it. Instead, she set herself the goal of the dreaming spires and had to work hard at the crammer to get herself accepted. Her determination could not be doubted. Her motivation was less clear. The years to date had been predictable and planned, but now uncertainty, change, and also opportunity were in the air.

Notes

1. Cicely Saunders interview with David Clark, 25 September 2003.

2. Dauntsey's War Memorial, http://www.dauntseys.org/news/news-archives/autumn-term-2010/remembrance-sunday-service/dauntseys-war-memorial, accessed 21 April 2016.

3. Bourke J. 'Another battle front'. *The Guardian*, 11 November 2008. Available at: http://www.theguardian.com/world/2008/nov/11/first-world-war-changing-british-society, accessed 21 April 2016.

4. du Boulay S. *Cicely Saunders: The Founder of the Modern Hospice Movement*, 2nd ed. London: Hodder and Stoughton; 1994: 20, 208.

5. The house was subjected to a bomb attack by the 'Angry Brigade' in January 1971, when it was the home of Conservative Cabinet Minister Robert Carr.

6. du Boulay, *Cicely Saunders*, 21.

7. See Inside Story, http://www.telegraph.co.uk/finance/property/4809953/Inside-story-Monkenholt.html, accessed 21 April 2016.

8. du Boulay, *Cicely Saunders*, 21–22.

9. History of Roedean, http://www.roedean.co.uk/senior-school-history-of-roedean/, accessed 25 April 2015.

10. The word usually denotes a long, collarless coat or smock, specifically worn by Muslims.

11. Cicely Saunders interview with David Clark, 25 September 2003.

12. du Boulay, *Cicely Saunders*, 23.

13. Cicely Saunders interview with Neil Small, Hospice History Project, 24 October 1995.

14. *Roedean School Magazine*, November 1935, 8.

15. *Roedean School Magazine*, November 1936.

16. *Roedean School Magazine*, November 1936.

17. Lion A. A. *The Pedigree of Fascism: A Popular Essay on the Western Philosophy of Politics*. London: Sheed and Ward; 1927.

18. *Roedean School Magazine*, November 1937.

19. Roedean School, *Leavers' Book*, final report, March 1937.

20. This was Bendixen, in Baker Street, London — and close to the fictional home of Sherlock Holmes. Novelist and biographer Antonia Fraser, born fourteen years after Cicely Saunders, describes going there in the same circumstances, when she too, despite her privileged upbringing, was struggling to get into one of the women's colleges at Oxford to read Politics, Philosophy, and Economics. See Fraser A. *My History: A Memoir of Growing Up*. London: Orion; 2015.

21. Roedean school history, http://www.roedean.co.uk/senior-school-history-of-roedean/, accessed 9 May 2016.

22. 'British History Online: Monken Hadley — An Introduction', http://www.british-history.ac.uk/vch/middx/vol5/pp260-263 and https://historicengland.org.uk/listing/the-list/list-entry/1188803, accessed 25 April 2016.

23. Cicely Saunders interview with David Clark, 16 May 2000.

24. *The Dauntsey Agricultural School Magazine*, Midsummer, 1905.

25. *The Dauntsey Agricultural School Magazine*, Midsummer, 1906, 6–7.

26. *The Dauntsey Agricultural School Magazine*, 32.

27. *The Dauntsey Agricultural School Magazine*, Midsummer, 1905, 13.

28. Christopher Saunders interview with David Clark, 1 May 2015.

29. Company history, John D. Wood and Co., http://www.johndwood.co.uk/content/aboutus/, accessed 4 May 2016.

30. du Boulay (*Cicely Saunders*, 17–18) is the main source, with some references in interviews with Cicely Saunders and Christopher Saunders.

31. 'My mother always used to say that she came from a good thing and had a great family tree, which was meant to go right back to somebody who came over with William the Conqueror, but I don't know that I believe that. I don't think it matters very much'. This dismissive comment hints at some understanding of the possibly fictitious character of the 'Strode' connection on Cicely's part (from Cicely Saunders interview with David Clark, 25 September 2003).

32. Durrell G. *My Family and Other Animals*. London: Rupert Hart-Davis Ltd; 1956.

33. du Boulay, *Cicely Saunders*, 25.

34. Christopher Saunders interview with David Clark, 1 May 2015.

35. See http://www.companydirectorcheck.com/john-frederick-stacy-saunders, accessed 16 May 2016.

36. See *The Gazette*, https://www.thegazette.co.uk/notice/2426600, accessed 16 May 2016.

37. du Boulay, *Cicely Saunders*, 26.

38. Cicely Saunders interview with David Clark, 16 May 2000.

39. Christopher Saunders interview with David Clark, 1 May 2015.

40. Cicely Saunders interview with David Clark, 20 September 2000.

41. Glenquoich Lodge, http://exceptthekylesandwesternisles.blogspot.co.uk/2016/08/glenquoich-lodge.html, accessed 7 August 2017.

42. du Boulay, *Cicely Saunders*, 27.
43. Bunyan J. *The Pilgrim's Progress from this World to That Which Is to Come*. 1678.
44. Cicely Saunders interview with David Clark, 15 December 1999.
45. Cicely Saunders interview with David Clark, 20 September 2000.
46. Cicely Saunders interview with David Clark, 20 September 2000.

2 | Social Science, Nursing, Social Work (1938 – 1951)

It seemed obvious to read Philosophy, Politics, and Economics, and I took the exam and got into Oxford and settled down to working, but of course had to give it up because it didn't seem the right place to be during wartime.

But I really enjoyed nursing. I felt just absolutely in the right place.

As a lady almoner, I had been sending patients to one of the homes for end-of-life care in London, and there was one very near where I was living in Bayswater – St Luke's'.

The First Oxford Interlude

The University of Oxford is the oldest in the English–speaking world. Teaching has gone on there since the late eleventh century. Cicely's new academic home had a more modern cast, however, and can be traced back only to 1879, when the Society of Home Students was founded at Oxford with the aim of bringing educational opportunities to women, with the option for them to live across the city at home or in boarding houses, rather than in the colleges, thereby catering to those of more limited means. This did not apply to Cicely and she viewed the prospect with some ambivalence. She was conscious, too, that the Society of Home Students had not been her first choice and, more important, it had not yet been given full college status. That took a step forward when the Society adopted the name St Anne's College in 1942 and was concluded a decade after that when it received its Royal Charter. Meanwhile, and notwithstanding the rivalry among the women's colleges, it seemed a lesser place to study and was not the preferred destination of her Roedean school friends, who set their sights on Lady Margaret Hall or Somerville, that had been founded around the same time as the Society as women's colleges, but enjoyed their own premises and offered accommodations to their students, albeit at a distance from that of the men. At the same time, the Society had radical roots and represented 'a standing challenge to the assumption that an Oxford education could only be delivered in a college'[2]. It was a 'manifesto rather than a location'[3]. Cicely was at Oxford, but not wholly conventionally, and it would be the first of two periods of study there.

She arrived in 1938, at age twenty-one, for the Michaelmas term. In that year, there were 850 women studying at the University, making up a record 18.5% of the student body[4]. Cicely elected to read Politics, Philosophy, and Economics (P.P.E.). This programme of study had been established at Oxford in the 1920s as an alternative to 'Greats' or Classics. It was generally known as 'Modern Greats'. Oxford defined the degree as being 'the study of the structure, and the philosophical and economic principles, of Modern Society'[5]. Cicely was therefore in the vanguard of a new interest in social science which was entering British academic life. According to du Boulay, her tutor, Miss C.V. Butler, did not think Roedean was preparing its pupils well for this line of study, though she did single out Cicely for an excellent grounding in economics[6]. Christina Violet Butler was a noted scholar and social reformer who trained a generation of social workers and administrators. She had published a well-received[7] survey of housing in Oxford in 1912, and from 1919 to 1948 was director of Barnett House, the seedbed for later social administration and policy studies at the University. Her interests in social disadvantage and poverty had focused on the overcrowded conditions of working-class housing in Oxford neighbourhoods like St Clement's, St Ebbe's, and Jericho, where the parents of older children were advised to send them to sleep with neighbours to relieve pressures on space at home[8]. It was a long way from the conditions in which Cicely had grown up in Monkenholt and Hadley Hurst. It seems C.V. Butler, building on the influence of Mlle Lion at Roedean, was awakening an active social conscience in her student, and indeed this would soon find tangible expression.

P.P.E. at Oxford was designed with preparation for the Civil Service in mind, though it subsequently became a proving ground for many eminent British politicians of the twentieth and twenty-first centuries. At the time, Cicely had the idea of being 'a secretary to a politician or something like that'[9]. This was a gendered assumption which reflected the period and the context. Although women made up almost a fifth of the undergraduate body at this point, they continued to be heavily discriminated against. Yet, Oxford had already seen some remarkable female graduates, including Gertrude Bell, Vera Brittain, Winnifrid Holtby, and Dorothy L. Sayers. The name of Cicely Saunders would eventually be added to that list[10]. Notwithstanding, in 1938 the Oxford Union again voted to deny women access to full debating rights. Until 1934, women students studying medicine had to make use of their own anatomy laboratory. Oxford's conservatism and privilege would have been at once familiar to the undergraduate Cicely; but, the intellectual and moral foment, the daily engagement with world politics, and the constant discussion at meals about the prospects of war, were new and enervating.

Entering into War

On 29 September 1938, days before Cicely arrived among the 'dreaming spires', British Prime Minister Neville Chamberlain signed the Munich Agreement, handing over the Sudetenland to German control. Her first term at University therefore had as its signature theme the growing spectre of war. The new vice-chancellor, George Gordon, president of Magdalen College, took the initiative and quickly began making contingency plans, that were finalised in early 1939, providing for University premises and laboratories to be switched to government work in the event of conflict. A historian of Oxford later remarked: 'As war approached, the University was asserting its identity as a national institution and an integral part of the state. There was no one in Oxford to stand up for the lost cause of 1939 — peace'[11].

With turmoil all around, Cicely applied herself to her pass moderations. These were the first set of examinations at Oxford and would determine her onward progression to Modern Greats. Her year was enjoyable. She settled to her work but also joined the Bach choir, did Scottish Country Dancing, and made some friends[12]. At the end of the year, her results were sound and they allowed her to continue. The detailed focus on the core elements of P.P.E. was about to begin. Meanwhile, she went back to Hadley Hurst, took a holiday in the Scottish Highlands, and pondered what might lie ahead.

On 3 September 1939, Neville Chamberlain announced that Britain was at war with Germany. The assurances of Munich had fallen apart. Oxford students flocked to volunteer for officer training — despite the controversial debate of 9 February 1933, condemned by Churchill, when the Oxford Union had carried the motion 'This House would not in any circumstances fight for King and Country'[13]. Now a new patriotism was emerging, less jingoistic than in the Great War, and heavily focussed on the scourge of fascism. In due course, the exodus of undergraduates to the war would be matched by an influx of evacuees from London and elsewhere. Grace Hadow, Principal of the Society of Home Students, commented on their presence in the streets[14] and evocatively described the beauty of the Oxford skyline under wartime blackout. As Vera Brittain points out in her study of *The Women at Oxford*, it seemed somehow a eulogy, and — following an extensive lecture tour to Australia, America, and Canada in late 1939 — Hadow died of pneumonia the following January at age sixty-four[15].

In late 1939, Oxford was filling up with military personnel and civil servants, and the women's colleges were each adopting one of the nineteen London schools evacuated to Oxfordshire, where the undergraduates worked with the children at weekends. Precious items from the colleges were stowed away for safekeeping, and the college 'scouts' doubled up on their housekeeping duties to serve as air-raid wardens. By September 1940, the long-expected Blitzkrieg arrived, and London and many other towns and cities came under heavy bombardment (but never Oxford, though it was thought a likely objective for the 'Baedeker' raids that were targeted on cities of historical interest).

Making a Decision

During her second year at Oxford, Cicely watched these events unfold for just one more academic term before resolving to leave and get involved in the war effort. The decision seems to have been finalised towards the end of 1939, and it took her tutors and her family by surprise. An article she had written for the *Roedean School Magazine*, published in December 1939, gives only the mildest hint of it[16]. This elegantly written piece, seemingly composed in the months of autumn, begins by referring to the outbreak of war and 'the first unthinking moment, when a large proportion of the female population of England said "I shall give up everything, and either nurse, or drive enormous army lorries"' but after which 'most of us resigned ourselves to a thoroughly dim term, with nothing and nobody the same as before'. In the main, Cicely strikes a tone of normality. Lectures continue, the daily routine remains unchanged, and the city looks 'much the same as usual', apart for the sandbagged windows and bright orange signs denoting the air-raid shelters. She majors on the continuities — 'Christ Church Meadow, where the leaves are turning; the group of spires and towers across Merton fields; the river by Port Meadow; and the three college Chapels, where choral evensong is sung every day, Magdalen dimly lit by rows of tall candles placed along the pews'. She explains that most of the women students had taken up war-related interests — attending Red Cross lectures, organising sewing and knitting groups, helping with evacuees, and doing part-time ambulance work. Yet the article makes clear these remain secondary to the main purpose of being in Oxford: 'working for as a good a degree as possible, in the hope that nothing will happen to interrupt this'. Indeed, continuing with the life of Oxford she regarded as 'a National Service of the greatest value'.

These words may have been written to placate her teachers at her old school and also to reassure her parents that she was not about to make any rash decisions. They may also have been an exercise in self-deception, knowing all the while that her intentions were the reverse. For whilst they seem deeply felt, they were not enduring. Even by the time they appeared in print, Cicely had made the decision to foreshorten her Oxford studies, to leave the University, and to apply for training as a nurse. Certainly a plan seems to have been at work earlier that summer:

> I came down in 1939, deciding this was really no place for one to be in wartime, and decided that I wanted to nurse . . . I thought sitting at Oxford reading for a degree just wasn't a contribution to the war effort. A friend had gone off to do nursing and I thought, 'Goodness that's right. That's what I ought to be

doing, but I must train. I mustn't just be a V.A.D.[17] '. And my father wasn't all that pleased when my headmistress wrote some reference for me and wrote to me saying, 'What about your back? Is it going to manage?'[18]

Equally concerned was Eleanor Plumer, Acting Principal of the Society for Home Students. She wrote, dismissing the idea of nursing, when, she asserted, her student had made progress with her academic studies and the ranks of nurses were already filled beyond the level of need. Churlishly, she insisted that fees be paid for the forthcoming Hilary Term, as notice to leave had been served so late. Miss Butler, however, took a different view and felt that practical work would be eminently more suited to Cicely, who, despite her grounding in economics, had not impressed her as a student. On this basis, the transition to nursing was getting underway, but the gears were grinding in the process.

Nurse Training in Wartime

Things took time. In early 1940, Cicely made an application to London's St Thomas's Hospital to train as a nurse in the Nightingale Home and Training School. References had to be secured, then each suitable candidate was interviewed in turn at the hospital — on a Tuesday morning — by Miss G.V. Hillyers (matron from 1937 – 1945). Sometimes this was in the presence of the candidate's parents. The matron of the hospital had sole discretion over who was admitted. Matrons were known to look for a particular social type. At interview, Cicely was asked if she had any brothers and which schools they attended[19]. St Thomas's was associated with middle-class nurses from respected and prosperous families. In turn, the nurses had a strong esprit de corps and thought themselves special, if not rather superior to their counterparts at the other London hospitals. It was known as the most difficult hospital in the country to get into. Standards were high; discipline was strict. The training school was the first of its type in the world and was named after its founder. The nurses themselves were known as 'Nightingales'. But the 1940 intake of nurses would face an added layer of demands. Britain was at war and the London Blitz was about to get underway, which would continue for years, constantly disrupting everyday life, and wreaking death and mass destruction across the city.

The Influence of 'John Hadham'

During the wait, and as the 'phoney war' began to transition into something all the more tangible, Cicely stayed at home, taking Red Cross courses and working as a V.A.D. There was time to read, to reflect, and to contemplate the implications of nursing as a vocation, something containing an ethical stance towards others which would become a lifelong preoccupation. She also began to turn her thoughts more to matters of faith and religious belief. She came across a new book by 'John Hadham' called *Good God* [20], published that year in a classic orange and white paperback cover by Penguin Press. It was quickly followed by a companion volume, *God in a World at War* [21]. 'Hadham' was in fact the 'arch-liberal woolly thinker' [22], the Reverend Dr James Parkes [23]. Originally from the channel island of Guernsey, Parkes served during the First World War, was ordained into the Church of England in 1926, and then spent a dozen years working on the continent in organisations which promoted international co-operation. He became active in the Student Christian Movement and was a tireless campaigner against anti-Semitism. Parkes was prolific as a writer, historian, and social activist. In *Good God*, he was not concerned with whether God exists. He assumed the existence of God and proceeded to explore the character and activities of God and their implications for the world He had created.

It was like flipping a switch: 'there wasn't really anything, until I picked up this little book . . . I can't really quite think why, in the summer of 1940. So it was really starting from scratch'. Now she made the transition from atheist to theist. She became convinced 'there must be a God and this makes some sense' [24]. It is relevant that Parkes was the catalyst. Whether she was aware of the details of his life, we shall see so much of its influence in Cicely's later work. It is not difficult to understand how, as a woman of twenty-two, she could be drawn to his approach, not only to satisfy a spiritual yearning, but also to discover a template for faith-led action in the world. In time, this framework would deepen into a matter of profound personal conviction, but this was not to be for another five years. Meanwhile — and suitably strengthened — she could move on to her chosen métier in nursing.

It was in November 1940 when Cicely was finally able to begin her training at St Thomas's. Years later, she was still remembering with pleasure Shirley du Boulay's description of how she took to her first profession: 'like a book finding its right place on the shelf' [25]. In truth, this was a moment of transformational change for her. Brought up in the comforts of Hadley, educated in an elite school, and briefly exposed to the rhythms of undergraduate life in Oxford, now everything was altering. She was entering into a new, completely different, and more visceral world [26]. It was a world at war, a place of death and suffering, and an environment of endless physical labour coupled with the constant personal and psychological demands of giving nursing care in extreme circumstances.

St Thomas's Hospital

When the war started, extensive discussion had got underway at St Thomas's about whether it should evacuate to a safer, more rural location. The loyal patients were against this and preferred to take their chance with the threatened Blitzkrieg. St Thomas's became part of the Emergency Hospital Service, with two hundred beds reserved for air-raid and war casualties and 120 beds for sick civilians. At first, with no significant military operations on the Western Front, there were few consequences. But, on the night of Saturday, 7 September 1940, the Luftwaffe's terrifying bombing of inner London began. Two nights later, heavy ordinance fell on the hospital, hitting Medical Outpatients and the doctors' accommodation in College House. Two nurses and four physiotherapists were killed, and three floors of the hospital were destroyed. Three members of the hospital staff were subsequently awarded George Medals for their actions that night, rescuing buried casualties and working through fires made worse by burning alcohol and acid. From 7 September onwards, the first wave of bombing continued for fifty-six of the following fifty-seven days and nights.

Something had to be done quickly, and the hospital management began looking for rural properties in earnest. Soon, only 120 beds were left at the hospital, now located in the basement — about a quarter of the pre-war number. Despite the torment of aerial bombardment, however, St Thomas's never closed during the war and no patients died in the air raids, though on several occasions there were fatalities among members of staff. Located opposite the British Houses of Parliament, close to Waterloo Station and on a bend of the river Thames, St Thomas's was an easily visible target for German bombers, even under the blackout. In consequence it suffered more damage during the Second World War than any other London hospital[27]. One year after Cicely, another V.A.D., Lucilla Andrews, attended for interview at St Thomas's. In her memoir, she describes the scene:

> I did not know that St Thomas's had started the war with eight individual blocks . . . . I saw a jumble of three blocks standing close together and one of these looked less than intact. All three had bricks instead of glass in the upper windows and their ground floors were hidden by anti-blast walls and stacks of sandbags. On either side of the standing blocks were the now omnipresent in London blackened, roofless buildings, jagged walls, gaping, glassless windows, piles of rubble and grime, and one semi ruined block . . . still smouldering. A crowd of begrimed men were busy clearing the chaos, and there was a line of ambulances outside a heavily sandbagged entrance marked 'Casualty Department'[28].

Rural Relocation

To escape such surroundings, the preliminary training programme of the Nightingale nurses was moved in 1940 to a large country house in the village of Shamley Green, near Guildford, in Surrey, about thirty-five miles to the southwest of St Thomas's. There, the routines and traditions of the main hospital and its destroyed nurse training school were maintained as far as possible. Nevertheless, for Cicely and the other new recruits, the early days were bleak. Winter was on its way and their accommodation was unheated and devoid of comforts. They lived under blackout conditions at night, and stumbled around after dark with no illumination to guide them. They had a limited number of clothes coupons, some of which had to be used on their uniforms. Although they were provided with board and lodging, beyond that they received only pocket money, which amounted to £20 in the first year. The work routines were harsh and exhausting. They did domestic duties between classes, and those of privileged backgrounds, like Cicely, were initiated into important new skills, like 'damp' and 'dry' dusting, cleaning toilets and baths, and learning to use the ubiquitous abrasive pink cleaning paste called 'Gumption'. Strict inspections followed all their efforts. They learned their nursing skills on life-size mannequins, to which they administered 'blanket' baths. There were morning and evening prayers, and lights out occurred at 10:30 pm. On top of all this, there was talk and speculation everywhere about how the war was proceeding and where it would lead.

But Cicely was fortunate with her companions. Grouped in a 'set' of about twenty nurses in training, they bonded together and formed what became lifelong friendships. Cicely was slightly older than about half of her peers. Those of her age had come in through the V.A.D. route and were only drawn to nursing to be part of the war effort. She stood out in other ways. She had more expensive and stylish clothes, and her parents' money eased the inconvenience of wartime restrictions. If they didn't want her away from home, sleeping five to a room in makeshift beds and eating pilchards on toast as a main staple, they could supply her with desirable cosmetics and the all-important stockings that she must wear when on duty. On her days off, she and a friend would hitchhike from Basingstoke to Barnet, stay overnight at Hadley Hurst, and go back the next day. At a time when they were 'endlessly hungry', the larder at home was a wonderful respite from the iron rations of the Nightingale Home and Training School.

Gaining Confidence

Cicely won a measure of esteem among the set. She had a photograph of the handsome and uniformed R.A.F. serviceman Tony Holland by her bed. She told improbable stories, was a good mimic, and poked fun at the nursing es-tablishment. When she organised a comedy sketch about the esteemed found-ress, she was in trouble with Matron: ' "You'll never be a really good nurse, Nurse, unless you realise some of the things that are really important and some of the things that must not be joked about, and one of those, Nurse, is Miss Nightingale" '[29]. She gained a caché which she had not known be-fore. The tectonic plates of her self-esteem were shifting and, quite quickly, she became incredibly happy. Though only twenty-three years old, she found herself thinking that nursing could be something she could do all of her life — not just for the duration of wartime — and in turn that it could even compensate for other things, like not getting married[30]. She was 'absolutely in the right place'[31].

At the end of the first year came the Preliminary Training School final examinations. One person failed to make the grade at this point and two or three others had to leave when they got married. On successful completion, the 'Staff Nurses' moved from Shamley Green, proud of their new probationer status — they were referred to as 'pros' — and were about to come to grips with the detailed realities of hospital nursing. This began at Park Prewett, near Basingstoke, in Hampshire, where Staff Nurse Saunders was elected as the set representative. She had to take responsibility for the work of six or seven other probationers on the ward. She became efficient with her own tasks and was a good overseer of others. She got into the way of playing the piano for hymn-singing with the patients on Sundays and conducted a carol service at Christmas. Park Prewett Hospital was an asylum that had opened in 1917 and was re-purposed for military use at the start of the war. The pioneering plastic surgeon Sir Harold Gillies was based there at that time and had a special unit for teaching and clinical work.

Stresses and Strains

The conditions were basic. Crumbling wards, bars on windows, padded cells, and toilets without locks made up the defining features of the environment. The 'pros' were assessed and marked on everything they did in the wards, including their personal disposition as well as their practical skills. They were required to remember and be able to recite every detail about the patients they looked after.

The second year also brought some major clinical and personal challenges. Cicely was put in charge of a children's ward with twenty cots. Babies could die of diarrhoea and vomiting. There was a little boy called Reggie, very unwell, who she would feed at night. He was fond of pulling off her glasses as she cared for him. When he died she couldn't bear for the porter to take him to the mortuary, so she carried him there herself to steady her emotions and pay tribute to his short life. The next morning at eight, she had to break the news to Reggie's parents over the telephone that their only child had died.

The stooping, lifting, and long hours without sitting down also took their toll at this time. Quite early, she put out a spinal disc. It was a warning sign of problems to come, albeit obscured for the moment by the deep satisfaction of working at something where she could excel, and which was meaningful and rewarding.

At Hydestile

From Park Prewett it was on to Hydestile, near Godalming. There, the King George V Hospital had been created around 1921 by the Metropolitan Asylums Board as a tuberculosis (T.B.) sanatorium and, adjacent to it, was a more recently built hutted hospital, newly vacated by the Australian Imperial Force. Beginning in 1940, this too became part of St Thomas's. Extensive conversions were made and 260 beds were in use there after 17 April 1941. It comprised a series of single-storey buildings laid out in a star formation and linked by covered walkways, giving protection from the elements. It was set among low, rolling hills topped with mature trees, and patients could be brought out in their beds in fine weather to enjoy the air and the views.

The new facility was established not a moment too soon. On the night of 16 April 1941, the main hospital in London suffered its worst attack of the war. Incendiary bombs did untold damage and a further explosion the next morning destroyed most of Nightingale House. To add to the drama, the day after operations began at Hydestile, a German bomber crashed in the field opposite and the severely injured crewmen were taken in and cared for by the newly opened facility. In the recollections of the surgeon, Hugh Romanis, who worked there from 1941, Hydestile provided good care, managed to accommodate a large number of medical and nursing students, and by the time peace came, was also highly valued by the local populace as well as by those who had been brought in from London. In time, the numbered wards were re-named after their bombed counterparts in London: Christian, Victoria, Beatrice, George Makins, Arthur Stanley, George, and Adelaide. Unless in mufti, the nurses were required to wear their full uniform dresses at all times, correctly buttoned and belted, along with their caps. The culture and ambience of the great St Thomas's was being actively re-created, even in the rural setting of a former military hospital.

There, Cicely and her set worked a duty of twelve nights on, followed by two nights off, for three months at a stretch. Daytime nursing was based on split shifts with a break in the middle. She would often spend this time laying on her bed, easing her sore back. They got one day off each week, beginning at 5 pm the previous afternoon. There were a lot of soldiers and sailors to care for, particularly sailors. They were receiving treatment for injuries as well as for regular medical and surgical problems. It was apprenticeship nursing, and attention to detail was scrupulous. Some sixty years later, Cicely could still remember particular patients. One had made her a model ship. There was another man with neurological problems who couldn't speak, but in the course of an afternoon conveyed to his wife he was sorry Staff Nurse Saunders was going to another ward. She 'specialled' another, Cecil Tonsley[32], who was an expert on beekeeping and with whom she made contact again via the B.B.C. years later when she learned about an honour he had received. He had a pulmonary embolus, treated at the time with complete bed rest. He was so attached to her that he would repeat to himself 'Nurse Saunders to feed Tonsley, Nurse Saunders to feed Tonsley' in the hope that he would see her[33]. When he recovered, Mr Tonsley and his wife gave her a volume of poems by Browning, in appreciation. There were also patients with cancer, but no anti-cancer drugs, and a very timid approach to the management of cancer pain. Looking back, she recalled 'we really had nothing to offer but ourselves and meticulous nursing, and so that really made me realise how important relationships are in any medical sphere'[34].

She cared for a boy of five or six who had a cerebral tumour and was greatly distressed. One day, when the Professor of Paediatrics came down to do his weekly round, he heard the child crying — a high meningeal wail. Turning to the houseman he declared imperiously: 'I do not expect to see that child when I come back next week'. This egregious command and the actions that followed lived on in Cicely's memory half a century later:

> That night the houseman came in and wrote up a large dose of an opiate and, between the two of us, we gave it. I mean, Night Sister knew about it . . . I don't remember which of us gave the injection. But I knew it was wrong. I felt helpless and I really had to back up the houseman. We were just stuck; but, of course, thinking about it now, there was no alternative. There was no palliative medicine. It didn't exist. The child didn't, in fact, die that night. We had to re-peat it and he died the second night. It's extremely vivid to me now. I can place that cot exactly where it was in the ward. I think it may have been one of the roots of why I wanted to do something about palliative care[35].

Cicely became aware of other cases where doctors were intervening to end a patient's life and, on one occasion, wrote to a friend saying: "I think the doctor's got tired of looking after Mrs X. It wasn't that Mrs X was tired of life" [36]. It was wartime. These things happened; no one wanted to talk about it.

Her own health began to suffer. She had a bad attack of bronchitis and was sent home sick for a period. When she got back she had lost contact with her set, whose members had moved on in their training. She was getting run down and suffered from sties and whitlows. Still missing her set, she succeeded in making new friends with another group. For the final year, she moved to Botley's Park in Chertsey, Surrey, just over twenty miles from London. It had been founded in 1932 by Surrey County Council as 'a colony for mental defectives'[37]. The inmates had been housed in villas grouped around the Botley's Park eighteenth-century mansion. Now in wartime, two thirds of the patients were military casualties; the rest were civilians injured in the London air raids.

Despite her fatigue, Cicely got on well with some of the officer patients. They asked her to sing 'One Fine Day' from Madame Butterfly in a show they were planning. She loved to sing and readily agreed to a practice run. The result was well received by the officers, but Sister Tutor was not impressed and warned her against fraternising with patients. When Cicely referred to one of them, Peter, by name, this was further evidence of her misdemeanour. She was told in no uncertain terms 'that is not the relationship that a nurse should have with a patient'[38]. She had to withdraw from the show. Peter seized the moment and appeared onstage in his wheelchair, where to everyone's amusement he paraphrased a popular song of the day[39] and trilled: 'No Nightingales sing in Botley's Park!' Such episodes she later put down to being tall and a tendency to trip over herself in the atmosphere of the moment. She was enthusiastic, slightly irreverent, and increasingly capable of absorbing any criticisms that might come her way. After three years, she took her finals and gained a good result, but it was at a price. One night she could barely walk up the hill to the nurse's home, such was the pain in her back. She was sent home and saw an orthopaedic surgeon: 'He took one look at me and my back and said, "You're going to have to stop nursing"'[40].

Time to Stop

This was no surprise. The warning signs had been building, so much so that she had already written to Oxford asking about the possibility of returning to complete a war degree. She was also beginning to consider what might lie beyond that. If it was not to be nursing, she was drawn to other areas of work that would afford her a similar level of human contact with people, and with those who were suffering and who needed care. It was the summer of 1944. She spent a further period in the country helping Sister Tutor with some non-clinical and educational duties, and made ready for a return to academic study: 'I was determined to turn into a medical social worker and get back into hospital as fast as I could'[41]. If leaving Oxford and enrolling as a V.A.D. had been a spontaneous demonstration of conscience in a time of war, now she was laying out the path of her career for times of peace. The world of her father was receding fast. Profits, deals, and major-league commissions on big sales were not to be part of her life. Instead, she took the entrepreneurial flair which they required, and which she had gleaned from him, and applied them to people with illnesses and disabilities. In time, she began to define a new area of care, one that would eventually become a field in its own right of specialist practice, education, and research.

Second Oxford Interlude

The war was coming to an end. In August 1944, the Warsaw Uprising was underway, American forces were turning over the government of France to Free French troops, and the Soviet army was entering Bucharest. Month after month, the bloody liberation of Western Europe continued. Meanwhile, there were continuing reports of massacres, rebellions in many parts of the world, and the ongoing threat in Britain of Hitler's flying bombs, the 'doodle bugs', that were now reaching ever farther north in a desperate attempt by the Luftwaffe to inflict further damage on provincial Britain. Yet, despite the carnage, there was a growing optimism about peace. There were hopes — not to be realised — that the fighting would be over by Christmas. The Dunbarton Oaks conference had laid out the foundational basis of the United Nations. Plans were well underway for the era of reconstruction that would accompany the peace; in Britain, detailed provisions were being made for the creation of a welfare state that would care for its citizens 'from the cradle to the grave'.

The Socratic Club and C.S. Lewis

In the autumn of 1944, amidst these mixed emotions and expectations, Cicely returned to Oxford for 'three really good terms' of study[42]. Now she seemed to breathe more deeply from Oxford's rarefied air. Her brother Christopher was at New College and she spent time with him and his younger friends. She re-joined the Bach choir, where they were rather short of tenors, and sang in the College chapel. At that time, C.S. Lewis had been installed as president of the Socratic Club, that had been founded in 1942. It built on the foundations of the Oxford Pastorate and had the aim of providing students with a more intellectually challenging environment in which to explore matters of Christian faith. It began to focus increasingly on questions of how Christians should engage with the major issues of the day and how Christian students could find intellectual stimulation beyond the reassurances of doctrinal teaching. Lewis had been encouraged by Stella Aldwinckle of the Oxford Pastorate to be the 'senior member' — a don — taking responsibility for the organisation of the Club. He brought with him the reputation of a rising star among the Christian apologetics.

Lewis had been born in Northern Ireland in 1898. His mother died when he was nine years old and he later attended boarding school in southern England. An Oxford undergraduate, he had served, seen battle, and been injured in the Great War. In 1925, he took up a fellowship in English Language and Literature at Magdalen College, and from 1929 onwards, he developed a deep and lasting friendship with J.R.R. Tolkien, Professor of Anglo-Saxon, Fellow of Pembroke College, and later the famed author of *The Hobbit*[43] and the three-volume *Lord of the Rings*[44]. Their friendship appears to have been crucial in Lewis's conversion to Christianity. In 1933, Lewis and Tolkien had formed the nucleus of The Inklings — a fabled club and loose all-male amalgam of those wishing to explore, broadly defined, the subjects of literature and Christianity. By 1936, Lewis's book *The Allegory of Love*[45] was sealing his reputation with its learned exploration of courtly love in the medieval world and its subsequent literary unfoldings. He went on to become one of the most important

British writers of the twentieth century — as an essayist, critic, and, above all, children's novelist. By the time Cicely went to Oxford in 1940, Lewis was already forming his ideas for a globally acclaimed work of seven volumes, *The Chronicles of Narnia*, that commenced publication with *The Lion the Witch and the Wardrobe* in October 1950[46].

The Socratic Club met on Monday evenings during term time and those attending were primarily women. In 1944, the female members numbered 109, of a total of 169. The newly named St Anne's Society accounted for nineteen of them. Cicely Saunders was one. Atheists and Christians would meet for discussion and mutual challenge. The invited speakers came from the ranks of Oxford luminaries as well as distinguished visitors. Lewis spoke only once each term, but almost always present, he exerted a powerful moral and intellectual influence over the proceedings. There, led by him, Christians threw down a challenge to those of other beliefs and none[47]. Evidence and argument were the principles of engagement[48], and in most instances two speakers led the discussion, one by reading a paper and the other by critiquing it. In 1944 and 1945, no doubt with Cicely enthusiastically engaged, the Club considered such topics as the Grounds of Modern Agnosticism, Marxist and Christian Views of the Nature of Man, and Has Psychology Debunked Sin?

Cicely drank it in. She was moving forward on an accelerating spiritual path which had begun to unfold in 1940 with John Hadham. In her time away from Oxford, she had already been drawn to the thinking of C.S. Lewis. Whilst training as a nurse, she had enjoyed his live B.B.C. radio programmes of 1941 and 1942, and she had got to know his book *The Problem of Pain*[49], with its wider exposition of the meaning of evil in the world, and God's purpose for human suffering. Listening to Lewis across the airwaves she experienced something 'good, sound, beautifully expressed, basically coming to believe in the possibility of a new way of living. I remember one of his illustrations was of lead soldiers suddenly coming alive and the difference between one kind of life and another kind of life'[50].

It is not surprising that this happened. Lewis had been chosen by the B.B.C. explicitly to offer a calming voice on its newly established Home Service. He was there to reassure, to mollify doubts, and to give meaning and hope in times of war. He was all the more effective because he was not a clergyman, was outside any denominational position, and had only recently espoused the Christian faith. A learned academic, he was the establishment's 'voice of faith', much as others were 'the voice of medicine' (Charles Hill) or the 'voice of digging for victory' (C.H. Middleton)[51]. Lewis became an instant success as a broadcaster and reached a large audience.

Airing on Wednesday evenings at 7:45, just after a news bulletin, and therefore likely to attract lots of news-hungry wartime listeners, Lewis's first four talks in August 1941 were titled 'Common Decency', 'Scientific Law and

Moral Law', 'Materialism or Religion?' and 'What Can We Do About It?' The whole was held together under the headline *Right or Wrong: A Clue to the Meaning of the Universe*. In total, he did four series of talks, thereby laying the groundwork for his subsequent book *Mere Christianity*[52]. His listeners heard him espouse a consensual view of the Christian faith. His concerns were not with factions and divisions within the church, but rather with 'the difficulties that ordinary people feel about the subject'[53]. Whilst yet to be felt at a deep and spiritual level, these sentiments struck a powerful chord with Cicely's developing religious outlook. She was reassured that if Lewis could find a way out of unbelief, then she too could do the same. During the early 1960s, she returned to his work, when his pseudonymously published personal memoir, *A Grief Observed*, attracted widespread interest[54]. His books were on her shelves and easily to hand until the day she died.

Dorothy L. Sayers

Oxford was the source of another inspiration. As Cicely developed her thinking and reading in wartime hospitals, she was drawn to the writings of Dorothy L. Sayers, who had won a scholarship to Somerville College in 1912 to read Modern Languages and Medieval Literature. By 1915, Sayers had passed with first-class honours, but had to wait until 1920, when women were first allowed to gain their degrees, matriculate, and become members of the University. In 1935, with a growing catalogue of popular crime novels under her belt, Sayers had written a mystery novel set in an Oxford College. But she had other interests and talents — as a translator, poet, and playwright. She wrote several works on Christianity, was a good friend of C.S. Lewis, and was a sometime attender at the Socratic Club. In December 1941, sandwiched between the first two series of Lewis's radio talks, the B.B.C. began to broadcast a drama Sayers had written for radio titled *Man Born to Be King*.

Sitting in her quarters at Park Prewett on Sunday, 21 December, Cicely had tuned into the first broadcast with eager anticipation. The play was already provoking a storm of controversy. A human actor would take the part of Christ and speak his words. This alone was considered blasphemy in some quarters, but as the twelve-part series unfolded, in one broadcast per month, there were also criticisms from Christian conservatives who objected to Sayers's humanistic portrayal of the bible story, to the use of colloquial language, and also to her focus on the personal character of the figures within it. Conversely, there were charges that the B.B.C. was engaging in wartime Christian propaganda. Despite all this, the overall judgement on the drama was positive and the B.B.C. went on to repeat it in different versions for many decades afterwards. It was also published and widely read[55]. In a remarkable testimony to the play, almost sixty years later,

Cicely could vividly remember the original broadcasts, even recalling accurately the name of the central actor:

> Well, the Sunday Observance Society, or somebody like that, said 'This is terrible; they are going to have an actor being Jesus'. And she writes terribly cleverly . . . I've got a couple of copies, and so it turned into something in the 'Children's Hour' time, but something much more adult. And it was beautifully done, with a rare bell quartet, very emotive music, and Robert Speaight was Jesus, and there were twelve plays and they're really superb, and she absolutely wore out a Greek Testament in doing it. I remember organizing my nights off so I could listen to it[56].

Searching

By her own account, Cicely was seeking Christ at this period. She was convinced of the existence of God. She attended church and chapel. She read widely in religious works. In addition to Hadham, Lewis, and Sayers, she was also drawn to William Temple. Like her other influences, he was Oxford educated and connected. His book *Christianity and Social Order*[57] appeared in 1942, the year before he became Archbishop of Canterbury (he died two years later). He believed strongly that the most effective theological writing sometimes came from those who were working in other genres — an idea that sat well with Cicely's emergent thinking.

Despite all this, she was not yet a Christian: 'I was going through the motions . . . I was still really searching'[58]. The search had continued through nurse training and was still ongoing when she returned to Oxford. By now she was steeped in Christian intellect, in her own words to the point of 'brainwashing'[59], but still a 'lead soldier' yet to come alive spiritually. No matter. There was work to be done and a heavy academic load to shoulder if she were to leave fully qualified and ready to take the next step in her vocation.

Pedagogically, the second sojourn at Oxford was focussed and instrumentally oriented towards a clear endpoint. There was a strong sense of purpose in being there. St Anne's had advised her to take two 'sections' in the social sciences to complete her degree, towards which her wartime nursing service would also contribute. Because she was inclining towards hospital social work, she would also study for a Diploma in Public and Social Administration at the same time. It meant two years of studies in one year. Her back was, by now, so painful that she did most of her reading laying down. But she worked assiduously. Her 'war degree' included a distinction in political theory, in addition to which she gained a distinction in the Diploma. By now, her tutor, C.V. Butler, who had thought her mind would probably have atrophied during the years of nursing, was much more impressed. She found Cicely altogether sharper and more alert in this final year at Oxford — so much so that the two subsequently became lifelong friends.

The Oxford examination results in 1945 coincided with the end of the war in Europe. On 8 May, Prime Minister Winston Churchill announced that hostilities had ceased on the European continent. Crowds quickly flocked to the centre of the nation's capital. Cicely and a friend were not going to miss out. They hitched a lift to London on a meat lorry to join in the V.E. Day celebrations. The streets were awash with jubilant crowds. A speech from the King was relayed to the masses that gathered in Trafalgar Square and Parliament Square. The restaurants were sold out, people picnicked in the streets, some churches held thanksgiving services every hour. By early afternoon, there was a shortage of flags; by 5 pm, the city was in a state of triumphal gridlock[60]. 'We went all around, shouting for Churchill and saying thanks in Westminster Abbey. It was absolutely brilliant wandering around London on V.E. Day and shouting for the King outside Buckingham Palace, and then we finally went up and stayed the night at home'[61]. It was a joyous moment. The war was coming to an end, studies at Oxford were complete, but despite all this, turbulent personal waters lay ahead.

The Separation of Gordon and Chrissie

As military conflict subsided and as Cicely contemplated her next steps, there was still much to burden her spirit. It was this summer in which she took the remarkable step of intervening in the fate of her parents' marriage. Whilst nursing she had seen physical and mental suffering as never before. She had also been dragged low by the demands of the hospital routine in wartime, aggravated by the terrible state of her back. Her desire for the love of a man remained unfulfilled. Her spiritual yearnings had not been resolved. It was a critical moment when her conversion to Christianity, if not the precise manner of it, might indeed have been predicted. But first, and extraordinarily, she was emboldened to be the catalyst in her parents' separation. She seemed somehow open to new possibilities, prepared to take on new challenges. The one before her was hugely consequential.

Gordon and Chrissie Saunders had been married at the height of the First World War, but by the end of the Second World War, they were on the point of separation. Global war had formed the bookends to their life together as a couple. In the interim, they had endured their own private conflicts. Contained within the conventions of good manners, their problems could nevertheless sour the atmosphere, dampen the spirits, and produce in the children a whole host of coping and avoidance strategies whereby they insulated themselves from the marital pain of their parents. The inter-war years saw Gordon and Chrissie prosper hugely in their material life, but emotionally the marriage was increasingly impoverished. As the eldest, Cicely is likely to have seen most and to have more fully appreciated what was happening between Gordon and Chrissie. Christopher appears to have been often ignored by his mother, and took to schoolboy pursuits and reveries fed by his sharp intelligence. John probably sought the line of least resistance, avoided emotional labour, and cocooned himself in sport and his social activities, though later and once married himself, he and his wife, Barbara, did most to befriend Chrissie when her own life was in crisis[62]. Cicely recalls:

> My mother was a tense and rather unhappy person, but very good at caring for people and very good at superficial relationships. But she'd been bullied by her mother and was very much the inferior to her two brothers, and so she wasn't very good at relationships herself. But she was very good if any of us were ill, so she had a talent[63].

Cicely was the first to depart Hadley Hurst, followed by John, and then Christopher. With their adult children away from home, the cracks in Gordon and Chrissie's marriage began to open up into huge fissures. It took its toll on both of them. Chrissie (Figure 2.1) appeared deeply unhappy much of the time and Gordon was finding her more and more difficult to tolerate. Her depressive tendencies and migraines fuelled his exasperation. They could barely be in the same room as each other. By the summer of 1945, after twenty-eight emotionally precarious years of marriage, the end was coming. Just two years before she died, Cicely explained her role in the process:

> Things were alright as long as there were plenty of people around, but when it came to the war and they were left, just the two of them, then it broke up . . . . My mother went down to stay with my sister-in-law's parents, just to go away

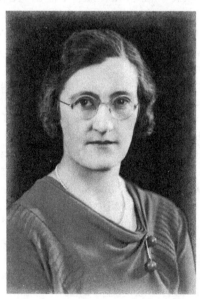

FIGURE 2.1 Chrissie in the days at Hadley Hurst. *Source: family album.*

for a few days because the atmosphere in the house was pretty poor, and rang up to say she was going to stay another day. And that absolutely sparked my father, who threw something across the room and said, 'This is it. I can't take any more . . .'. And we talked and talked until he said, 'I can't leave Chrissie here. She'll never run Hadley Hurst'. And so I said, 'Well, you know, she's the one that's got to move and I'm the one that's got to tell her'. So I did[64].

A few days later, Chrissie was back at Hadley Hurst. At this time, the Second World War was hurtling towards its conclusion — from Berlin to Hiroshima. But here was a piece of deeply personal history, set in stark contrast to the backdrop of global events. Cicely took her mother out to do something in the garden. In the warm, dull weather, the borders were ablaze with the purples and deep pinks of aster and Japanese anemone. They picked some late raspberries. Cicely was candid: 'Do you realise how awful things are being? You know you just can't go on like this. It really is . . .'. She hesitated and then made things abundantly clear: 'The time has come to split'[65]. 'You've really got to leave home. My father won't and you can't possibly run this huge great house'[66]. It seems a remarkable thing for a daughter to say to her mother. It was done with all the skill Dr Cicely Saunders would later deploy when she broke bad news to her patients or confronted their false hopes with compassion and a startling honesty. They had crossed the Rubicon, but it happened, as she put it much later, with 'the maximum amount of trauma'[67].

Practical arrangements were quickly made. Aided by a lack of financial constraint, Chrissie would leave and Gordon would stay. Like a cork bobbing on water, Chrissie was then pushed to and fro by plans and living arrangements made by Cicely and Gordon. She had accommodation in Bedford and then St Albans, and money was passed to her each week by a bank manager intermediary. At one point she shared a house with one of his family. It was a miserable state of affairs for Chrissie, and Cicely was afraid she might have to take in her mother, just as she herself was beginning to enjoy life in the second half of her twenties. Chrissie had lost status, felt ashamed, and was rudderless and prone to threatening suicide. Then Gordon had a brainwave. He bought a big house in Highgate and offered it to Chrissie's former companion Lilian, who was now married, along with her husband Bill and their son and two daughters (Cicely's god-daughters). This would be in exchange for providing support to 'Aunty Chrissie', who would live with them. There were even a few rooms set aside for students, to provide some income. Lilian's children had access to good schools. The setting was busy and bustling. It seems to have worked.

For Chrissie, happier times ensued. She did voluntary work with the Red Cross, took up gardening, and enjoyed the modest pleasures of her private sitting room, bathroom, and comfortable bedroom in a house which, for all its scale, was a far cry from Hadley Hurst. Lilian was kind to her. They played Scrabble together in the evenings and, from the early 1950s, became devotees of 'The Archers' radio serial. Despite the annoyances between them, Cicely and Chrissie also gradually got on better and later went on holiday together[68]. But Chrissie and Gordon did not divorce. That was a step too far for her, even when he produced trumped up 'evidence' to bring it about. Chrissie made a lot of friends, who could not understand why her daughter found Chrissie so difficult. But there was never any question of another man in her life.

It didn't seem to matter. Gordon began to spend more and more time with the widowed Dee Diamant, who had come as a housekeeper to Hadley Hurst from Bromley to escape the 'doodle bug' flying bombs that menaced Kent, Surrey, and Sussex during the last year of the war. Dee was musical, sociable, and the life and soul of the party. Though Chrissie, in a sustained state of animosity, habitually referred to her as 'The Snake', Dee and Gordon were themselves companionable with one another. They took to spending time at the Lodge in the Highlands, and hosting fishing parties as in the pre-war years. Eventually, Hadley Hurst was sold and they moved into the more modest Hadley Chase, with its nineteenth-century façade, just adjacent. Cicely didn't see evidence of romantic love between Gordon and Dee. It was as if her parents couldn't bear to be together, but would never countenance being fully with someone else. The ambivalences and sorrows of all this stayed with Cicely. Eventually, as we shall see, they resurfaced during the 1960s, the decade when both of her parents died. As Cicely put it, so alliteratively and late in her life, she was caught up in the 'terrible tangle of being the person between the two'[69].

The Evangelical Almoner

Exhausted after an exceptional year of study, upset and drained by her parents' separation, and relieved that war had ended, in the late summer of 1945, Cicely invited herself on holiday to Cornwall with a group of friends. The venue was the village of Trevone, near Padstow on the north Cornish coast. She was in a county familiar to her from childhood. The group of six or seven had taken a bungalow for two weeks, close to two sandy beaches surrounded by high cliffs on one side and big rocky ledges and outcrops on the other. Meg Foote was the leader of the trip; she was secretary for the Inter-varsity Fellowship and later vice-president of the All Nations Bible College. The days were focussed around daily bible reading, prayer, and earnest discussion among a group chiefly comprised of evangelical Christians.

Conversion

Cicely had somehow been drawn to the group, but it seems they were less keen for her to join them, fearing she might prove intellectually challenging, rebellious, and intolerant of the mood. At the same time, they all knew and had been praying for her. On this basis, the members might well have been keen to welcome someone whose past record suggested the likelihood, in such a regulated setting, of a conversion to faith. Her request to come along was therefore, on balance, accepted[70]. At first the group's fears were borne out as she railed against its prevailing norms and values. She deliberately went swimming on Sunday to offend them. She challenged their assumptions and their tenets of faith. But, privately she prayed and then, quite suddenly, she felt that God had answered her. Years later she likened the experience to the words of Charlotte Elliot's hymn[71]: 'Just as I am, without one plea, But that thy blood was shed for me, And that thou bidd'st me come to thee, Oh lamb of God, I come, I come'. As she became fond of saying, in a habit for self-referential aphorisms that would grow over time, suddenly: 'the wind that had so long been in my face was now at my back'[72]. The lead soldier had come alive.

In the circumstances, it might be said that she was 'vulnerable' to an evangelical conversion. Yet the motivations were clear, fully understandable, and are captured in detail here:

> There was a sense of guilt, of being not good enough, and snapping at my father, and things like that. There was a considerable amount of lack of self-worth. You see, I'd been unpopular at school. I was very popular as a nurse, the first time I really got happily together with lots of friends, but I wasn't a particularly sought-after girl. I had one or two rather nice boyfriends, but not much. So I wasn't all that pleased with myself, and it was a change into feeling that you really mattered to the real meaning of things[73].

Meg Foote quickly got Cicely established on the prayer diary known as *Daily Light*. It contained, for every day of the year, a short set of scriptures from the King James Bible, devoid of commentary and with full license for the reader to connect the verses to their own preoccupations of the moment. She followed it diligently for the rest of her life. As she herself later remarked, she had been 'soundly converted'[74].

Not everyone was so enthusiastic. Aunt Daisy seemed uncomfortable with the drama of it all. Her father was rather indifferent, pre-occupied with remaking his own life in the aftermath of the separation from Chrissie. As Cicely threw herself wholeheartedly into bible study, prayer, and the earnest pursuit of her faith, some friends were also troubled. Later, colleagues would be uneasy over her tendency to start the working day with a round of prayers. Evangelicals during the post-war years were, in fact, a broad constituency, loosely divided between 'liberal' and 'conservative' orientations. The former gave birth to the Student Christian Movement and was the pole towards which Cicely generally gravitated. But she was also attracted to the stance of Billy Graham and attended some of his crusade-style meetings where the focus was on mass conversions and more simplistic acceptance of Scripture and its social correlates. The evangelical culture she was embracing was variously intense, literal, high-minded, and not at all hedonistic. She was to make this culture her 'home' for the following, lengthy period.

If Cicely was entering such a world, it nevertheless seems at odds with her Oxford education, her wide reading, her solid experiences on the wartime wards of St Thomas's, and, above all, her social class. Dramatic conversion, the literal interpretation of the Bible, and a narrowness of moral parameters are often associated sociologically with dispossessed social groups who find in such belief systems a way out of worldly and material suffering, through what E.P. Thompson famously called 'a chiliasm of despair'[75]. None of this sat with Cicely's privileged upbringing, the sense of social order which had prevailed at Hadley Hurst, or the solidly upper-middle-class elite cultural world to which she had been given easy entry. It is therefore hard to see such a religious worldview enduring over time in the context of Cicely's whole life. Rather, it matched a phase in her life, albeit an extended one. From 1945 right into the early 1960s, the evangelical orientation would persist, eventually falling away in a shedding that revealed something altogether deeper and more profound.

Service

For now Cicely was eager to 'say thank you and serve'[76]. Within weeks of the conversion, she was embarked on training as a lady almoner. During the mid 1940s, the term 'social worker' had not yet come into common use. The almoners, as the name implies, were historically linked to the disbursement of alms to the poor, usually on behalf of an institution of some kind — in early times, often a monastery or church. Almoners in Britain were an element in the growth and expansion of hospitals during the nineteenth century. Almost always women, they started to appear in the 1880s, when major hospitals found increasing numbers of patients were too poor to pay for their treatment and were often discharged quickly and in unsuitable circumstances. Almoners were particularly engaged in organising aftercare and convalescence, and in mitigating the effects of poverty, poor housing, and over-crowding. They worked in groups that were the forerunners to the hospital social work departments which were established during the 1950s, following the creation of the National Health Service.

Bolstered with a glowing reference from St Anne's and guided by her Oxford tutor, Cicely moved to live at the Lady Margaret Hall Settlement. It had been established in 1897 by members of Lady Margaret Hall, the Oxford women's college. Its purpose was to carry out religious, social, and educational work for the benefit of the deprived London community of Lambeth and adjacent areas[77]. It was part of a wider 'Settlement' Movement in which university students, motivated by Christian values, lived together in poor areas and undertook charitable work in the local community. At first a preserve of males only, as women entered into the universities, they too became active in the movement. Lady Margaret Hall Settlement established clubs for young people as well as for the elderly and the sick. It took over a disused public house as a centre for local people to use. It assisted with the consequences of slum clearance during the 1920s and 1930s. During the Second World War, it ran a nursery on the newly created Cowley Estate. Some of its members died in the bombings of 1940. The Settlement was closely associated with the development of sociology as a subject of study, and later played a key role in the formation of social work as a profession. It was a fertile context for Cicely to sharpen her social awareness, outside of the institutional hospital setting, and to get close to the ordinary lives of working-class people in inner London, albeit just a short distance away from St Thomas's Hospital.

Her formal training was under the auspices of the Institute of Almoners in Tavistock Square. Newly created in 1945, it was an amalgam of two other hospital almoner associations, the origins of which went back to before the First World War[78]. From 1948, and as an expression of its expanding purpose and professionalism, the Institute had its own journal, *The Almoner*. Cicely's newly chosen profession was entering into a period of consolidation at this time. The training programme was essentially one of practical learning in various settings, one of which, to her delight, was St Thomas's. There were also examinations of a more theoretical nature, and these she negotiated with ease. At the Institute, her tutor was the watchful and supportive Betty Read, who in 1949 moved to St Thomas's to take up the position of head almoner. Cicely was enjoying direct contact with those whose medical problems rendered them in need of social support. She found these people inspiring, and enthused about them to her colleagues. But she also considered the work less fulfilling than nursing, and some of those around her wondered if she would continue as an almoner once qualified. As Betty Read later noted, Cicely 'needed a much broader canvas'[79].

Despite her wider reservations, Cicely was enthusiastic about the teaching she received and was eager to connect it with her practical training in the hospitals. Miss Peggy Gibbs gave a lecture to her group that prompted Cicely to choose the Royal Cancer Hospital (re-named the Royal Marsden Hospital in 1954) for her special elective. Amongst the first of the patients she met was a Mrs Chester Fox, who introduced herself with the words: 'Yes, it's me — the lady with the horrid face'. She had a facial tumour and died soon afterwards. When her body was about to be taken away, Cicely called to see her: 'The door was open and I went in. I can still remember the impact. It was not only a bit of a cancer smell, but also a *terrible* feeling of loneliness'[80]. She was quite quickly beginning to see not only the physical consequences of serious illness, but also its social and emotional sequelae.

New Friendships

It was in September 1945 that Cicely met and established an important friendship with Rosetta Wray (later Burch). They first encountered each other through St Margaret's Settlement. Cicely was newly embarked on her almoner training; Rosetta was just completing hers and about to take a job at the Middlesex Hospital. Attending the same church, they quickly became good friends. Rosetta's fortunes had not been as favourable as those of Cicely. Rosetta had a sister, Isobel, two years younger. Their father had died when Rosetta was fifteen. The two of them then nursed their mother through Addison's disease. After her death, they were taken in by a strict Plymouth Brethren family. When the family's son died in an accident, Rosetta, close to a breakdown, suspended her studies as an almoner and took refuge for seven months near Barnstaple, in Devon, at a Christian guesthouse run by one Madge Drake, who Cicely would also later get to know. At the end of that time, Rosetta emerged much improved and resumed her training.

Along with Cicely, Rosetta and Isobel (a medical student) were all 'without a perch'[81] and seeking somewhere to live in London. Gordon, the well-connected estate agent, stepped in and did the needful, finding them a flat with a telephone in 7 Leinster Gardens, Bayswater, London W2. It was still being repaired from bomb damage. Along with two other medical student friends, they moved in from early January 1946 as a group of five and set in train a riotously happy time together, living in conditions of post-war austerity, but relishing everything they did. There were three pious ones, all Christian. They gave each other sobriquets: Woozle (Rosetta), Wizzle (Isobel), and Winkle (Cicely), from Winnie the Pooh. And the other two were 'splendid atheists'[82]. Cicely paints a vivid picture of the arrangements:

> I don't know if you ever met an Ascot heater – but it's a sort of modern gas geyser for hot water – and there were two Ascot heaters waiting to be fitted and they got stolen. So we moved in with no hot water. We were on the third and fourth floors. Below us was 'Captain Cricket' and 'the Countess'. It was an extraordinary set-up. We none of us had ever done any shopping because we'd all been living in hospitals or things. We went to Whites for food and almost said, 'What is a [ration] point?', because everything was on ration. The one bit of heating we had was a sort of coal-burning, slow-burning stove which was on the top floor; there was a big room which we called the 'tablinium room'. That was some Latin name and it was known as the 'blin'. And we had to go and fetch coal in a taxi [chuckles] from the back of Paddington Station to get something to heat ourselves, and then we had gas fires in our bedrooms and a sixth person joined us, so there were about six bedrooms and the big 'blin' and a bathroom which had no hot water, and the kitchen. And I was the one who always got up and got the early-morning tea and made the porridge. And my

father produced a bucket of eggs in that sort of glutinous stuff that you could keep eggs in and we had a bucket of eggs. And we lived for £2 a week each — rent and food and everything [chuckles]. And it was absolutely hilarious and glorious. We all bathed in our respective hospitals, Rosetta took the laundry to a laundry office at the Middlesex, and I was, by that time, a student at St Thomas's. We got a small Ascot heater for the kitchen after three months and we got the big Ascot heater for the bathroom after six months, and we had an absolutely gorgeous time entertaining friends and making a terrible amount of noise. I don't know how the Countess and Captain Cricket ever coped with us. And there was a lovely couple called Mr and Mrs Hastings who lived at the bottom and who were meant to be sort of looking after the house. It was three lovely student years, at the end of which Rosetta got married, the two girls qualified, the fifth one disappeared, and I was left sort of alone and they started doing some more bomb damage and I moved around, living out of a suitcase, staying with various friends for a few weeks and then another girl came and joined me[83].

Cicely and Rosetta got into the habit of undertaking bible study on a daily basis. Rosetta's friend Joan (whom they knew as 'Bridget', for some reason) also came along. Attending each day before work, they were diligent in their task and, as a result, read the whole Bible in considerable detail. They went initially to the chapel of St Peter in Vere Street, Marylebone. A charming brick building with a clock tower, at the time it was serving the congregation of All Souls, an Anglican evangelical church in Langholm Place, Marylebone, that had suffered war damage. All Souls, a striking spired building designed by John Nash and located right opposite the headquarters of the B.B.C., came back into use in 1950 and was then Cicely's regular place of worship during that decade. Both churches became important contributors to her support networks and to her sense of identity.

When Rosetta married in 1948, Cicely helped her choose the wedding dress and held a 'spinster's commiseration party' afterwards, following which she and her friends went to see the film *Scott of the Antarctic*, with its gloomy conclusion after so much early hope and optimism perhaps reflecting their lugubrious mood. Rosetta wrote from honeymoon, recognising that Cicely had come off worse and was now left alone. It was Rosetta who was tuned in to Cicely's sensibilities about men. She noticed when Cicely took a shine to the choirmaster at St Thomas's, the Vaughan Williams enthusiast Wilfred Dykes Bower. 'She seemed to just know me falling in and out of love and being, you know, wildly enthusiastic and so on'[84]. She was 'a lovely, warm, gentle-looking person, with a spine of steel'[85]. Rosetta Burch also had a significant role to play in Cicely's later deliberations and experiences with St Christopher's. Summing up her friend's character at one point, Cicely drew on George Eliot's *Middlemarch*[86] and described her as one of those who have 'an incalculable effect on people around them, who live a hidden life and rest in unvisited tombs'[87,88].

Along with the fun and the earnest religious activity of the immediate post-war environment, Cicely's back was continuing to cause problems. Things came to a head again. She had a damaged inter-vertebral disc and was soon offered one of the first laminectomies ever to be performed. Conducted by an orthopaedic surgeon in July 1946, it was a 'quite a manoeuvre'[89] which blew a six-month hole in her almoner training. Whilst convalescing towards the end of the year, in a period of warm weather which preceded the bitter cold that was to come, Cicely spent time with a group of friends at the ivy-clad Willesleigh House in Goodleigh, that was Madge Drake's place near Barnstaple (Figure 2.2). Madge was quite a lot older than the rest of Cicely's circle. Her older sister Eileen married a widowed missionary doctor who had six children, and they went on to run an old people's home at Reigate, where Cicely's Aunt Daisy was eventually one of their first residents. Cicely also went on holidays with Madge in the New Forest, and it was Madge who later introduced her to the pleasures of bird-watching. Cicely described her as 'lovely company and an awfully good listener'[90]. The frail-looking Madge, sensitive and slightly neurotic, presided over the earnest discussions that took place amongst her visitors. An arthritic doctor and his frail old mother

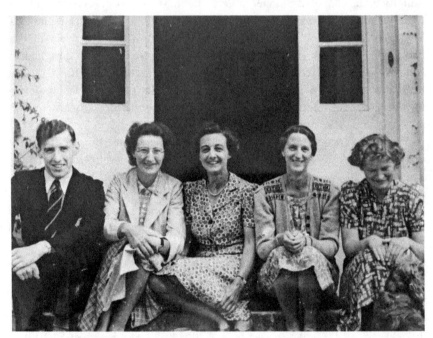

FIGURE 2.2 At Willesleigh House in Goodleigh, Devon, late 1946. L to R: Dr Malcolm Brown, Cicely Saunders, Margaret Dyke, Madge Drake, not known. *Source: courtesy of David Allbrook.*

were also in residence. Cicely recalled it as 'a lovely place which just sort of gathered us all in'. Amongst them was the medical student David Allbrook, who many years later was a professor of medicine and hospice physician in Australia. In September 1946, he had been rusticated to Devon due to a small T.B. lesion he had contracted. He later recalled from his diary at the time, that on Sunday, 6 December 1946, the residents gathered round the fire in the drawing room and Madge Drake asked the keen group of young evangelicals how they planned to spend the rest of their lives. 'I remember very clearly Cicely saying she was going to look after people who were dying'[91]. If accurate, this suggests that, through the disruption of her back problems and the painful surgery that followed, and despite the ambivalences about almoner training, a clear pathway was already opening up in Cicely's mind. What could not be known was that she was only one year away from a crucial encounter that would set the seal on this and change everything.

Qualifying as an Almoner

Cicely returned to complete her course with a placement in Bristol during the sub-zero weeks of early 1947. Britain froze to a halt. By now something of an expert on heating devices of the time, she recalled: '*Never* have I been so cold. I had nine blankets on my bed and a Valor Vector convection heater'[92]. Returning to London, her immediate goal was in sight. By July 1947, she was qualified and had begun work as a lady almoner at St Thomas's Hospital. She was one of twelve in the Northcote Trust Team, founded in 1909 and which was then headed by Betty Read. At age twenty-nine, Cicely had at last obtained full-time, paid employment.

Great change was in the air. In 1942, economist, progressive, and reformer William Beveridge had published his report *Social Insurance and Allied Services*[93]. It launched an attack on five 'giant evils' in society — squalor, ignorance, want, idleness, and disease — and proposed widespread reforms to the system of social welfare by which to address them. Then, in 1947, as part of the unfolding welfare state, the creation of the National Health Service was only months away. Because medical care would soon be free at the point of delivery, the work of the almoner would cease to be about assessing how much patients could afford to pay for their treatment. From there on, almoners would concentrate more on casework and would focus on the social and psychological dimensions of patients' health-related problems. This appealed to Cicely enormously. The department at St Thomas's kept a cancer register and had a home visitor who followed up on those discharged home. There was greater scope for assessing problems in their context and for reaching out beyond the hospital walls. It was to be the dawning of the era of 'medical social work', with greater freedom to undertake casework and to offer patient and family support. Looking back on those times, many years later, Cicely observed: 'In the days of cash-strapped voluntary hospitals, we had to collect vouchers and suggest possible contributions to patients. It was a huge relief when the National Health Service was introduced in 1948'[94].

David Tasma

In the first ward she visited at St Thomas's, Cicely found Mr David Tasma, a forty-year-old Polish man with inoperable bowel cancer[95]. He had just had a colostomy and his prospects looked poor indeed. After having migrated from Poland to Britain, he was now succumbing to cancer of the rectum, far from home in a country where he had hoped to build his future. In the chaos of the war he had lost contact with all three of his brothers. Cicely immediately sensed he was in trouble and so kept in touch, following up with him in the outpatient clinic during the ensuing months.

Returning to work on Monday, 5 January 1948, after the Christmas and New Year holidays, Cicely received a call from David Tasma's landlady, Mrs Spreadborough of 17 Scala Street, in the Fitzrovia district of London. She explained that Mr Tasma had collapsed at home and was very unwell. Cicely's response was immediate: 'I'll come and see him tonight; but, meantime, get his family doctor in'. By the time Cicely arrived, Dr Pipka of Gower Street, a few blocks away, had moved swiftly. His patient was ready to go to hospital and a decision had been made not for St Thomas's, but for the Archway, in Highgate, North London. Tasma was ambivalent about this, having felt very well cared for by the nurses during his previous stay at St Thomas's. As they waited for the ambulance to arrive, Tasma asked Cicely if he was going to die. Apparently confident in her judgement, but nevertheless at odds with usual procedure for an almoner, she told him of his advanced cancer and confirmed his fears. There was no question of dishonesty or dissembling. He asked her to visit him. Again, breaking with due process for a lady almoner, she told him she would: 'I knew I couldn't do anything else'.

During the next two months, at the start of 1948, Cicely made twenty-six visits[96] to ward 12 at the Archway Hospital, each recorded in the briefest of notes in her small, red appointment diary. There he is listed at first as 'Tasma', but then after the eleventh visit, more tellingly, as 'David'. She made her first visit to him the day after his admission to hospital on 6 January. The Christian feast day of Epiphany was unequivocally to bring a sense of sudden and striking revelation. During the following visits, Cicely began to piece together the elements of his life.

Ela Majer ('David') Tasma had been born into the Jewish quarter of Warsaw in 1907. His mother died when he was quite young. His grandfather was a rabbi with whom he had engaged in argument and disputation as he grew up, sometimes long into the night. Tasma was agnostic and something of a rebel. He left school and started work at a young age. Later, he fell in love with the wife of a friend. Here, as elsewhere, the record is unclear. In her article of 2004, Cicely states that the issue about his friend's wife occurred when he was age twenty-two, and this impelled him to leave Poland. That would have been around 1929. In an interview[97], she says David had left in his late twenties, which could push the date back to around 1936. In either case, his departure was before both the Nazi invasion of Poland in 1939 and the 'unbounded inhumanity and sorrow'[98] of the Warsaw Ghetto from 1940 to 1943, neither of which he experienced first-hand. Though Cicely seems to have thought he spent the war in France, his personal papers reveal a different story. In fact, he was given leave to land at Dover on 5 June 1938, on condition that he did not enter employment. His registration certificate describes him as Polish, but with Russian as his previous nationality. On arrival in England, he went to live at 26 Smithy Street, in the East End of London, but his former address is given as Warsaw. There is no reference to time in France. Then, on 14 September 1940, permission was granted for his employment as a waiter at the Wardour Restaurant in London W1. His photograph, thought to have been taken before he left Poland (Figure 2.3), shows him well dressed, groomed, with just the suggestion of a smile as he gazes, eyes sparkling, at the camera.

Why he moved to London is also unclear. Born on 26 October 1907, he must have been thirty years old at the time. On arrival, he appears to have adopted the name David and, from the time he was able to work, he found lodgings in a run-down property, closer to the restaurant, in a street near London's West End. He was living in an area which was home to bohemians,

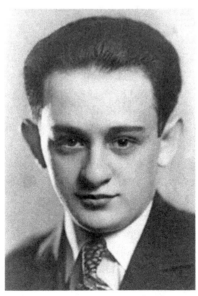

FIGURE 2.3 David Tasma, probably circa 1930 in Poland. *Source: unknown, kept by Cicely Saunders.*

writers, musicians, and actors — and nightlife. After working at the Wardour Restaurant, on 6 June 1941, he was given leave to work at the nearby Kosher Restaurant run by a Mr Biedak at 14 Denmark Street. Permission to work there was renewed in January 1945 and he was still employed with Mr Biedak when he first encountered Cicely. He seemed to have few acquaintances beyond his workplace and his lodgings. There is no hint that he had any close personal relationships. According to Cicely:

> The most important thing for him was to find somebody who would listen because he had the strong feeling that here he was, dying at the age of forty, and it made no difference to the world that he'd ever lived in it . . . . His past was less important than where he was at that moment . . . it was just our exchange in the present moment[99].

As the visits proceeded, they moved beyond the narrative of what he regarded as a wasted life. She found him, 'sad, unfulfilled . . . but ready to be interested'. She recorded in the briefest fashion the essence of their encounters. To read these diary entries, notwithstanding their brevity, is to reach into an intensely private space where a dying Jewish agnostic and an evangelical Christian found a deep mutuality, snatched from the jaws of death itself. The entries were later enhanced by Cicely in her subsequent commentaries, where more interpretation, if not detail, is revealed.

She must have known she was skating on thin ice. Her heart and body were telling her she was falling in love with this 'rude sort of fellow'[100] more than ten years her senior, who had enjoyed none of the advantages of her privileged upbringing. Most of all, she was playing fast and loose with protocol. Admonished as a nurse for calling a patient by his first name, now as an almoner she was visiting a patient in her own time and coming perilously close to transgressing the boundaries of professional distance, objectivity, and, not least, discretion. On one occasion he told her, 'I've waited all my life to find a nice girl, and here you are, and look at me'. She was sorrowful for him and was, herself, deeply moved. She too had been looking for love. Now, on finding it, she knew it would soon be taken from her. She had fallen for someone older, from a different world, and, through his imminent death, unattainable.

After each brief encounter, Cicely made her journey home on the number 27 bus to her flat in Bayswater. There, she shared her thoughts and feeling with Rosetta, Isobel, and the two medical students. They were knowledgeable about the issues and empathetic about the implications. He was in a 'very, very busy' surgical ward of sixty beds. There was little indication that he was in pain or suffering from other physical symptoms, but it didn't seem the right place to die. There was hubbub and activity. There was no privacy. Aneurin Bevan, one year earlier, had starkly captured the context when, as Minister of Health in the post-war Labour government, he introduced the National Health Service Bill to the British Parliament and stated he would 'rather be kept alive in the efficient if cold altruism of a large hospital than expire in a gush of warm sympathy in a small one'[101]. The setting at Archway echoed these tensions. It had been opened in 1879 as the Holburn Union Infirmary on the west side of the Archway Road in Highgate, a four-storey building with 625 beds. In 1930, it came under the control of the London County Council and was renamed the Archway Hospital. By 1948, as part of restructuring associated with the new National Health Service, it merged with St Mary's and Highgate Hospitals and became the Archway Wing of the newly constituted Whittington Hospital[102]. It was therefore a place caught up in a modernising and bureaucratising ethic, and no doubt lacked the facility to support someone at the end of life who was engaged in a process of reflection and seeking solace in the presence of a stranger. There should be a better place to die and 'the idea of somewhere that could have been more appropriate for him sort of came as we were talking'[103]. She shared with David the notion of some alternative home for the dying. Soon she would return to this in much more detail.

When David asked for help with making a will, a solicitor was found through the hospital. Because Cicely was visiting him in the evenings and could be deemed 'off duty', she was appointed as his sole executrix. It was a delicate judgement call. David had an insurance policy. He told Cicely he would leave her some money and said, 'I will be a window in your home'. When his liabilities had been cleared, a significant sum was left. How a policy of this nature could have been arranged by an immigrant to Britain and someone working in a low-paying job is another one of the mysteries of the Tasma story. However, and it would seem surprisingly, Betty Read agreed that the balance of the money after disbursements could be retained by Cicely for some future use. At this point, Cicely was a decade away from formulating her vision for hospice care, so the notion of a future purpose for the money — even allowing for the conversations she had with David — seems remote indeed, and the manner of its acceptance is unorthodox. In later anecdotes and writings, Cicely elaborated more on this part of David Tasma's legacy. In time, he became the 'first patient' of St Christopher's and the centre of a complete foundation myth for the hospice. In these later accounts, she says far more than is noted in her diary. 'I'll be a window in your home' became an oft-repeated phrase, though it is nowhere recorded at the time. It provided Cicely with an image to take her forward, an offer to accept and a vision to fulfil. The window brings light into the building. At night, the light shines out from it. The window can also be an opportunity. It provides air and ventilation. It is the meeting place of the inner and the outer, the private and the public. 'Window' comes from the Middle English *vindauga*, meaning literally 'eye of the wind'. The window frames something, as in a painting. Yet, it also reveals an openness to the wider world outside. Tasma (or perhaps Cicely) chose the metaphor well. It is rich in symbolism and yet mundane and familiar. It also ensured he would live on. Disarmingly, Cicely would observe in later life: 'I mean, it's very poetic to say, "I'll be a window in your home", and it was a lovely key phrase which was awfully good when I was talking about it afterwards'.

Another time, David asked, 'Can't you say something to comfort me?' Respecting his Jewish heritage, she said the 23rd Psalm: 'The Lord's My Shepherd'. He asked her to go on. She said the Venite, Psalm 95, that is also used as a canticle in Christian liturgy, typically at Matins: 'Oh come let us sing unto the Lord'. She knew this well from singing in choirs. She went on to Psalm 121: 'I will lift up mine eyes to the hills', that she also knew by heart. He asked for more. She was unsure, considered something else, hesitated, and asked if she might read to him, reaching into her handbag for a copy of the Psalms. He shook his head, demurred, and with deliberation replied, 'I only want what is in your mind and in your heart'. The statement and the distinction immediately resonated, but it was only later that they came to embody the two dimensions of 'hospice' care at the end of life — the application of the knowledge and wisdom of the mind, sitting alongside the care and vulnerable friendship of the heart. It was, again, a moment to which Cicely would return many times in the future[104], though, sorry to say, it is unverified in the contemporary record.

She explained to him the basis of her Christian faith. He explained to her how he had turned away from the faith of his fore-fathers. There is just a hint she might have been hoping that, on his deathbed, he was open to Christian conversion. She even played something of the coy female: 'I remember saying to him one day, "But you mustn't say you believe just because you like me"'. But Tasma was having none of that and replied, 'I like you too much to say I believe just because I like you'. Thus dealt with, the matter was quickly 'put on one side'. Cicely's diary entries remain cryptic and tantalising: 'I knew you wouldn't' (Monday, 13 January). 'I said it' (Wednesday, 22 January). 'She had' (Sunday, 2 February). 'How we really feel' (Thursday, 20 February). On Monday, 24 January, he was 'well'. On Friday, 7 February, he was 'ill'. On Monday, 24 February, he was 'weak'. There are four references to the Gospel or the Bible. Sunday, 23 February, was the 'best ever' visit. Shirley du Boulay elaborates the scene[105]; it was an afternoon of laughter, a perfect afternoon, something to cherish even if nothing else remained.

On the evening of Tuesday, 25 February 1948, Cicely left him drifting into unconsciousness. 'I said good night to him and he closed his eyes'. Next morning, to safeguard her privacy, she called the hospital from Bayswater underground station rather than from the flat. He had died at 8.40 pm, one hour after she had left the previous evening. When she arrived at St Thomas's, she explained to Betty Read that she would need to assist with the legal and funeral arrangements. Cicely returned to the ward at Archway Hospital. As she collected what there was of his things — a watch and a dressing gown — the nurse told her, 'You were the last person he saw. He didn't open his eyes again after you left'[106]. It meant so much for Cicely to know this, then and into the future, when it was always remembered. Miss Murray, the Ward Sister, showed no disapproval of what had happened. Indeed, she and Cicely kept in intermittent contact for many years afterwards, bound together by the experience with David.

Two days later, Cicely and Mr Biedak were the only people to attend the funeral of Ela Majer (David) Tasma. In some 'sort of hut, it wasn't a chapel really', they said the 91st Psalm: 'Under his wings you will find refuge'. He was buried in Streatham, in the Rowan Road Jewish cemetery. Afterwards, there was still much for Cicely to do. As executrix she had to ensure the beneficiaries of the will were all contacted and the debtors were paid. She approached this with characteristic attention to detail, writing out more than a dozen cheques and many more letters, and receiving extensive correspondence from Maffey and Brentnall, Tasma's solicitors. The total sum paid out by the Prudential Insurance Company was £1,020. Various people at Scala Street received money, as did the cook at the Kosher Restaurant and Mr Biedak himself, amounting to £170 in total. They all wrote subsequently to thank Cicely, and one of them, Mrs Massacé, explained she would use the money to make a visit home to Morocco, her first in twenty-three years. Less clear, and never referred to elsewhere, is why Cicely gave Madge Drake in Devon a cheque for £200. There were legal fees (£43-7-7), funeral costs (£47-2-0), and an amount to London City Council for seven weeks and two days 'maintenance' (£43-1-6). A balance of £527 was left to Cicely as executrix, as the will stated, 'absolutely'; it became the later and much-quoted £500 for a 'window in your home'.

Sociologist Yasmin Gunaratnum has written eloquently about David Tasma, Cicely Saunders, and the significance of their shared story[107]. Gunaratnum makes an important assumption. She takes the view that all of David's family had been killed in the Holocaust. Consequently, his death would bring to an end the family line, as his 'inconsequential' life disappeared into 'nothingness'[108]. She frames him as the migrant who, newly arrived in London (albeit, as we now know, that was some ten years before), would have been struggling with language and with finding a place to live and a place to work. In these circumstances, she considers, he might well have neglected or even overlooked his own illness, though in fact it is now clear he was in settled employment and seems to have found a surrogate family among his fellow residents at Scala Street, to whom he left various parcels of money when he died. She points to the trust that grew between him and Cicely as his situation worsened, but is puzzled by Cicely's failure to describe more fully and chart the 'dark coordinates'[109] of his life, whilst at the same time being faithful to his memory. David's trust in the face of his own death came in the light of not knowing fully what he himself had survived. Gunaratnum asks, 'Who were you David?'[110] Perhaps the question is wrongly worded. It might better be phrased as, 'Who were you Ela?'

Further questions remain unanswered. We have so few details of Ela Majer 'David' Tasma. Cicely is inconsistent with the small number of facts she lays out. She gives differing ages for when he left Poland. Did his relatives all perish in the Holocaust? Did she correctly recall that a brother had gone to South America? After his death, and the profound influence of what they had shared together, why did she never visit his burial place until decades later, when she was even unsure where the grave was located? It was just four miles from St Christopher's Hospice and her nearby place of residence. Even then, she didn't go to the grave, but placed a stone in the garden, in the Jewish tradition. More puzzling is why she remained permanently sketchy about his circumstances after leaving Poland. As his executrix, Cicely had in her possession his registration documents, clearly stating his date of arrival at Dover, the details of his employment, and the places where he subsequently lived in London for almost a decade.

We have only shards of evidence about these things, and they cannot be pieced together to make a convincing case. It would be possible to think the story was an invention if the documentary record did not tell otherwise. Yet, David was far from alone in his experience. In 1940, the Polish government in exile had transferred to Britain. Some two hundred thousand displaced Poles were living there in 1945. The Polish Resettlement Act of 1947 gave them leave to stay. The Poles had made a significant contribution to the war effort; they would now (it was rationalised) also be useful in the process of post-war reconstruction[111]. Tasma was perhaps inclined to stay on in this context, optimistic about creating a new life and a better future, maybe even with a wife and family. His death at the age of forty put all that to an end.

Aftermath

A couple of evenings after David Tasma's death, Cicely was in a prayer meeting at All Souls church in Langholm Place. They started to sing 'How sweet the name of Jesus sounds . . .' and she thought to herself, 'But it didn't for him'; it was as if God was saying to her 'He knows me now far better than you do'. After that, she never worried about him again or about anybody else who died angry, sad, bitter, or unbelieving, because she was sure that, in death, they would be met with total understanding and love, and be safe[112]. It was a conviction which would support her through the deaths of countless patients in the years to come. But for the moment, it was incompletely revealed. She was sorrowful and cleaved to a grief which must remain private and unspoken. She had sailed close to the wind of professional misconduct, perhaps saved only by the wise and indulgent stance of Betty Read, who seems to have made an understanding and measured response to the events that occurred. What got underway on 6 January 1948 had indeed been an epiphanal moment. To mask her grief, she kept up the intensity of her appointments and social activities. In May she was at a Yehudi Menhuin concert and a meeting of the Nightingale Fellowship. There was 'singing' every Wednesday night and bible study next evening at St Peter's. There were suppers with Chrissie, lunches at Hadley. She read John Buchan novels voraciously and listed them all in the back of her 1948 appointment diary. Perhaps the improbable plots, the rumbustious adventure, and sometimes the Highland settings brought solace and escape, coupled with reassurance in the simplicity of the author's well-known sense of sexless romance.

A deeper release came in the summertime. On 4 June 1948, she took the night sleeper to Inverness and travelled on to meet her father and friends at Glenquoich Lodge. Rising early one morning in glorious weather, she sat where a small burn ran into the loch, the peat-stained water rippling over shining pebbles. At that moment, she slipped into the 'timeless now'. This is something neither past nor future, and yet something much more than the present moment. It is the changeless or eternal now. In that 'now', David was present somewhere. She knew David was all right and that this 'now' was also all right. 'It was *so* strong and comforting'[113].

Even by this point, Cicely had embarked on a strategy of practical action. Following David Tasma's death, the evenings were empty and listless. On 15 March she telephoned Miss Pipkin, a member of the Salvation Army and matron at St Luke's Home in Bayswater, just near the flat where Cicely and her friends were living. She asked if she could volunteer her services. She could take the number 12 bus there from St Thomas's and walk home afterwards. From the start of April she was visiting regularly, and soon settled into a steady pattern of being there on Sunday and Monday evenings. When Miss Pipkin observed her skills as a registered nurse, she quickly gave Cicely the role of Sister for the evening rotation. The commitment was to last seven years. She 'loved it there'[114]. In addition to her practical nursing, her clear soprano voice was popular with the patients, to whom she sang Victorian melodies and folk songs, accompanying herself at the piano. Later, Miss Pipkin found her a dedicated accompanist. Their renditions always finished the evening. Her time in this home for the dying, tucked away in a Bayswater street and proclaiming itself to nobody, felt worthwhile, even formative.

For something deeper was also going on. After the death of David Tasma, she had asked herself, 'What should I do?'[115] The answer was almost immediate; she should find a way to work with the dying, just as she had told her friends in Devon at the end of 1946 and just as she had expected something would be revealed to her after her conversion in 1945. But she was still unsure about how this would be realised[116]. 'I still didn't know what to do, other than go on doing what I was doing. They say "testing your vocation", but I didn't have that vocabulary'[117]. 'I really went there to see whether I was right in that slot, and they said that I slotted in straight away'[118].

This was how Cicely became familiar with a handful of terminal-care homes that existed in London during the late 1940s. In some cases, as an almoner, she had arranged to send patients to them following discharge from hospital. They represented what the American writer Grace Goldin and later friend of Cicely called the 'proto-hospices'[119]. They came before the wave of modern hospices that began with St Christopher's in 1967. They were all deeply rooted in religious values and usually linked to one or another branch of institutional Christianity. Their focus was on those imminently dying, chiefly from T.B. and from cancer. The first, founded by the Scot Frances Davidson and known as The Friedenheim, had opened in Islington in 1885. After that came The Hostel of God, founded by Anglican nuns in Clapham in 1892 following an appeal in *The Times*. Next, in 1893, came St Luke's Home for the Dying Poor in Regents Park, founded by Dr Howard Barrett, the medical superintendent of the Methodist West London Mission. Like the other two establishments, St Luke's had comfortable amenities and facilities. With accommodation for fifteen or sixteen beds, it also had pleasant corners, enormous potted plants, easy chairs, and sofas. In 1901, it moved to bigger premises in Hampstead, but had to relocate again when problems arose with the lease and when neighbours complained that the home's presence prevented other properties in the street from being let. It reopened in early 1902 in Pembridge Square, before moving to purpose-built accommodation in nearby Hereford Road, Bayswater, in 1923. Barrett retired in 1913, and from 1917 onwards St Luke's became a 'Hospital for Advanced Cases'. The early religious influences began to wane. By the time Cicely arrived there, with the National Health Service then in the process of formation, its management was about to be absorbed into St Mary's Teaching Group of Hospitals. But for a while at least, it maintained its special character and its careful approach to the regular administration of pain relief. In 1974, the building was renovated and the hospital was re-named Hereford Lodge (thus avoiding the depressing connotations of advanced cases and dying). It had forty-two beds for pre-convalescence and terminal care. But as the National Health Service underwent further changes, Hereford Lodge eventually closed in 1985, and its functions were reallocated to St Charles Hospital and the Paddington Community Hospital.

In Cicely's time at St Luke's in Hereford Road, there was a twelve-bed ward, a three-bed ward, and a single room, to which patients were moved when they were imminently dying. Although it had suffered no damage during wartime, it had been reduced in capacity due to staff shortages. In 1945, it was back to full strength[120]. There, Cicely made a profound and consequential observation. It concerned the St Luke's approach to pain control, that was based on the regular and routine giving of narcotics. By such means, the idea was to prevent the onset of pain, rather than to attack it once it was established. It was an important principle which she would later elaborate in detail. The concept was attributed to Miss Pipkin, who had joined St Luke's in 1935, but she in turn suggested that it was the nurses there who had developed it before her arrival. It was seen as a nursing, rather than a medical, innovation, and that idea appealed to Nurse Saunders too. Later in the decade, the approach was described by visiting physician Dr J. Cameron Morris in an article which appeared in the *St Mary's Hospital Gazette*: 'Our experience is that repeated quite small injections of morphine never — or very seldom — fail to relieve otherwise intractable pain of terminal Ca., and that they never lead to the necessity for immense single doses'[121].

Despite the demands of the long days working as an almoner at St Thomas's and the evenings spent as a volunteer nurse at St Luke's, Cicely was becoming more and more drawn to the needs and care of dying people. As her understanding advanced and as the 1940s came to an end, she was convinced that she should get more involved in terminal care. It seemed the only way to do so would be to resume her full-time nursing career, for all the attendant risks to her own health. She was keeping an eye out for possibilities. She could not know that, in 1951, a chance remark from a senior colleague would change everything and plunge her into a completely new direction of travel.

Notes

1. Cicely Saunders interview with David Clark, 2 May 2003.

2. Prochaska A. Reflections on the history and identity of the former women's colleges. Paper presented at The History of Oxford Colleges Conference, Trinity College Oxford, 15 November 2014, http://www.some.ox.ac.uk/research/research-profiles/alice-prochaska-womens-colleges/, accessed 19 May 2016.

3. *St Anne's College: Our History*, http://www.st-annes.ox.ac.uk/about/history, accessed 19 May 2016.

4. Addison P. Oxford and the Second World War. In Harrison B., ed. *The History of the University of Oxford: Volume VIII: The Twentieth Century*. Oxford: Clarendon Press; 1994: 167–188.

5. University of Oxford. *The Examination Statutes, Together with the Regulations of the Boards of Studies and Boards of Faculties for the Academical Year 1926–1927*. Oxford: Clarendon Press; 1926: 149–154.

6. du Boulay S. *Cicely Saunders: The Founder of the Modern Hospice Movement*, 2nd ed. London: Hodder and Stoughton; 1994: 31.

7. There was a favourable review in *The Spectator*, 'Social conditions at Oxford', 28 June 1913, 10.

8. Butler C.V. *Social Conditions in Oxford*. London: Sidgwick and Jackson; 1912.

9. Cicely Saunders interview with Neil Small, Hospice History Project, 24 October 1995.

10. See, for example, Famous Oxford Alumni, http://www.biography.com/people/groups/famous-alumni-of-oxford-university, accessed 21 May 2016.

11. Addison, Oxford and the Second World War, 169.

12. Cicely Saunders interview with David Clark, 2 May 2003.

13. Ceadel M. The 'King and Country' debate, 1933: Student politics, pacifism and the dictators. *The Historical Journal.* 1979; 22(2): 397–422.

14. Addison, Oxford and the Second World War, 171.

15. Brittain V. *The Women of Oxford: A Fragment of History.* New York: Macmillan; 1960.

16. Saunders C. Oxford in war-time. *Roedean School Magazine.* 1939; December: 104–106.

17. This was the scheme for voluntary aid detachments (V.A.Ds.) which offered first-aid and nursing care to civilians injured by air raids as well as injured servicemen.

18. Cicely Saunders interview with Neil Small, Hospice History Project, 24 October 1995.

19. David Clark interview with Christopher Saunders, 1 May 2015.

20. Hadham J. *Good God: His Character and Activities.* Harmondsworth: Penguin; 1940.

21. Hadham J. *God in a World at War.* Harmondsworth: Penguin Books; 1940.

22. Watson G.C. Review of Hoover A. J. *God, Britain, and Hitler in World War II: The View of the British Clergy, 1939–1945* (Westport, CT: Praeger; 1999). *Anglican and Episcopal History* 2001; 70(1): 136–138.

23. The Parkes Institute, http://www.southampton.ac.uk/parkes/about/jamesparkes. page, accessed 16 June 2016.

24. Cicely Saunders interview with David Clark, 15 December 1999.

25. du Boulay, *Cicely Saunders,* 35.

26. We have two excellent accounts of this period, first in du Boulay (*Cicely Saunders,* 33–39) and also in the first paragraphs of Saunders C. A personal therapeutic journey. *British Medical Journal.* 1996; 313: 1599–1601. I draw on both of them here, along with interviews conducted by myself and by Neil Small.

27. Romanis H. *The Compleat Surgeon: The Autobiography of the Surgeon WHC Romanis.* Bury St Edmunds: Arena Books; 2013.

28. Andrews L. *No Time for Romance.* London: Corgi; 2007: 187. First published by Harrap and Co Ltd in 1978.

29. Cicely Saunders interview with Neil Small, Hospice History Project, 24 October 1995.

30. Cicely Saunders interview with David Clark, 20 September 2000.

31. Cicely Saunders interview with David Clark, 2 May 2003.

32. For an obituary, see Cecil Tonsley BEM FRES 1915–2003, http://www. tandfonline.com/doi/abs/10.1080/0005772X.2003.11099593, accessed 20 June 2016.

33. Cicely Saunders interview with Neil Small, Hospice History Project, 24 October 1995.

34. Cicely Saunders interview with David Clark, 2 May 2003.

35. Cicely Saunders interview with Neil Small, Hospice History Project, 24 October 1995.

36. Cicely Saunders interview with Neil Small, Hospice History Project, 24 October 1995.

37. Botley's Park Hospital, Chertsey Records, http://discovery.nationalarchives.gov. uk/details/rd/6bc62d5e-ecf2-46e0-a87e-fd70eb8e6f24, accessed 1 June 2016.

38. Cicely Saunders interview with Neil Small, Hospice History Project, 24 October 1995.

39. 'A Nightingale Sang in Berkeley Square', song written in 1939 with lyrics by Eric Maschwitz and music by Manning Sherwin.

40. Cicely Saunders interview with Neil Small, Hospice History Project, 24 October 1995.

41. Cicely Saunders interview with David Clark, 2 May 2003.

42. Cicely Saunders interview with Neil Small, Hospice History Project, 24 October 1995.

43. Tolkien J.R.R. *The Hobbit*. London: George Allen and Unwin; 1937.

44. Tolkien J.R.R. *The Fellowship of the Ring, The Two Towers, The Return of the King*. London: George Allen and Unwin; 1954, 1954, 1955.

45. Lewis C.S. *The Allegory of Love*. Oxford: The Clarendon Press; 1936.

46. Lewis C.S. *The Lion the Witch and the Wardrobe*. London: Geoffrey Bles; 1950.

47. The Socratic Club—Religious Debate at Oxford, http://www.scriptoriumnovum.com/l/club.html, accessed 16 June 2016.

48. McGrath A. *C.S. Lewis: A Life*. London: Hodder and Stoughton; 2013.

49. Lewis C.S. *The Problem of Pain*. London: Geoffrey Bles and The Centenary Press; 1940.

50. Cicely Saunders interview with David Clark, 15 December 1999.

51. McGrath, *C.S. Lewis*, 205.

52. Lewis, C.S. *Mere Christianity*. London: Geoffrey Bles; 1952.

53. Lewis C.S. Preface. In *Broadcast Talks*. London: Geoffrey Bles; 1943: 1–2.

54. Clerk N.W. *A Grief Observed*. London: Faber and Faber; 1961 (later, Lewis C.S. *A Grief Observed*. London: Faber and Faber; 1964).

55. Sayers D.L. *The Man Born to Be King: A Play-Cycle on the Life of Our Lord and Saviour Jesus Christ, Written for Broadcasting*. London: Wm. B. Eerdmans; 1943.

56. Cicely Saunders interview with David Clark, 15 December 1999.

57. Temple W. *Christianity and Social Order*. Harmondsworth: Penguin; 1942.

58. Cicely Saunders interview with David Clark, 15 December 1999.

59. Cicely Saunders interview with David Clark, 15 December 1999.

60. V.E. Day, 8 May 1945, as it would have happened. http://www.telegraph.co.uk/history/world-war-two/11591735/VE-Day-8th-May-1945-as-it-happened-live.html, accessed 20 June 2016.

61. Cicely Saunders interview with Neil Small, Hospice History Project, 24 October 1995.

62. du Boulay, *Cicely Saunders*, 45.

63. Cicely Saunders interview with Neil Small, Hospice History Project, 24 October 1995.

64. Cicely Saunders interview with David Clark, 25 September 2003.

65. Cicely Saunders interview with David Clark, 25 September 2003.

66. Cicely Saunders interview with David Clark, 15 December 1999.

67. Cicely Saunders interview with David Clark, 19 February 2003.

68. For example, in October 1963, they stayed in the Hotel Poort von Cleeve in Amsterdam and Cicely was able to arrange a meeting with F.J.J. Buytendijk, the doctor and phenomenological scholar whose book *Over de Pijn* (Utrecht, 1943) had appeared in English as Buytendijk F.J.J. *Pain: Its Modes and Functions*, trans. Edna O'Sheil. London: Hutchison; 1961. See more on this in Chapter 4.

69. Cicely Saunders interview with David Clark, 15 December 1999.

70. du Boulay, *Cicely Saunders*, 47.

71. 'Just As I Am Without One Plea', http://www.oremus.org/hymnal/j/j257.html, accessed 20 June 2016.

72. Saunders C. Consider Him. In Saunders C., ed. *Watch with Me*. Sheffield: Mortal Press; 2003: 40, 39–50.

73. Cicely Saunders interview with David Clark, 15 December 1999.

74. Cicely Saunders interview with David Clark, 20 September 2000.

75. Thompson, E.P. *The Making of the English Working Class*. London: Victor Gollancz Ltd; 1963.

76. Cicely Saunders interview with Neil Small, Hospice History Project, 24 October 1995.

77. Lambeth Archives. Records of Lady Margaret Hall Settlement, http://discovery.nationalarchives.gov.uk/details/rd/bad738d3-4687-4399-b178-57d793f2c10b, accessed 27 June 2016.

78. The Institute of Almoners eventually became the Institute of Medical Social Workers in 1964 and was part of the formation of the British Association of Social Workers in 1970. See Archives of Institute of Medical Social Workers, 1895–1971, http://web.warwick.ac.uk/services/library/mrc/ead/378IMSW.htm, accessed 27 June 2016.

79. du Boulay, *Cicely Saunders*, 41–42.

80. Cicely Saunders interview with Neil Small, Hospice History Project, 24 October 1995.

81. Cicely Saunders interview with David Clark, 20 September 2000.

82. Cicely Saunders interview with Neil Small, Hospice History Project, 24 October 1995.

83. Cicely Saunders interview with David Clark, 20 September 2000.

84. Cicely Saunders interview with David Clark, 20 September 2000.

85. Cicely Saunders interview with David Clark, 20 September 2000.

86. Eliot G. *Middlemarch: A Study of Provincial Life*. Edinburgh: William Blackwood and Sons; 1872.

87. Cicely Saunders interview with David Clark, 20 September 2000.

88. Rosetta Burch (nee Wray) died on 18 February 2009 in Chiswick House, Norwich. As we shall see, her daughter Rosemary Burch, a breast-care nurse specialist, looked after Cicely Saunders at St Thomas's Hospital in the final phases of her illness.

89. Cicely Saunders interview with David Clark, 20 September 2000.

90. Cicely Saunders interview with David Clark, 20 September 2000.

91. Professor David Allbrook, pers. comm., 7 October 1998.

92. Cicely Saunders interview with Neil Small, Hospice History Project, 24 October 1995.

93. Beveridge W. Social insurance and allied services. Presented to Parliament by Command of His Majesty, November 1942. HMSO Cmd 6404.

94. Saunders C. Social work and palliative care: The early history. *British Journal of Social Work*. 2001; 31: 791–799.

95. I base my account of David Tasma here on some key sources. First, two interviews (Cicely Saunders interview with Neil Small, Hospice History Project, 24 October 1995, and Cicely Saunders interview with David Clark, 2 May 2003), the un-referenced direct

quotations come from the interviews. Second, I draw on the six-page chapter in du Boulay (*Cicely Saunders*, 54–59). Third, I make use of pieces written by Cicely Saunders herself: two letters to Professor I. Ta-Shma dated 3 February 1987 and 6 March 1987 — reproduced in Clark D. *Cicely Saunders: Founder of the Hospice Movement: Selected Letters 1959–1999*. Oxford: Oxford University Press; 2002: 291, 295; and the article Saunders C. David Tasma. *Hospice Information Bulletin*. 2004; 6–7. Fourth, I draw on various files from the Cicely Saunders archive at King's College London, particularly K/PP149/1/1/4, which includes Cicely's own appointment diary kept at the time. I return to the importance of David Tasma in later chapters.

96. du Boulay (*Cicely Saunders*) states there were twenty-five visits; Saunders's article of 2004 (see footnote 95) states twenty-eight. Close scrutiny of Cicely's diary kept at the time (see footnote 95) indicates twenty-six.

97. Cicely Saunders interview with David Clark, 2 May 2003.

98. Davies N. *Rising '44: 'The Battle for Warsaw'*. London: Macmillan; 2003: 98.

99. Cicely Saunders interview with David Clark, 2 May 2003.

100. Diary, 11 February 1948. It was Ash Wednesday.

101. Quoted in Abel-Smith B. *The Hospitals 1800–1948: A Study in Social Administration in England and Wales*. London, UK: Heinemann; 1964: 481; and Murphy C. From Friedenheim to hospice: A century of cancer hospitals. In Granshaw L., Porter R., eds. *The Hospital in History*. London, UK: Routledge; 1989: 221–241.

102. Lost Hospitals of London, Archway Hospital, http://ezitis.myzen.co.uk/archway.html, accessed 29 June 2016.

103. Cicely Saunders interview with Neil Small, Hospice History Project, 24 October 1995.

104. The first written record appears to be in 1974: Saunders C. A place to die. *Crux*. 1973–1974; 11(3): 24–27.

105. du Boulay, *Cicely Saunders*, 57.

106. Cicely Saunders interview with Neil Small, Hospice History Project, 24 October 1995.

107. Gunaratnum Y. *Death and the Migrant: Bodies, Borders and Care*. London: Bloomsbury; 2013: especially 34–40.

108. Gunaratnum, *Death and the Migrant*, 34.

109. Gunaratnum, *Death and the Migrant*, 38.

110. Gunaratnum, *Death and the Migrant*, 35.

111. Kay D., Miles R. Refugees or migrant workers? The case of the European Volunteer Workers in Britain (1946–1951). *Journal of Refugee Studies*. 1998; 1(3–4): 214–236.

112. du Boulay, *Cicely Saunders*, 55–56.

113. du Boulay, *Cicely Saunders*, 59.

114. Cicely Saunders interview with Neil Small, Hospice History Project, 24 October 1995.

115. Cicely Saunders interview with Neil Small, Hospice History Project, 24 October 1995.

116. Cicely Saunders interview with Neil Small, Hospice History Project, 24 October 1995.

117. Cicely Saunders interview with David Clark, 15 December 1999.

118. Cicely Saunders interview with David Clark, 2 May 2003.

119. Goldin G. A proto hospice at the turn of the century: St Luke's House, London, from 1893 to 1923. *Journal of the History of Medicine and Allied Sciences*. 1981; 36(4): 383–415.

120. Lost Hospitals of London, Hereford Lodge, http://ezitis.myzen.co.uk/ herefordlodge.html, accessed 30 June 2016.

121. Cameron Morris J. The management of cases in the terminal stages of malignant disease. *St Mary's Hospital Gazette*. 1959: 65(4): 4–6.

3 | Becoming a Doctor (1951 – 1957)

So I read Medicine entirely to do something about pain at the end of life[1].

The Influence of Norman Barrett

At the start of the 1950s, the capacity of Britain for post-war optimism was beginning to wane. The Labour government under Clement Atlee was re-elected in February 1950, but only with a slender majority which soon proved unworkable. By November of the following year, the people were back at the polls and this time a Conservative government came to power, led by a resurgent Winston Churchill. Cold War tensions were mounting. Then, in February 1952, King George VI died suddenly in his sleep after a day's shooting. Age fifty-six, he had been suffering from lung cancer for some time, but his end, when it came, was unexpected and shocked the nation. The country was at odds with itself. On the one hand there was a desire for progress, change, and modernisation — a spirit that the Festival of Britain, held in 1951, had sought to promote. On the other hand, there was a longing for stability, for the privacy of family life, and the assurance which could come from a settled economic outlook and an ordered approach to morals, culture, and values.

Cicely was now in her early thirties. She too seemed torn. Her parents' marriage had broken apart and she had yet to find a romantic love of her own that would sustain her into the future. She was still clinging to an evangelical version of Christianity, as practised at All Souls, Langham Place, but was also possessed of a growing commitment to her work and, in particular, to the care of those who were close to the end of life. She fitted in well with the institutional environment of hospitals and homes for the elderly and sick. She seemed to have more to offer than her role as an almoner could fulfil, even with an expanded brief to undertake casework. Like the country as a whole, she was suspended between tradition and change. She was holding on to deep and long-held beliefs about death and its meanings, the virtues of family care at the end of life, and the power of religion to make sense of suffering. Yet, she was also looking for new approaches, dissatisfied with established medical practice, and cultivating an appetite for advocacy and innovation. One key person was astute enough to see where this could lead, if suitably harnessed.

In 1950, an opportunity arose for a change of tack. Staying under the umbrella of St Thomas's and without entirely losing direct contact with patients and families, Cicely engineered a hybrid role for herself: part caseworker and part medical secretary. She was to report directly to surgeon Norman Barrett.

Born in Australia in 1903, but brought to Britain at the age of ten, educated at Eton School and Trinity College Cambridge, Barrett had been at St Thomas's since 1928, when he commenced his training. His reputation was phenomenal. On 7 March 1947, he had performed the first successful repair of a ruptured oesophagus. Of ruddy complexion as a child, he had been known ironically since schooldays as 'Pasty'. He was a mine of aphorisms, opinions, and eccentricities. Cicely admired his bluster, but knew it was backed up by rigorous methods, surgical skill, and a passion to improve the lot of his patients. She was drawn to his approach, and he in turn seems to have sensed her potential.

During the early 1950s, part of Barrett's work still involved the surgical treatment of people with T.B. He had also described the case of the oesophagus lined with columnar epithelium, a condition with which his name became synonymous. He practised across several hospitals and homes, and consulted to the Royal Navy and the Ministry of Social Security. In her new hybrid role, Cicely accompanied him on ward rounds, dealt with his medical records and correspondence, but also followed up with patients and families in need of social work help, visiting them on the wards and at home. The work was adding to the stock of her experience and honing her administrative skills, but despite her inspirational boss, she remained unsure of her direction and was contemplating a return to nursing. In the summer of 1951, Cicely noticed that a position had come up as Night Sister at St Columba's, one of the London homes for the dying. She thought it might be manageable for her despite her back problems.

Contemplating Change

A few days later, she and Barrett were driving along from London to Midhurst in Kent, to the King Edward Sanatorium, where he was to perform an operation. Ruminating on the need to make a decision about her future direction and focus, she told him: 'I think I'm going to have to go back and nurse, because I've really got to get on with this.'[2] He was swift to disagree. As Cicely often recalled subsequently:

> He said 'No. Go and read Medicine. It's the doctors who desert the dying, and there's so much more to be learnt about pain and you'll only be frustrated if you don't do it properly, and they won't listen to you.' And he was right[3].

She did not linger over his advice. Within weeks she was embarked on an application to medical school.

Norman Barrett's influence on Cicely Saunders has been underplayed. Even before she began to work for him directly, he had been interested in her involvement with St Luke's hospital for 'advanced cases'. Impressed by the pain control methods she was observing there, Cicely invited him to make a visit and to see one of the patients. In another instance, and unusually, she took him to the home of one of his own patients, where he was able to see more fully the wider context of family, illness, and distress. This urbane and patrician surgeon must have seen some special dimension in Cicely Saunders's enthusiasms. Eponymously, she 'winkled' him out of the hospital and his natural environment and into the terrain of the almoner and the wider community. His interest built her confidence. More important, though she may not have realised it at the time, it was a dry run for many future encounters with doubting members of the medical establishment who would have to be won over to her ideas if her goals were to be realised. One patient and his wife particularly caught their imagination.

Mr and Mrs S.

Mr S., from Brixton in south London, had been operated on by Barrett for thoracotomy in September 1950. Age forty-six, he was found to have advanced lung cancer. At this point, like many others in similar situations at that time, he would have received the baleful message: "There is nothing more that we can do". He was discharged home and left to get on with things. Except that in this instance, he was fortunate to have Cicely as his almoner, and she was growing more and more curious about what could be done to help such patients and their families. A successful publishing manager, involved with the Rationalist Press, and a convinced atheist and member of the Secular Society, Mr S. could often be found on a soapbox at Hyde Park Corner. He was outward-going and had strong opinions. Now his world was collapsing inwards; he was becoming anxious and was desperate not to be abandoned by his doctors. His wife was finding it hard to look after him and — as his pain and distress increased — so, too, did the tension between them as a couple. In February 1951, Mr S. was admitted to St Luke's, where he again encountered Cicely, there during one of her volunteer sessions. Responding to the regular giving of narcotics that was practised there, he improved somewhat and was able to return home. But, within a fortnight, Mrs S. called St Thomas's, distressed for her husband and anxious for herself about how to cope. Cicely began visiting on a weekly basis. She organised a regular regime of medication through the local panel of family doctors. His pain was contained by a mixture of morphine, alcohol, codeine, and sodium amytal — the famous 'Brompton Cocktail' which was commonly used in London and elsewhere at that time, and which took its name from the Brompton Chest Hospital, where it was used to ease the suffering of people with advanced T.B.

Cicely's visits boosted the morale of Mrs S. and provided an opportunity for her to get out of the house for a while. Mr S., for his part, enjoyed a friendly argument with his Christian almoner and looked forward to her visits and the disputations they generated. For a time, the couple were able to keep going. Although his pain was never completely absent, Mr S. preferred to remain alert and to withstand it, rather than to become woozy with medication. He maintained a sense of dignity and his wife, too, found satisfaction in her ability to look after him in their home.

But when Cicely and Mr Barrett visited in August 1951, their patient was deteriorating significantly. He had lost weight and his pain was no longer being kept at bay. This time, he was admitted to St Columba's Hospital. Originally known as The Friedenheim, it was the first dedicated home for the dying in London when it opened its doors in Mildmay Road, Islington, in 1885. Now it was located in Hampstead, in rather palatial accommodation that was somewhat at odds with the ethos of the National Health Service, into which it had just been assimilated. There were open fireplaces in the wards at Hampstead, and comfortable furniture that fostered a homely atmosphere. When the weather allowed, patients could sit outside and enjoy the air in the pleasant grounds. In 1949, the newly retired resident doctor at St Columba's had written an extensive account of the care that was practised there[4]. It was a place where staff were familiar with patients like Mr S. Drugs for pain and symptom relief were freely given, not held back out of caution or fear of addiction. Mr S began receiving morphia by injection, up to a whole gramme every four hours, as his condition worsened. Sedatives settled him at night and, on his last day, he was also given the anti-spasmodic drug hyoscine to relieve cramps in the stomach, intestines, and bladder. Even up to his final hours, he was alert and fairly comfortable.

Mr S. died after six weeks in the supportive atmosphere of a home that specialised in caring for people at the very end of life, particularly those with T.B. and cancer. Apparently unperturbed by the prevailing atmosphere of re-ligious solicitude and the Christian imagery around the place, he was also reassured that everything had been done for him and his wife, and that he had not been rejected by St Thomas's. When he died, Mrs S. was left with no regrets about his care. The couple's last few months together had been a time of great closeness and reward. Having known him for a year and seen the pro-gression of his illness, the worsening of his prospects, and then the manner of his dying, Cicely was again inspired by what could be achieved in this kind of setting — so much so that she had actively considered going to work at St Columba's.

Sowing Seeds

Barrett sensed her motivations and could see she had found a strong sense of calling to work with the dying. His encouragement was crucial to Cicely's next steps. It was typical of his interest in his colleagues and their potential to work together. As one commentator noted: 'Many years before this would be standard practice, he promoted the development of a skilled and harmonious team, with nursing, social work, physiotherapy and clerical staff all accorded attention and importance'[5]. There was much in this which Cicely would later emulate as she too became a leader and fostered the multi-disciplinary approach which was a hallmark of St Christopher's Hospice. Barrett had spent a year in the United States and came back richly enthused by the experience of meeting like-minded colleagues in other settings, discovering the high value given to medical research, and building professional links and friendships that lasted for decades. It is no accident that, by 1963, as we shall see, Cicely herself embarked upon a string of extensive visits to the States, where she too found the stimulus that Barrett had encountered. Yet, her mentor also cautioned against an overly scientific approach to medicine. In a speech given in 1962, he coined an oft-repeated phrase and condemned the tendency to 'publish or perish', one often resulting in immature works in which wisdom was over-ruled by knowledge[6]. These were issues with which Cicely would also grapple later on, as she embraced the need for research into terminal care, but held fast to the importance of compassion, understanding, and human empathy when caring for patients.

Barrett's advice to her on the car journey to Midhurst, just days after Mr S. had died, was loaded with import. Medicine was defined as the highest of the caring professions. Anyone outside would find it hard to bring about change and could easily be ignored by those on the inside. Medicine was the route to understanding pain, a sub-field of specialisation that was soon to open up under the leadership of John Bonica and his associates in the United States, whom Cicely would in due course come to know and admire. Above all, in Barrett's view, medicine had turned its back on the dying patient. Enthused by new possibilities for cure and rehabilitation, doctors — and the language is strong here — were *deserting* their dying patients. It is perhaps a perspective tempered by Barrett's experience in the metropolitan and elite setting of St Thomas's, but it was not a lone view. Others also considered that medical neglect of the dying had become pervasive during the first half of the twentieth century. The American family physician Alfred Worcester had bemoaned the tendency more than fifteen years earlier when, in his book, *The Care of the Aged, the Dying and the Dead*, he observed:

> Many doctors nowadays, when the death of their patient becomes imminent,
> seem to believe that it is quite proper to leave the dying in the care of the

nurses and sorrowing relatives. This shifting of responsibility is unpardonable. And one of its bad results is that as less professional interest is taken in such service, less and less is known about it[7].

In such a context, Barrett was throwing down both a personal and professional challenge. He wanted Cicely not only to take up this line of interest by training as a doctor, but also he was provoking her to make bigger changes which would have wider effects. She responded in spades.

Getting into Medicine

Apart from the temporal advice from Barrett, Cicely felt that she had also received spiritual guidance with her decision to read medicine: 'One minute you don't know and the next minute you do'[8]. 'God tapped me on the shoulder and said "Now you've got to get on with it"'[9]. The world of medicine and the world of her religious life were becoming linked in a way that would continue to reverberate in the work that was to come — not least when she began to formulate plans to establish her own hospice.

On talking to her father about the latest course of action, Gordon Saunders's response was immediately positive. He had indeed suggested the same idea after her first spell at Oxford, and also when she had to give up nursing. Quizzical at first about the preoccupation with the dying, he nevertheless seemed relieved that his daughter had at last opted for a profession that was commensurate with her status in society. Money would not be a barrier. He would support her through medical school. Cicely's brief days of financial self-sufficiency as a hospital almoner were therefore soon to be at an end, but first there were applications to be made and the required qualifications to be confirmed. Albeit with training and experience in nursing and social work, Cicely was a graduate in Modern Greats. At Oxford she had studied politics, philosophy, and economics. She now needed to look to the scientific basis of her knowledge if she was to proceed. It seemed logical to apply to St Thomas's, but that great institution would have to be convinced of her suitability. The initial response was not favourable. Her application, made in the summer of 1951, when 'Pasty' was away on holiday, received a lukewarm reception. At interview she was told she must gain her first Medical Bachelor (or M.B.) before she could be considered.

The solution, as it had been for Oxford entry, would have to be a 'crammer'. It seemed a ridiculous prospect. Tall, imposing, and mannered in speech, she stood out among her fellows. One eighteen-year-old boy was overheard remarking to his pal: 'She'll be ninety before she qualifies!'[10] Fortunately Barrett came to her assistance. Returning from holiday, he quickly intervened with the Dean of Medicine at St Thomas's. At the same time, the hospital matron wrote a letter of strong recommendation. A second interview was hastily arranged. One interlocutor asked if she would struggle with exams. Another answered on her behalf, pointing to her record at Oxford and the Nightingale School. After a few days' agonising wait, a letter came through offering her a place. To seal her good fortune, the same post brought a cheque from her father for £500. He had sold some shares and got his daughter off to a solid start with her new direction. She embarked on her first M.B. — 'an elderly medical student at the age of thirty-three'[11].

Sancte et Sapienter

The medical student years stretched from autumn 1951 to spring 1957. She had been employed full time as an almoner for exactly four years and was on the move again, but still dependent on her father's largesse and still located in the heart of London. His influence and that great city would be an alternating drum beat throughout her life. This next spell of training at St Thomas's echoed some of the nursing school years, but now it was accompanied by a level of personal maturity that came with added years and experience. There was pleasure in the institutional life and culture of the hospital, its camaraderie, gossip, and routines. There was the sense of belonging that came from the Christian Union. New friendships developed, several with fellow believers. Faith and works intertwined in her life. Cicely continued to worship and to pray, but she also buckled down to the rote learning of the early years, then the clinical work, and eventually the enormous challenge of final examinations. By the time Cicely began her training, the medical school at St Thomas's had recently (in 1948) become a part of King's College London. Given her strengthening belief, growing knowledge, and maturing life experience, she was, in a sense, living up to the challenge of the college motto: *With holiness and wisdom.*

Moving in New Circles

St Thomas's Hospital was founded in Southwark during the twelfth century and was named (or possibly re-named) after St Thomas Becket. Closed by Henry VIII during the Reformation, it reopened under Edward VI and was dedicated to Thomas the Apostle. The hospital therefore had its roots deep in history and in religious tradition. But it did not have a tradition of caring for the dying. Indeed, in 1721, one of its governors, Sir Thomas Guy, had established an alternative in his own name to the take the 'incurables' from St Thomas's. During the nineteenth century, it was closely linked with Florence Nightingale, who established her Nightingale Training School and Home for Nurses there in 1860. It was on her advice that the hospital began its relocation, in 1862, to nearby Lambeth, where it subsequently remained. Later buildings were constructed according to Nightingale's 'pavilion principle', at right angles to the river, maximising light and ventilation. It was some of these that were destroyed in the London Blitz. St Thomas's was a citadel of prestige and influence, with a glittering array of medical alumni. Its medical school had begun about 1550 and later merged with Guy's, though the latter became independent in 1825 and the two eventually reunited in 1982[12]. The St Thomas's medical school was four hundred years old when Cicely began her studies there.

She stood out as the tall, mature female medical student. She was also comfortably off. By 1952, she was living in a smart mews-type flat at 5 Pembroke Court, Edwarde's Square, in Kensington, London W8. Beginning in 1955, she was at 60 Ashley Gardens, in Westminster. There were no others like her in the set. A few of the men had done a period in the army, but St Thomas's recruited only small numbers of mature students to medicine, and just fifteen per cent of the intake at that time was female. So Cicely was doubly unusual. At times, she was desperate for adult conversation, but in due course she was drawn towards two students who, whilst not equivalent to her in age, did have some wider life experience. Both had served in the armed forces, both struggled with the basic science that was so key to the early medical curriculum, and both, by their bearing and background, seemed likely to go on to greater things.

She soon bonded with A.G. (Tony) Brown. They taught each other physics in the Flower Walk in Kensington Gardens, at the western extent of London's Hyde Park. He later went on to specialise in community medicine. Her busy social calendar, kept assiduously in small Letts pocket diaries, shows lots of appointments with Tony Brown. For example, in January 1952 they were shopping together on the 9th, at church on the 13th, and having tea with one another on the 16th. On the 23rd, the entry reads 'Tony supper and *work*' as if there might have been other distractions. On the 26th, they were out for a walk together before having tea at Hadley. The following month he stayed the night. In March there was another session marked 'Tony, supper and work!' and on the 29th they went to the Oxford and Cambridge boat race on the Thames[13].

More substantial and enduring was the friendship with Tom West, though judging by the appointments diary for 1952, he was at that time playing second fiddle to Brown and, in some instances, Cicely alternated on a daily basis as to with which of them she was having tea or dinner. Public school educated, West had failed to get into Lloyds, had then tried farming for six months without success, before undertaking national service in Europe. Whilst he was in Germany, his parents had been interviewed on his behalf and he had gained entry to read Medicine at St Thomas's. Three months at the crammer was his preparation[14]. At St Thomas's he and Cicely were labelled 'elderly students' (though he, in fact, was twelve years younger than she). Both were challenged by their degree of scientific acumen. Desperate to get through to a point where they could move to the patients' bedside, they laboured during the first three years at what Cicely called 'the pigsty end' of the physics and chemistry laboratories. But whilst Cicely gained confidence in her studies, West was less successful. He struggled through his work and adopted an orbiting pattern around Cicely, who clearly eclipsed him. That said, they shared particular student enthusiasms, as he recalled some sixty years later: 'Books were important. We wrote to Tolkien begging him to hasten publication of the third volume of 'Lord of the Rings'. We had tea with Stevie Smith . . . not drowning but waving!'[15] Cicely visited his home for weekends and became friendly with his mother. She was halfway in age between Mrs West and her son. A solid pianist, Tom would accompany Cicely in performances she gave for the Hospital Musical Society. She had a lovely soprano voice, always eased by a glass of champagne before she took to the stage. If they became good friends, it was platonically.

> I mean, I remember my father's housekeeper saying to me, 'You two together are really as close as lots of married couples', and we had an awful lot in common — I mean spiritually and musically and fun and the holidays we had and so on, that were lovely, that made it all the more disappointing when it simply didn't work out[16].

The relationship was complex. Each may have wished it to become deeper, but although they later became close colleagues at St Christopher's (where he eventually succeeded her as medical director) and continued to spend free time together, Cicely's opinion of Tom West seems to have deteriorated over the years.

Meanwhile, her wider social, cultural, and intellectual life stayed in high gear. In 1953 she was at the Chelsea Flower Show before heading off on a month-long holiday in Switzerland and Italy, that proved a judicious mixture of walks, shopping, and gallery visits. She had weekends at Poole for birdwatching with Madge Drake, and regular lunches and outings with Rosetta Burch (Figure 3.1). There were frequent Saturday afternoon gatherings of the Nightingale Fellowship. She delved into the writings of philosopher Bertrand Russell on science and society[17] and physicist Erwin Schrödinger on the physical aspect of the living cell[18]. In October 1953, she heard the guitar maestro Segovia in a concert at the Royal Festival Hall. She was a regular at Covent Garden. In the summer of 1954, she had a long touring holiday with Tom West in Scotland and then spent a month travelling around Switzerland. She also kept busy that year with large-scale evangelical rallies in Haringey, White City, and Wembley. There were visits to her father (Figure 3.2) at Hadley and to her mother in Hampstead, and weekends spent with like-minded Christians, which was how she met solicitor Jack Wallace, who would prove so important to her in later years. By any stretch of the imagination, it was a full and varied existence, underpinned by equal measures of material good fortune and spiritual certainty.

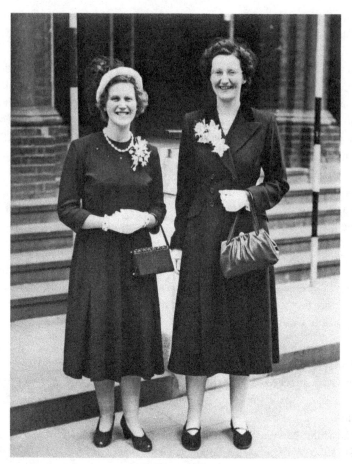

FIGURE 3.1 Cicely and Rosetta Burch, early 1950s. *Source: family album.*

Others came into the medical school circle, with lasting consequences. Mary Silver (later Baines) had done her pre-clinical medical training at Cambridge, gaining a first-class honours degree. She arrived at St Thomas's in 1954 and, during the next three years of clinical training, got to know Cicely and Tom through the Christian Union[19]. They were all in the same clinical year group and they would each go on to practise medicine at St Christopher's Hospice. Another friend was Christine Dare, who trained as a physiotherapist at St Thomas's Hospital and attended the Christian Union. She subsequently read Medicine in South Africa and was instrumental in the development of St Luke's Hospice, Cape Town. In later life, Cicely could look back on being 'the centre of quite a busy group. I had great fun, and those two [West and Brown] were really fairly devoted to me, I think'[20]. In the summer of 1952, a group of them had gone off to 'surf bathe' in North Devon, staying at the home of Madge Drake. There, Tom West and Tony Brown ('my two boyfriends') both

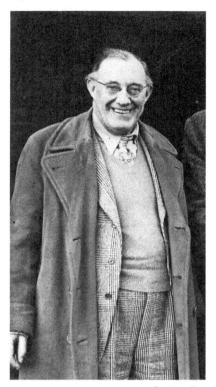

FIGURE 3.2 Gordon Saunders in later years. *Source: family album.*

underwent a conversion to Christianity, just as Cicely had done in Cornwall six years earlier. Also present was twenty-year-old Stephen Smalley, who likewise 'found Jesus' at the Christian guesthouse and was ordained eight years later; in time, he became a noted Johannine scholar and dean of Chester Cathedral. Cicely's world was not only heavily populated with people of faith, these were also people from privileged backgrounds who would later be recognised and honoured by the British establishment. This was not the peer group of her father's business friends. Rather than the conjoined worlds of landed money and entrepreneurial flair, she was finding a home among the thoughtful, even self-denying, upper middle classes — Oxbridge educated and en route to lives of leadership and service in the public sphere. It was a world in which, despite her reputed shyness and lack of self-esteem, she also would later move easily.

Patients and Their Worlds

By the end of 1954 and the beginning of 1955, Cicely was coming into clinical contact with cancer patients at St Thomas's who made a great impression upon her. As an almoner, she had seen such patients before, but now with the growing insights of the physician, she began to understand their problems in a different light. Building on her three levels of training, she could identify their nursing, social, and medical needs more clearly. It was a powerful and rare combination. The patients who seemed to impact most on her thinking were women and men in their forties, still with responsibilities for children and grappling with an illness that was replete with negative associations, fear, and stigma.

People with Cancer

Cancer at this time was widely seen as a 'death sentence'. In the absence of screening tests, detection was poor. Late presentation was common and survival rates were low. For those who received treatment, damaging surgery and unsophisticated radiotherapy were the main options. In 1950, the Registrar General had stated that cancer (at around fifteen per cent of all deaths[21]) killed nearly as many people in a single year as all the men who died during the six-year conflict of the Second World War. The disease was clearly becoming a growing burden for the National Health Service, and the prevalence of many forms of cancer was set to increase[22]. In 1953, James Watson and Francis Crick discovered the structure of D.N.A. It was to kick-start a revolution in molecular biology that would fundamentally change the understanding of cancer — but the effects of those discoveries were still some way off. Chemical treatments for cancer (chemotherapy) had been the subject of much interest since the late nineteenth century, but the early 1950s were characterised by a pessimistic attitude as these ideas continually failed to bear fruit. In the United States especially, significant resources were being invested in a controversial effort to develop cancer drugs, 'yet there was no evidence that the new drugs could cure or, for that matter, even help cancer patients in any stage despite some impressive antitumor responses'[23]. At the same time, there was nervousness among clinicians when treating the symptoms of advanced cancer. Dying from malignant disease was synonymous with pain, but there was a pervasive hesitancy about the use of morphine, with widespread fear of addiction and unwelcome side effects. Likewise, the wider symptoms of cancer such as breathlessness, weight loss, oedema, and fistulae were poorly controlled and frequently caused great distress to patients, their families, and the professionals who looked after them. Capping it all was widespread public silence about the disease that prevented its name from being spoken and which led to concealment, guilt, and secrecy.

In this context, it is clear Cicely was moving into a challenging and, at the time, less-attractive field of medicine. Not only was she concerning herself with a group of patients for which medical science had little to offer which was definitive, she was doing so in a way which recognised the widespread social and personal consequences of disease, and acknowledged that the relief of suffering depends on engaging with these aspects as well as with the underlying physical causes and their symptoms. As a doctor-in-training, she was starting to see the issues close-up and in graphic detail.

Mrs A. was a London housewife, age forty-three, with five children. She developed a lump in her breast in 1952. In August 1953, she had a radical mastectomy, followed by radiotherapy. A year later she began suffering chest pains and, in October 1954, she was found to have rib secondaries. Aware of the seriousness of her condition, she accepted another course of radium treatment and went home to celebrate Christmas as best she could. By the start of April 1955, she was very ill, cyanosed, and breathless, with a large pleural effusion on the left side and a bronchial spasm. She then had a hypophysectomy — the surgical removal of the pituitary gland. After discharge to a convalescent home, she was soon back at St Thomas's. She became extremely distressed and anxious; the pleural effusions were now bi-lateral and she was terribly breathless. She was given oxygen and sedated at night, but became still more distressed when her cortisone was stopped. She felt the hospital was giving up on her. Within a week, she too seemed to give up the battle and was dead. Cicely was troubled by those patients who found it hardest, and whom she felt should be protected for as long as possible — in particular, those leaving children behind. In this case, it was a woman dealing with cancer whilst bringing up a large family. Mrs. A. endured a protracted period of illness after initial treatment, then the distressing symptoms of breathlessness and anxiety which seemed in some ways more challenging than the problem of pain. Always wanting to know what was happening, and fearing concealment, she struggled to interpret the doctors' intentions in her course of treatment. Cicely could tell there was a complexity there which needed deep reflection, clear thinking, and confidence in the approach. But, in the hurly-burly of the hospital, these ingredients were often lacking and rarely found in combination.

During the same period, another forty-three-year-old woman, Mrs R., described by Cicely as 'educated and intelligent', had an excision of the rectum for adeno-carcinoma. For a while she was able to maintain her part-time teaching job, play tennis, and organise things at home. She then began suffering from abdominal pain and urinary problems. A laparotomy involving a large incision into the abdominal wall revealed a mass of cancer that was breaking down. After the operation, she was continually vomiting and nauseous. The drug chlorpromazine gave help for a few days, after which she felt able to go home. But she soon returned to the hospital as the abdominal pain took hold. She battled against it, trying to be brave and not wanting to accept strong medication, but she was experiencing unending nausea and was increasingly distressed. There followed the indignity of intubation and continuous suction to remove her bowel obstruction. But, one third of a gramme of morphia, given every four hours, did help, as did the surgeon's daily visits, that boosted her spirits. Her intense period of distress had lasted five weeks, but had been preceded by a year of some normality in which she resumed her everyday activities in the face of a life-threatening condition. Now she knew she was dying and she said goodbye to her husband. Her death was calm, despite the suffering that led up to it. But to Cicely, the general hospital ward — with its flimsy screens and lack of privacy — seemed ill-suited to the care of someone with such distressing problems.

Cicely was moved by what she saw in these patients, whether they were the parents of young children battling to stay alive or lonely, tired older people who sensed their struggle would not last much longer. She learned to document these things in a medical language which would be credible within her profession. She became proficient at listing the symptoms, the treatments, and the drug regimes. Yet, she was also starting to capture the social and personal circumstances of the 1950's cancer patient, for whom optimism so often gave way to doubt, then to resignation, and often to despair. There were those who sought to understand their condition but feared to ask too much, and who often felt immensely dependent on the doctor or surgeon looking after them. There were others who seemed to know the 'truth', but were determined not to discuss it. Cicely also saw that dying patients were rarely alone. Very often they were part of a family, whose members were also suffering. Here, sympathy needed to be backed up with practicalities. Suitably supported, it seemed to Cicely that family members could surprise themselves with their achievements in caring for a person who was dying.

Mrs G.

Deep observation of patients and families in this way was laying the foundation for a set of ideas that would come to fruition in the next decade. Nor was this completely restricted to those with cancer. Between 1954 and 1961, Cicely came to know someone struggling with a rare and non-malignant condition. A friendship developed between them that grew under the shadow of illness and eventual death. It was not like the situation with David Tasma — intense, private, and, above all, short-lived. This time it was something protracted, shared with others, but still deeply enriching. Cicely had encountered another 'foundational' patient for her thinking and, as before, she was able eventually to share with that person her now-growing thoughts about what care at the end of life might be like if approached differently.

It all started one Sunday in July 1954. At evensong, the Hospital Chaplain asked if anyone present would like to spend time reading to one of the patients. In Cicely, the call fell on fertile ground. She was not particularly enamoured with her first six months of clinical training, that were confined to the Casualty Department, where she had started on 20 April. As she observed some years afterwards, 'I was an idle student at that time, pining to meet patients again after the arid wastes of first and second M.B., so I went to find her'[24]. Her name was Barbara Galton, 'but she was known as "Mrs G." to all the staff and she remained "Mrs G." and I was "Miss Saunders" until she died seven years later, and she was very, very special'[25].

Mrs G. had first been admitted to St Thomas's in September 1953 with a sudden onset of transverse myelitis, a rare condition first described in 1948[26] and caused by inflammation of the spinal cord. By November, she was recuperating in a convalescent home, but was suddenly re-admitted with a severe relapse. The worrying pattern of recovery and relapse continued until April 1954, when she had severe optic neuritis and lost movement and sensation in her arms. She was diagnosed with a condition called 'Devic's disease'. This was first described by French doctor Eugene Devic and his doctoral student Fernand Gault in 1894 amongst sixteen patients who had lost vision and then developed severe weakness of the limbs and loss of sensation[27]. Later known as 'neuromyelitis optica', the condition is a type of inflammatory demyelinating disease that occurs when the myelin sheath, a protective covering that surrounds the brain and spinal cord nerves, is damaged, leading not only to spinal cord inflammation but also to inflammation of the optic nerve. It was devastating to Mrs G.

An only child herself, she had a husband, and one son who was two and a half years old. Mr G. and Mrs G.'s mothers both had jobs, but they visited assiduously on alternate evenings. Each would be first onto the ward and they were always interested in Mrs G.'s life there — a stance they were to maintain for seven years. Initially, Mrs G. was kept at St Thomas's for investigations and specialist consultations. But, as hopes for curative treatment failed, and as her condition worsened, she was moved rather suddenly in the summer of 1956 to a long-stay accommodation in St Thomas's 'country branch', at Hydestile in Surrey, where Cicely had undertaken part of her nurse training. There, Mrs G. was dreadfully homesick; but, in September, after some lobbying, she was brought back to London and to the Royal Waterloo Hospital, that was part of St Thomas's. She felt immediately content there and remained in the same ward until her death in 1961. As her condition allowed, there were visits home for an afternoon or an occasional weekend. The core years of her son's childhood were marked by his mother's confinement to these hospital wards, brief home visits, and, once in a while, an outing to Kew Gardens or a tea party.

Cicely first found Mrs G. on 'Charity' ward. She was thirty-three but looked younger, and was recovering some movement and sight at that time. The previous afternoon, Mrs G. had been sleeping when a visitor came from the London Flower Gift Mission, leaving behind a bag of lavender, attached to which was a text from the Bible: 'I am the light of the World. He that followeth Me shall not walk in darkness but shall have the light of life'. Cicely read it to her. A lengthy discussion followed. It seemed to Mrs G., whose sight was fading, to carry a special message about her situation. Cicely sensed that here was a person who might be open to the Christian path, though she was clearly untutored in matters of religion. Cicely, like others, was quickly drawn to this woman, who was facing so many medical and personal challenges, yet maintained an enquiring air, and — for much of the time — an enthusiasm for the life she had, whatever its constraints. Cicely brought in a copy of the J.B. Phillip's translation of the New Testament and began reading it to Mrs G. She also introduced her to *Daily Light* with its selected bible readings for morning and evening. Cicely covered the first reading and one of the nurses would usually read the second as Mrs G. was 'tucked down' at night. By now, Cicely was visiting Mrs G. every day: 'Sister often let me feed her, more and more often the ward fed me as well .... Sometimes I read, usually we discussed, always we gossiped'[28]. Their friendship grew. When Mrs G. was unhappy in the country, she asked the nurses to keep it from Cicely, who by then was doing her part-one final examinations. In turn, it was Cicely and others who urged hospital management to return Mrs G. to London and the Royal Waterloo Hospital. If Mrs G. made many friends and dependencies in her seven years in hospital, it was nevertheless only one — Cicely Saunders — who went on to write about her in a journal article containing four pages of closely observed detail[29]. It was a narrative that riveted those who read it.

Cicely's account of Mrs G. has a good deal to say about the complex medical and personal problems she experienced. During the early years, loss of sensation in her limbs and intermittent blindness brought a roller coaster of despair followed by optimism. In 1955, however, neurosurgeon Dr Ludwig Guttman, a spinal injuries specialist and founder of the Paralympic Games, was brought in (from Stoke Mandeville Hospital) for a second opinion, but had to deliver the bad news that nothing could be done to reverse her condition. In that same year, Mrs G. suffered when her beloved Ward Sister moved to another position. The following winter, Mrs G. nearly died of a chest infection and spent time in an 'iron lung' to keep her alive. In time, 'colours, shapes, and finally light, left her. Her hands got weaker, her left hand curled up and her right elbow stiffened'. She developed ingenious ways to scratch her nose; she learned to work a 'talking book'. She enjoyed the personal attention of hairdressing and nail polishing. But, she endured uncontrollable jerking and painful muscle spasms which were only partially held in check by intrathecal phenol. She suffered vertigo and, at one point, had an extended period of unconsciousness, from which she again recovered.

By August 1958, Mrs G.'s pain was increasing. She was given injections of methadone and, later, pethidine. She had sedatives at night and sometimes during a bad day. Routine was vital to her. Whilst she hoped for improvement, she became accepting of her condition. Harder to bear was absence from home and the inability to be involved in the daily care of her son. Cicely rationalised that Mrs G. could not feel a sense of loss for something she had not known. It seemed a clumsy observation. Mrs G. found it difficult to accept; though, in the end, she reluctantly did so. Over time, a Christian faith was kindled in Mrs G., no doubt encouraged by Cicely and some of the nurses who were believers. Eventually, she was confirmed into the Church of England. Her flow of visitors never reduced and her husband, as Cicely eloquently put it, fitted his life into the 'cramped lines' of her illness[30]. Her mother eventually retired early to be with her daughter in the final months, but continued to be supported by her employer, who ran a chain of restaurants and went on paying her wages until she reached age sixty.

The final weeks of Mrs G.'s life were challenging for everyone. She became paranoid and mistrustful at times, and those who had come to love her found this hard to bear. The beginning of the end came at Christmas-time. Calmer, she had enjoyed the quintessential 'half glass of sherry' during the celebrations. A few days later, in early January 1961, she slipped into a deep coma and died in the night-time.

Mrs G. seemed to cast a spell on those she met. She had a host of admirers. Above all, and despite her own lack of education, she was a teacher of others. From her, Cicely learned the power of family relationships, the effects which nurses and doctors and hospital staff can have on their patients, the ways in which profound disabilities can be overcome, and the indomitable nature of the human spirit. Cicely ended her account of Mrs G. with a stirring and fitting conclusion: 'She fought a very good fight, and she found and kept the faith'[31].

Evangelical Circles

Faith was, indeed, now a central aspect of Cicely's own world and would remain so — in differing manifestations — for the rest of her life. Shirley du Boulay describes a rumbustiously evangelical orientation in the medical student years. She links this to what she sees as a developing prowess for leadership in Cicely. The reality was more one of earnestness, a conviction about the world based on a highly coloured, born-again, and resurrectionist theology, and a moral world relatively easily divided between good and evil. It is summed up in Cicely's pre-occupation with the teachings of two evangelical men during a period that has been described as 'the age of Billy Graham and John Stott'[32]. The Christian Union was its organisational focus at St Thomas's, whilst in her world beyond the hospital, it was All Soul's, Langham Place, that gathered her in and occupied her attention.

Cicely's evangelical 'turn', however, that lasted from about 1945 to 1960, needs to be set in a wider context. Deeply personal and tied up with her own private troubles in the 1940s, it was also a public issue, a matter of wider import, and not something which could be circumscribed solely within the parameters of her own life. It needs a measure of sociological imagination for its interpretation, at a point where 'biography' and 'history' come together[33].

Billy Graham and John Stott

In Britain, the rise of the Evangelical Movement from the 1860s was closely tied up with Oxford and Cambridge Universities and with the student-led Christian Union, that broke with the more liberal and ecumenical Student Christian Movement during the early 1900s. We have seen that, as an undergraduate, Cicely was drawn towards these kinds of groupings, and in particular to the influence of C.S. Lewis at Oxford. By the middle years of the twentieth century, evangelicalism took diverse institutional forms but cohered around a particular consensus. This was about the importance of the individual's conscious turning to Christ in repentance and faith — and the need to awake this across the world. In the years after the Second World War, British evangelicals were in a state of ferment, anxious about a rising tide of secularism and convinced that the nation had lost its central and Christian ethos. They were divided, however, on how they should respond. For the more denominationally oriented, it was a time to bear witness to the God who would, in His own time, act to remedy the situation. For more liberal evangelicals, it was a call to action in which Christian doctrine should be actively presented across society to those of all beliefs and none. In both Britain and America, evangelical forces opted for this latter orientation and their target audience was often university students. In the United States, interest coalesced around evangelist Billy Graham, whose mass rallies began to attract significant press interest beginning in the late 1940s. By 1954, Graham was in London and, despite some initial local scepticism, his Greater London Crusade in the Haringey area attracted some two million participants and ran for three months before closing in Wembley Stadium in front of a crowd of 120,000 people. Over time, there were seven more Billy Graham 'crusades' in Britain[34]. Despite this, British evangelicalism at this time was struggling to define its own identity. Graham's success was, for some, at too high a price — the adoption of fundamentalist ideas in the absence of intellectual and theological rigour.

John Stott, the rector of All Souls, Langham Place from 1950, demurred from this viewpoint and was keen to defend Graham's approach and his call for a decisive commitment to Christ. But Stott also sought to distance himself from the wilder excesses of the North American Christian fundamentalists. His 1956 pamphlet, *Fundamentalism and Evangelicalism*[35], positioned him at the forefront of a 'new evangelicalism' which he sought to promote in 'the higher echelons of church and society'[36]. He fostered the revival of the Eclectic Society, originally an eighteenth-century group in London which brought together evangelical Anglican priests under the age of forty. Now re-constituted, they would be the driving force that would reshape the Church of England from within. In turn, Stott focussed his own efforts on universities, Christian Unions, and Missions, again seeking out tomorrow's leaders and capturing them for future influence. His books were widely read, sold in quantity, and translated into many languages. Within educated Christian circles with evangelical leanings, he was a dominant intellectual force and a person widely admired and emulated. He was a compelling writer, an expository preacher, and, amongst those to whom he reached out, was Cicely Saunders, who worshipped in his church throughout the evangelical reverberations of the 1950s. Her personal experience, her 'turning to Christ', the learning of Scripture, the readings of *Daily Light,* and the conviction that the world was ripe for conversion were formative to her years as an almoner and a medical student. The decade of her thirties coincided exactly with the ascendant years of Graham and Stott. But just as in the wider society, the revival in Cicely would eventually temper and, in her case, open out into a richer, more nuanced and multi-facetted religious worldview which would see her through to the end.

The Christian Union at St Thomas's, unlike others, was comprised of a mixed group of nurses, physiotherapists, and medical students. Cicely was never an office bearer, but was constantly active in the background. There were Sunday services in the wards, at which she was often found playing the piano for the hymns. She formed a Christian Union choir. The physiotherapists ran Sunday schools in the children's ward. They all took part in missions to bring in non-believers, and weekend discussions and house meetings to strengthen their faith and resolve. They organized what might have been one of the first 'come and sing the Messiah' events: 'I got about seventy people. I had a friend who was a very good pianist and she played the piano, and I had a friend who'd got a trumpet. Four of us each did a solo and then we sang the well-known choruses'[37].

Cicely continued to follow the advice of Meg Foote after her conversion in 1945, building on *Daily Light* and attending bible classes at St Peter's in Vere Street every Thursday night and, for some years, rarely missed a session. Switching to All Souls after its reparation, she continued as a medical student in 'all the usual evangelical inter-varsity fellowship-type ways of behaving . . . you didn't drink, you didn't smoke, you didn't dance, and you were *very* serious'[38]. She also trained as a parish visitor and called on people in their homes. At the time of the North London Billy Graham rallies in 1954, she saw how, at the public meetings, many of those attending were 'coming forward' when called out to declare their faith in Jesus. At this point they had to see 'trained' counsellors, who set them on the next steps in their journey. Churches like St Peter's and All Souls were asked to help and, in due course, Cicely took the training. In 1955, she received a certificate signed by American Dawson Trotman which confirmed her as a 'Navigator'[39]. The Navigators had been started by Trotman during the 1930s as a taskforce to help new converts to Christianity to find their way[40]. Cicely's certificate stated that she had acquired the 108 verses of the Navigators' 'topical memory system' — in short, she had memorized and been tested on each one of these passages from Scripture. These were then written on cards to be used as prompts with the newly converted. Counsellors attended the rallies, schooled in the 108 verses, and were then required to seek out one convert to whom they felt guided. Later in life, Cicely could still recall vividly what the counsellors had to do:

> And then there were various rooms and you sat and talked a bit with them and gave them one or two verses, where to start from, and then got their name and wrote to them and sent them a bit of literature and then did a certain amount of following up. And I went to the very big meeting at Earls Court, I think it was, when he [Billy Graham] came the second time[41]. You gave very simple instructions, four or five verses, for them, to say 'This is what Jesus has said, this is what He has done for you, accept that and know that you've made your commitment to Him and now you've got to move on from there and the best thing for you to do is to join your local Church', and I think they sent a list of names so that they knew how many people went on afterwards and how many fell away. So I was a pretty diligent evangelical in those days[42].

It was a disposition that was to last until the summer of 1960 and the death of a second Polish patient — Antoni Michniewicz. Evangelical Christianity brought many things to Cicely over a fifteen-year period. In those years she embarked on her work as an almoner, trained in medicine, and then began researching the terminal care of patients in a hospice. At its height — during her time as a medical student — it gave friendships, a social life, a sense of fellowship in shared activities with others, a measure of spiritual certainty, and a conviction that others should be brought into the same fold, including those facing death. Yet it was a world she would outgrow. Its theological strictures became too narrow. As her understanding of the nature of suffering deepened first-hand and then matured, the evangelical world appeared one-dimensional. In time, as her own personal relationships changed and she found love with a man who was not imminently dying, but was married to someone else, it became a moral millstone which she had to cast off.

Drawing Together Her Experience

As mentioned, the promise of Britain's post-war welfare state was to deliver care 'from the cradle to the grave'. Cicely's clinical observations were already revealing that this was going to be a challenge. She discussed some of the issues with her former tutor, Miss Butler, when she visited Cicely in London for tea and when the two spent time together in Oxford. Whether terminal illness arose in middle age or when death gradually approached at the end of a long life, too often the caring professions could be found wanting. A few places were making it their business to look after dying people, or 'the dying', as Cicely always called them. But the influence of these terminal-care homes seemed limited and was hampered by a smallness of scale and perhaps also by an off-putting religious orientation. Modern medicine was forging ahead as a scientific discipline with the potential to bring health and well-being to whole populations. A cure had been found for T.B., huge efforts were going into cancer treatment and research, immunisation offered protection against a range of diseases, infant mortality had decreased, and life expectancy was increasing. In this brave new world, who, then, would champion medicine's 'failures' — the patient who could not be cured, old people coming to the end of their days?

Evidently, in the Britain of the 1950s, this was not to be the National Health Service, or the wider welfare system of which it was a part. Change might eventually come within these great edifices, but Cicely could see, even as a medical student, this would require doctors, nurses, and the related professions of social work, physiotherapy, and chaplaincy all to work in new ways and to forge new priorities. But, to kick-start the process, it might be necessary, as she would later often say, to move outside the National Health Service to let new ideas come in.

Coming to Grips with the National Health Service

It was not just the culture of medicine that was at issue. Established in 1948, the British National Health Service was offering free medical care to the entire population. It was a comprehensive system of universal entitlement based on collective provision of health care through taxation, but within a market economy[43]. It was intended to replace charity, dependency, and moralism with a new ethic of social citizenship[44]. The creation of the National Health Service signalled the final phase in the expansion of the Voluntary Hospital Movement, which had first got underway two hundred years earlier and, by 1938, accounted for more than a half of all acute services[45]. But, as Cicely had seen in her work as an almoner, the voluntary hospitals were facing growing problems of financial viability and were increasingly reliant upon patient fees to survive. Their development had been piecemeal and administratively complex, and there was a sense that new scientific and technical knowledge in medicine was ill-fitted to the way they were organised. Now an intensely modernising ethic was in the ascendant; it entailed a deep ideological suspicion of charity and, in the clinical context, made cure and rehabilitation its goals.

Amidst such priorities, there was to be little attention to those in their last illness whose time was short. Accordingly, the early years of the National Health Service saw no strategic or operational guidance on terminal care and no systematic commitment to the subject as a clinical issue. Instead, a pattern emerged of modest and continued involvement on the part of the terminal-care homes and associated charities, together with isolated examples of interested clinicians, from whom a limited literature developed. It is upon these two rather fragile edifices that Cicely's work began to be established, starting with the appearance of her first publication on terminal care in 1958. By the close of her time at St Thomas's, she was reviewing what was known about her subject, tracking down the small number of publications that existed, and reading voraciously when she found material relevant to her interests. In this context, a major report published at the beginning of her medical student days gripped her attention.

Ronald Raven and the Marie Curie Memorial

The Marie Curie Memorial had been established as a national charity in 1948 and held amongst its objects the promotion of the welfare and relief of cancer patients. In 1950, it established a joint committee with the Queen's Institute of District Nursing, chaired by the surgeon Ronald Raven[46]. He had been at London's Royal Cancer Hospital (later the Royal Marsden Hospital) since 1939. Although he favoured the concept of 'rehabilitation and continuing care' rather than 'terminal care' for his patients, he was a staunch supporter of multi-disciplinary work and of the growing specialty of oncology. Involved from its inception in 1948, he also did much to further the interests of the Marie Curie organisation and was later its president[47]. The purpose of the joint committee was to collect information about people in Britain with cancer who were living at home. Its focus was on their social problems as well as their medical situation. The level of ambition for the committee was high and the amount of data collected was prodigious. The method involved sending questionnaires to district nurses across the country from February to August 1951, when 179 of the 193 local health authorities approached co-operated in the survey. In this way, information about cancer patients being seen by the district nurse was obtained for 7,050 cases in England, Wales, Scotland, and Northern Ireland. Nearly seventy per cent of the patients were age sixty or older and more than twenty-four per cent were seventy-five or older. It was amongst these older people that some of the gravest social problems were found.

The committee did not hold back in its descriptions of the conditions identified. It revealed cases of far-advanced illness accompanied by isolation from medical services, squalid conditions, and the personal neglect of the patients. It described people living alone, seldom visited by their adult and married children, relying on the goodness of neighbours, and receiving very little nourishment. In one case, the house was dirty because the patient was too ill to clean it, her clothing was filthy from neglect and the discharge from an ulcer, and yet the person in question gave food to her pets which she needed herself. There were numerous examples of delays in seeking treatment or even of the refusal to be treated. A high proportion of patients were considered gravely ill at the time of the survey, and the district nurses often believed they had been called in at too late a stage of the illness. More than half the patients were reported bedridden. The nurses likewise described the mental suffering of their patients, such as the man who was not depressed by the acute pain he endured, but had become despondent, losing faith in every possible way as he felt his condition gradually worsening, whilst no one took any interest[48].

Shocked by what had been learned, the committee concluded its report with a series of recommendations, including the need for more residential and convalescent homes; the importance of better information for cancer sufferers; and greater provision of night nursing, home helps, and equipment in the home. Some patients, the report indicated, were unaware of the provisions of the National Health Service Act or of their eligibility with the National Assistance Board. Stunned by the results, the Marie Curie Memorial alone was galvanized into action and, within a year of the report's publication, it had begun opening new homes for terminally ill cancer patients. Hill of Tarvit, established in Cupar, Fife, in east Scotland, was the first, in December 1952. The property was leased from the National Trust for Scotland and contained an array of antiques and fine furnishings. Over the next twelve years, nine more Marie Curie Homes opened, from Tiverton in Devon in 1953 to Solihull in the west Midlands in 1965. They were each housed in converted buildings, including a preparatory school, a railwayman's convalescent home, a police orphanage, and a handful of lavish mansions. In 1958, provision was further extended by the addition of a night nursing service which would take nursing care into people's own homes, offering security to patients in the night-time hours and a degree of respite for exhausted carers who could be left undisturbed to get some rest and repose.

Cicely obtained this ground-breaking report from Ronald Raven himself, whom she approached directly at Marie Curie. It was important source material as she began to prepare her own first paper on the subject of terminal care. The year was 1957. She was still a medical student, but now she began to piece together her accumulated wisdom and knowledge about the problems of patients, families, doctors, nurses, and social workers as they sought to respond to the challenge of advancing illness in the face of death. Her years of nursing, volunteering at St Luke's, and experience as a hospital almoner were combined with her more recent medical insights. The result was a robust piece of work. She was so pleased with her efforts that she submitted it for an undergraduate prize. Astonishingly, and by the judgement of history and the acknowledged later importance of the work, it was unsuccessful. But despite the knock back, Cicely was convinced it merited a wider audience and she went on to get it accepted for publication in the hospital's own *Gazette*, where it appeared the year after she graduated[49]. It proved to be a remarkably complete statement about the issue of terminal care in Britain at that time.

A First Medical Paper

Couched partly in the formal language of the medical case history, Cicely's article outlines the circumstances of four cancer patients with advanced disease whom she encountered during her days as an almoner (and already described earlier in this chapter). The discussion includes sections on general management, nursing, the terminal stage, and pain. She drew on her direct experience of care at two of London's homes for the dying: St Luke's and St Columba's. In 1955, she had also visited St Joseph's Hospice in Hackney for the first time[50]. The value of these special homes for terminally ill patients is brought out strongly by Cicely, refuting the notion that they are dismal and depressing places, and arguing for the importance of their specialist attention to complex problems, such as pain, fungating and eroding growths, mental distress, fear, and resentment. She also tackles the controversial issue of telling the patient and relatives about the diagnosis and prognosis. Her exploration of the importance of spiritual care contains the memorable phrase: 'The door of hope must be shut slowly and gently'. Nor was the subject matter of her article limited by its title: 'Dying of Cancer'. Presciently, she also teases out the problems of those with non-malignant conditions, that she conceded were often the most challenging of all.

The 1958 article is long for a medical journal — comprising ten pages of dense text. It is also well referenced, citing other publications on related subjects. That was unusual for the time, when articles which did appear from doctors writing about terminal care were heavy on personal anecdote and short on citation from elsewhere. The twelve references contain some gems. First amongst them is the work of American pain management pioneer John Bonica. His vast 1953 volume, *Management of Pain*[51], gained classic status and became the platform on which the whole pain specialty was later built. Like Norman Barrett and Ronald Raven, Bonica favoured a multi-disciplinary approach, captured in his idea of the 'pain clinic', where patients could be assessed in a rounded way and given a package of support for their problems. He also warned against the prevailing body of opinion in the United States by endorsing the use of powerful narcotics in the purpose of pain relief. His work had a strong influence on Cicely and, eventually, despite the vast gap in their professional life span, they came to know one another.

A similarly important citation in her article is to the work by Alfred Worcester, American Physician, Harvard Professor, Nursing School Founder, and sometimes called Father of Modern Geriatrics, titled *The Care of the Aged, the Dying, and the Dead*[52]. As we have already seen, Worcester's work bemoans the lack of interest in the care of older people and the diminishing interest of doctors in care for the dying patient. It is packed full of practical wisdom about the 'process of dying', its associated symptoms, the role of fluids, and the problem of restlessness. He attends to the environment of the dying person's room, to the need for light and ventilation. He too endorses the liberal use of opiates and considers morphine to have 'no rival'. He deals with the role of faith and religion, with visions and hallucinations, and with the question of uncertainty. Cicely first encountered Worcester's work in 1951 and later described it as an 'early inspiration', at a time when she had little material to feed her growing appetite for works on terminal care[53]. She was now building up some powerful influences and looking beyond the shores of Britain, in ways which she would later exploit to the full. Bonica and Worcester each played an important part in her thinking.

During the 1950s, even talks and publications on the care of the dying were rare indeed. At the British Medical Association's annual meeting held in Newcastle-upon-Tyne in July 1957 (just when Cicely was finishing her paper), a plenary session took place on the subject. One speaker, Dr Ian Grant, struck a typical tone. Drawing on more than thirty years of experience in general practice, he simply concluded that his dying patients 'require kindness most of all, and that they first and foremost wish and hope to find a comprehending and sympathetic friend in the physician'[54]. More worryingly, he asserted the 'first duty is to relieve pain and to induce merciful oblivion'. There is little sense in this material of an accumulated body of knowledge on the care of the dying which draws on sustained analysis of the medical literature. Cicely's first paper was to change that. Not only does the article describe the prevailing issues and problems, it also becomes a manifesto for future action. Condensed into its pages is the entire range of issues with which the subsequent field of palliative care would have to grapple. The dapper and forthright Raven must have been impressed and, as we shall see, was soon commissioning a chapter from Cicely for his six-volume encyclopaedic work *Cancer*, prepared between the years 1957 and 1963, that became the state-of-the-art benchmark for that time[55].

Decades later, Cicely could still give a religious rationale for her first publication. When asked how such a mature work could have emerged, fully formed, in the earliest stages of her career in medicine, she found her response in the divine. 'I mean, God wanted me to do it; so, you know, "As thy day is, so shall thy strength be." He doesn't give you the opportunities for you to take without giving you some of the capacity to deal with them'[56].

Examinations

During her years at medical school, Cicely had been building that capacity. She passed her first M.B. in nine months and her second M.B. at the first go. The array of specialisms she had to learn was dizzying, though she received no specific instruction in the thing that interested her most — the care of the dying. Rote learning and revision were never far away. At times, she had back problems to accompany them, with the most acute episode in 1953, when she had treatment for generalised arthritic symptoms. After completion of her second M.B. and a holiday, they never recurred[57]. Indeed, her tutors found her industry to be prodigious. From 1955 to 1956, she lived on-site in St Thomas's House, Lambeth Palace Road; but, for her final year of study — and to ensure a successful outcome — she went into purdah in a bed-sitting room in Ebury Street in nearby Westminster. No one had her telephone number, her breakfast was made for her each morning, and her only indulgence was a record player. She gained her reward. As du Boulay notes, she obtained honours in Surgery, was praised by her examiners, and was awarded the Beaney Prize for Obstetrics and Gynaecology. She qualified as a doctor in April 1957[58]. In her own words:

> I worked really hard, and two or three chaps that I knew best, I made them come and work with me and we used to go through old exam papers and answers and so on. And you have to pass everything all the way through to get honours because there were only about a dozen people who, at that time, got honours in the year and . . . I never went to see the list — somebody saw it for me — but I passed my pharmacology, that you take at the end of second M.B., as well as the other things. I had to be pushed through chemistry and physics for first M.B., and biochemistry for the second. I really had to be pushed through. I found it really difficult. I didn't even know how to look up a log, that we were still working with in those days. And to do physics with no maths, algebra, and things like that, absolutely non-existent, but we managed . . . and when I was taking pharmacology, that I hadn't really attended terribly well — to the lectures; they were the sort of questions that I could answer as a nurse so, of course, I got through and . . . I got a prize for gynaecology and obstetrics. So I am pretty tiresome in that I can pull it out for an exam[59]!

Tony Brown wrote to Cicely on 9 May 1957, thanking her for a record she had given him and 'more especially for everything you have done for me in the last five years. The fact that I am a doctor is on the whole due to you more than any other single person!'[60] She had helped him and West through the pressures of the examination system, but soon both of them had left the country and were working as doctors — one in Vietnam and one in Nigeria.

On top of all this, in the years just before and at the close of her medical training, Cicely had done another remarkable thing. She had inspired two hard-headed surgeons, each from one of London's most prestigious hospitals, to have confidence in her and to take seriously her interest in the care of the dying. If Barrett had seen the potential, then Raven was among the first to recognise the early work. In between had been the sheer grind of qualifying in medicine. The foundations were now laid for higher things in the coming decade.

Practical Applications

Flush with the excitement of her first publication and newly qualified as a doctor, Cicely was soon given a chance to hone her terminal care skills further. Against the backdrop of his final examinations, Tom West had received bad news. His father had been diagnosed with advanced lung cancer. Cicely was now good friends with Tom's mother. Newly qualified in medicine, she offered to come to help, eventually breaking off a holiday in Scotland to return south and spend three weeks with the Wests in the short time that remained. They lived on a small farm in the county of Kent. The local G.P. recognised Cicely's special interest and apparently accepted her involvement. It was another example of her unorthodox approach — moving in with friends and becoming the physician-in-attendance to someone for whom she had no formal clinical responsibility. Tom West considered it crucial in keeping his father at home for the last weeks of his life.

> Three weeks, so much better than expected . . . . The G.P.s listened to her: Regular adequate pain relief. Regular adequate whisky. Regular-ish bowel movements. We are proud of the fact that the very first terminal (horrible word!) cancer patient that Dr Cicely Saunders cared for was our Dad (and he was a home care patient too!)[61].

Or, as he put it on another occasion, his father was the 'first patient in the worldwide Hospice Movement'[62]. The claims are extravagant, but du Boulay quotes Cicely at length on what happened at the Wests in an unreferenced passage that must have been based on one of their conversations and which gives weight to the importance of the experience:

> I have a very good memory of helping friends to care for their father who was dying of carcinoma of the bronchus on a farm in the country. I remember that strong community — the family, the family doctor, the life of the farm, and the interest of the village. The whole thing was a pattern. The patient had the central place, very conscious of that, and rather enjoying it. In many ways, controlling the situation, and even planning ahead, sometimes looking sideways at us to watch our reaction to his more Rabelaisian remarks. He was neither uncertain nor fearful, but was typical of himself up to the last, although he well knew what was happening[63].

For Tom West, it was something to be remembered long after as the best weeks the family ever spent together, a time in which 'all sorts of things [were] put right that had not gone right in the previous thirty years'[64]. The care of Tom West's dying father and his family had placed Cicely in a pivotal position, one she would later relish in many other cases of care at the end of life. It enabled her to demonstrate her theoretical knowledge, built up and expressed in her student paper, along with a measure of *phronesis* which was born of her experience as a nurse, almoner, volunteer, and trainee doctor. It was also consequential in other ways which bear the imprint of Cicely's growing modus operandi. Her friendship with Tom West would continue, even when he departed for Nigeria to work on behalf of the Church Missionary Society. Later she would offer him a job at St Christopher's and, eventually, he would succeed her as medical director. Their friendship, his debt of gratitude to her for what she had done for his father, and the work-related tensions that later developed between them would prove a heady mixture. But this inter-weaving of the professional and the personal, the willingness to take risks, and then the need to live with the consequences were all becoming part of Cicely's approach. It was further enlivened by what she was beginning to get back — a sense of being needed, the visceral nature of being with people in some of their darkest hours, and the reward of being the one perceived to transform a desperate situation.

Notes

1. Cicely Saunders interview with David Clark, 16 May 2000.

2. Cicely Saunders interview with Neil Small, Hospice History Project, 24 October 1995.

3. Cicely Saunders interview with Neil Small, Hospice History Project, 24 October 1995.

4. Sprott N. Dying of cancer. *The Medical Press*. 1949; February 16: 187–191.

5. Lord R.V.N. Norman Barrett, "doyen of esophageal surgery". *Annals of Surgery*. 1999; 229(3): 428–439, 432.

6. Barrett N.R. Publish or perish. *Journal of Thoracic Cardiovascular Surgery*. 1962; 44: 167–179.

7. Worcester A. *The Care of the Aged, the Dying, and the Dead*. Springfield, IL: Charles C. Thomas; 1935: 33.

8. Cicely Saunders interview with Neil Small, Hospice History Project, 24 October 1995.

9. Cicely Saunders interview with David Clark, 15 December 1999.

10. du Boulay S. *Cicely Saunders: The Founder of the Modern Hospice Movement*, 2nd ed. London: Hodder and Stoughton; 1994: 63.

11. Cicely Saunders interview with Neil Small, Hospice History Project, 24 October 1995.

12. McInness E.M. *St Thomas' Hospital*. London: George Allen and Unwin; 1961; Agha R., Agha M. A history of Guy's, King's and St. Thomas' hospitals from 1649 to 2009: 360 Years of innovation in surgery. *International Journal of Surgery*. 2011; 9: 414–427.

13. King's College London Archives, SAUNDERS, Dame Cicely (1918 – 2005), K/PP149/1/2.

14. Tom West interview with Neil Small, Hospice History Project, 28 January 1997.

15. West T. Tom West's recollections. In Remembering Cicely — Founder of the modern hospice movement, https://eapcnet.wordpress.com/2015/08/05/remembering-cicely-founder-of-the-modern-hospice-movement-2/, accessed 24 August 2016.

16. Cicely Saunders interview with David Clark, 20 September 2000.

17. Russell B. *The Impact of Science on Society*. London: Allen & Unwin; 1952.

18. Schrödinger E. *What Is Life? The Physical Aspect of the Living Cell*. Cambridge: Cambridge University Press; 1944. [Based on lectures delivered under the auspices of the Institute at Trinity College, Dublin, in February 1943.]

19. Mary Baines interview with Neil Small, Hospice History Project, 10 July 1996.

20. Cicely Saunders interview with Neil Small, Hospice History Project, 24 October 1995.

21. Quinn M., Babb P., Brock A., Kirby L., Jones J. *Cancer Trends in England and Wales 1950–99: Studies on Medical and Population Subjects No. 66*. London: Office for National Statistics; 2001.

22. Cancer cases up but survival more than doubles in breast and bowel cancer, 3 July 2008, http://www.cancerresearchuk.org/about-us/cancer-news/press-release/2008-07-03-cancer-cases-up-but-survival-more-than-doubles-in-breast-and-bowel-cancer#K57jxYlImu4Egihf.99, accessed 26 August 2016.

23. DeVita V.T., Chu E. A history of cancer chemotherapy. *Cancer Research*. 2008; 68(21): 8643–8653.

24. Saunders C. A patient . . . . . *Nursing Times*. 1961; March 31: 394–397.

25. Cicely Saunders interview with Neil Small, Hospice History Project, 24 October 1995.

26. Suchett-Kaye A.I. Acute transverse myelitis complicating pneumonia: A report of a case. *The Lancet*.1948: 2(6524): 417.

27. Jarius S., Wildemann B. The history of neuromyelitis optica. *Journal of Neuroinflammation*. 2013; 10(1): 8.

28. Saunders, A patient, 394.

29. Saunders, A patient, 395.

30. Saunders, A patient, 397.

31. Saunders, A patient, 397.

32. Stanley B. *The Global Diffusion of Evangelicalism: The Age of Billy Graham and John Stott*. Downers Grove, IL: InterVarsity Press; 2013.

33. Mills C.W. *The Sociological Imagination*. Oxford: Oxford University Press; 1959.

34. Capon J. Sixty years on: Billy Graham's London Crusade. *Church Times*. 23 May 2014, https://www.churchtimes.co.uk/articles/2014/23-may/news/uk/sixty-years-on-billy-graham-s-london-crusade, accessed 25 September 2016.

35. Stott J. *Fundamentalism and Evangelism*. London: Crusade Booklet; 1956.

36. Stanley, *The Global Diffusion of Evangelicalism*, 42.

37. Cicely Saunders interview with David Clark, 15 December 1999.

38. Cicely Saunders interview with David Clark, 15 December 1999.

39. King's College London Archives, SAUNDERS, Dame Cicely (1918 – 2005), K/PP149/1/1-38.

40. Hankins J.D. Following up: Dawson Trotman, the Navigators, and the origins of disciple making in American evangelicalism, 1926–1956. Unpublished PhD thesis, Trinity International University, 2011, http://gradworks.umi.com/34/87/3487752.html, accessed 29 September 2016.

41. She seems to have mis-remembered the location. The second set of rallies to which she is referring was in 1955 and was held in Wembley Stadium. The rally of 1966 was in Earls Court, by which time she had left the evangelical fold.

42. Cicely Saunders interview with David Clark, 15 December 1999.

43. Klein R. *The Politics of the National Health Service*. London: Longman; 1983.

44. Harris J. 'Contract' and 'Citizenship'. In Marquand D., Seldon A., eds. *The Ideas That Shaped Post-War Britain*. London: Fontana; 1996: 122–138.

45. Webster C. *The Health Services Since the War, Vol II: Government and Health Care, the National Health Service 1958–1979.* London: The Stationery Office; 1996.

46. Joint National Cancer Survey Committee of the Marie Curie Memorial and the Queen's Institute of District Nursing. *Report on a National Survey Concerning Patients with Cancer Nursed at Home.* London: Marie Curie Memorial; 1952.

47. Royal College of Surgeons. Plarr's lives of the Fellows online: Raven, Ronald William (1904 – 1991), http://livesonline.rcseng.ac.uk/biogs/E008284b.htm, accessed 24 September.

48. Joint National Cancer Survey Committee, *Report on a National Survey,* 25.

49. King's College London Archives, SAUNDERS, Dame Cicely (1918 – 2005), K/PP149/7/1/1.

50. Saunders C. Working at St Joseph's Hospice, Hackney. In *Annual Report of St Vincent's, Dublin.* 1962: 37–39.

51. Bonica J. *The Management of Pain.* Philadelphia: Lea and Febinger; 1953.

52. Worcester A. *The Care of the Aged, the Dying, and the Dead.* Springfield, IL: Thomas; 1935.

53. Saunders C. Letter [Re: Alfred Worcester]. *The American Journal of Hospice and Palliative Care.* 1992; July/August: 2.

54. Grant I. Care of the dying. *British Medical Journal.* 1957; December 28: 1539–1540.

55. Saunders C. The management of patients in the terminal stage. In Raven R., ed. *Cancer.* Vol. 6. London: Butterworth and Company; 1960: 403–417.

56. Cicely Saunders interview with David Clark, 2 May 2003.

57. Medical report dated 1968 in King's College London Archives, SAUNDERS, Dame Cicely (1918 – 2005), K/PP149/1/1-38.

58. du Boulay, *Cicely Saunders,* 65–66.

59. Cicely Saunders interview with Neil Small, Hospice History Project, 24 November 1995.

60. King's College London Archives, SAUNDERS, Dame Cicely (1918 – 2005), K/PP149/1/6.

61. West, Tom West's recollections.

62. Tom West interview with Neil Small, Hospice History Project, 28 January 1997.

63. du Boulay, *Cicely Saunders,* 77.

64. Tom West interview with Neil Small, Hospice History Project, 28 January 1997.

4 | Learning the Craft and Crafting the Vision (1957 – 1967)

I keep finding new things in this work all the time[1].

A Decade of Change

Cicely had written her first medical paper on the care of the dying in the summer of 1957. By the summer of 1967, St Christopher's Hospice was ready to open under her leadership. In the interim were years of immense personal and professional transformation. This was also a period of enormous cultural change. In 1957, American Bill Haley had stormed London with the simple twelve-bar blues anthem called 'Rock Around the Clock'. In 1967, the Beatles released their British psychedelic epic 'Sgt Pepper's Lonely Hearts Club Band', to huge critical acclaim. These were the years of social reform, civil rights protests, the Cuban Missile Crisis, the assassination of President Kennedy, and the start of the war in Vietnam. They saw the emergence of the contraceptive pill, the spread of recreational drug use, the partial decriminalisation of homosexuality, and the legalisation of abortion. Of course, none of this over-turned the somewhat more conservative world inhabited by Cicely and her contemporaries. Her ideals were being shaped by her Christian beliefs, she was moving into the assured world of the London medical establishment, and she was continuing to benefit from her family background and the connections that came with it. She showed no interest in London's 'swinging sixties'; indeed, her social worlds were more akin in many ways to those of the 1940s. But change was in the air, and whatever one's personal or political orientation, it was a period during which it became commonplace to challenge prevailing orthodoxies, to de-bunk assumptions, and to project new ways of living, of being, and, ultimately, of dying. This was Cicely Saunders's contribution to the counter-culture of the times.

On a summer day in 1957, Gordon Saunders was at Wimbledon and ran into his old tennis partner, Dr Harold Stewart, who had been a regular player on the grass courts at Hadley and whom Cicely had known from her younger days. The two men had tea together and Stewart asked about Saunders's family. The proud father of a newly qualified doctor, Gordon explained that Cicely was about to do her house jobs[2] but eventually wanted to concentrate on problems of pain and pain relief. Stewart's interest was piqued. Since 1950, he had been head of the Pharmacology Department at St Mary's Hospital Medical School in London, where he had a programme of animal-based laboratory work investigating the actions of opiates. He asked for Cicely to contact him when she had finished her house jobs, and was confident he could help her ambitions by unlocking funding from the Sir Halley Stewart Trust, of which he was a family member. The remarks may have been made casually between two successful men enjoying time off at a major sporting and social event — part of the London 'season'. There is almost a filmic quality in the way the scene is described, yet it is hard not to see an old boys' network in evidence here. Cicely was not present. There was an ease about the encounter and its underlying assumptions which smacked of privilege and favour and of 'backs being scratched'. But however it is judged — and by the standards of the day, it would have been normal among men of that social class — it was nevertheless hugely consequential.

At St Joseph's

By the following summer, Cicely had completed two house jobs, at the Waterloo Hospital and Hydestile, both under the auspices of St Thomas's. Now a well-trained and more experienced doctor, she followed up the Wimbledon conversation, approached Harold Stewart, and they met at St Mary's. He told her, 'I can get money from the Halley Stewart Trust but I don't have access to patients', to which she replied, 'Well I think I could get access to patients but I don't have any money'[3]. The outcome was that, from October 1958, and with funding of £1,000 per annum from the Trust, Cicely was able to focus exclusively in the area of terminal care and to advance the breadth and depth of her ambition in that direction as a research fellow. After some casting around for suitable settings in which to work (a home in Bexley was an option but was too small in scale), it was agreed that her studies should be done at St Joseph's Hospice, Hackney, in East London, along with a link to St Luke's, in Bayswater. St Joseph's was not a familiar setting to Cicely. Although as an almoner she had been involved in the care of patients at the other London hospices, St Joseph's was not a place she knew well, though she had visited it in 1955. Run by Catholic Sisters, and heavily inflected with Catholic imagery and practises, it was a new and slightly bewildering environment for her. In any event, she received a warm welcome there, perhaps tempered by the knowledge that, with new beds just opening, St Joseph's was seriously under-doctored. She recalled:

> I went and talked to Mother Mary Paula at St Joseph's and she said, 'Well I desperately need more medical help because Dr Ross can pop in every day and Dr Browne does a very good round once a week and can come in occasionally, but that's all I've got, but I don't have money for it'. So I said, 'Well, you don't have to pay me'. So she said, 'Well meet the doctors. See what they say'. So I met them both and said I had this grant to do clinical research . . . but basically I wanted to really look after patients and look at the clinical scene of nature and management of terminal pain . . . . And they said 'Fine . . . come'. They would be delighted to have somebody to come and do the donkey-work . . . . And so I started out with a desk in the department at St Mary's, in what was then the animal house where they were working on cats and things, and it was just round the corner from where I was living in Connaught Square, and going over to St Joseph's three times a week and to St Luke's, which was part of St Mary's, a couple of times a week[4].

Her period at the desk in the animal house was short. Very quickly she began working from home. She also spent hours in the reading room of the nearby Royal Society of Medicine, where she would submit a list of requests and 'they'd pile the books up on one of the tables and you'd come in and everything you want is out for you, it was wonderful'[5]. St Mary's was generous and paid for Cicely to have a secretary, Jenny Powley, who began in late 1959. She helped with the punch-card system Cicely was to adopt for data storage, typed up notes and correspondence on the kitchen table, and transcribed many hours of dictation as Cicely shaped her thoughts and formed her strategy.

A New Home

On qualifying in medicine, Cicely had quickly moved out of St Thomas's accommodation and into more elegant surroundings. Her flat was at number 37 Connaught Square, London W2, near Marble Arch. The property was owned by Cicely's former housemate from Leinster Gardens, Isobel (now a consultant radiologist), and her husband, Cledwyn Lewis (a consultant anaesthetist). They wanted someone to live on the top floor for £6 per week, cash. Cicely stayed there from October 1958 to June 1967, when she moved to southeast London to be closer to St Christopher's. Up about seventy stairs, her accommodation in Connaught Square comprised two bed-sitting rooms, a kitchen, and a bathroom. Beginning in 1960, she shared the space with Gillian Ford, who she had met during Cicely's final year of medical school. Gillian would later go on to work for the Department of Health and have a key influence at St Christopher's as well as in the recognition of the specialty of palliative medicine. As a flatmate (on two occasions during this period) she was a good friend, a wise and thoughtful companion, and also a committed Christian. The two of them would work assiduously in the evenings, but then 'explode with a great noise at about ten o'clock at night', when they would prove 'absolutely maddening to the people downstairs'[6].

Whilst doing a house job at the Waterloo Hospital, Cicely had engaged the services of a Ghanaian woman to do occasional washing and laundry. The lady's name was Mrs Chrubim. Cicely asked her to take on some cleaning jobs at Connaught Square. A devout Christian herself, Mrs Cherubim 'used to come and sing good hymns around the place a couple of times a week and she used to go off and say: "See you Tuesday, if I'm spared", and off she'd go!'[7] When Jenny Powley's husband got a job farther afield, she left and was replaced for a short time by a young Polish woman, Harnia Tokirska. Then Peggy Nuttall introduced Cicely to 'a terribly bereaved widow who needed an easy secretarial job'. That was Kitty Cole, who was four years older than Cicely. They remained in contact for the rest of their lives and the secretarial job, all those years earlier, was — in Cicely's later view — life saving for Kitty. Cicely was beginning to build a small team and a sense of support around her. 'It was terrific. I'd never worked so hard in my life'[8].

The Culture of the Hospice

The setting at St Joseph's inspired Cicely. The hospice bought its supplies from local retailers, a nearby butcher donated meat to them, they ran a football pools scheme to raise funds, and there were money-raising flag days, concerts, outings, and bazaars — all organised with groups in the local community. She could see how such an organisation had to relate closely to the context and culture of the people it served and how, since its opening in 1905, St Joseph's had become a prominent aspect of life in Hackney. It had never stood still and was constantly adapting, expanding, and making the most of its generous portion of land. It admitted four hundred to five hundred new patients each year. Under the leadership of Mother Mary Paula, a new ward was built at the hospice and opened in 1957. The facility was light and airy, and looked out onto the bustling scene of Mare Street, one of Hackney's main roads. Named Our Lady's Wing, it 'majored on bright, spacious bedrooms that had large bay windows and balconies, echoing earlier exemplars such as the Peckham Health Centre'[9]. The wing had been designed by the firm of Stewart, Hendry and Smith, which Cicely later engaged for St Christopher's Hospice. Our Lady's Wing offered a strikingly modern hospital setting in which to practise terminal care. It had sixty beds in total, forty-five of them for cancer patients. In each bay of six beds there were usually four dying patients with cancer and two longer stay patients. In total, the hospice had 112 beds, many of them for long-stay patients. From the moment she began working at St Joseph's, Cicely was impressed by the environment which had been created there and also by the peacefulness of the setting and solicitude of the Sisters and caring staff:

> Every new patient is greeted by one of the Sisters: 'You're welcome, Mr X'. He is welcomed into a place that will be home rather than just another hospital . . . . He is welcomed by someone who is really interested in him as a person, in his soul and in his mind as well as his body. His physical burden will be lifted and his individual ways . . . will also be respected as far as possible[10].

At the same time, Cicely found St Joseph's 'virtually untouched by medical advance'[11]. There were no drug charts, no patients' notes, just a brief record of their status as temporary patients of a G.P. She immediately set to work to introduce more complete patient documentation and, in particular, to establish a regime that involved the regular giving of morphine — a practice observed at St Luke's but not in use in St Joseph's. As one of the nuns and Cicely's greatest ally there, Sister Mary Antonia, subsequently recalled, Cicely introduced the mantra 'constant pain needs constant control'. It meant the transformation from 'painful' to 'pain free'[12]. At first, Cicely was given four patients to look after in the men's ward on the ground floor. One of them was a former civil servant who kept a prayer diary, something that interested Cicely and was an immediate source of rapport between them. The other three had pain and were quickly put on regularly administered analgesia. The effect was dramatic. Everyone could see the benefits and Cicely's duties were quickly scaled up. She was soon responsible for each new admission to the forty-five available beds in the new wing[13].

It was there that she had the opportunity to learn more extensively about the little-explored field of terminal care, that had so captured her imagination at medical school. Over time, and from very modest beginnings, she built up a network of international contacts to strengthen her endeavours, some of whom visited her at St Joseph's. She also formed her own key ideas and specific approach to clinical practice, laying down what were to become the fundamentals of modern hospice care. In particular, Cicely was able to put into practice her enthusiasm for the regular giving of analgesics, and was also attracted to the pain-relieving mixtures that were in use in London at that time. St Joseph's gave her an opportunity to develop a wider view of pain in the context of the whole person's suffering. She realised too that something else was needed if this work was to gain more recognition and to reach more people who could benefit from it. She began forging her own vision of a new kind of hospice, one that would build on the legacy of St Joseph's, St Luke's, and St Columba's, but would also go beyond their approach to offer the vital additional components of *teaching* and *research*. She began to formulate her ideas about how all of this could be translated into a modern context which might have the potential for wider influence. By late 1959, she had resolved to establish her own hospice, built for the purpose and founded on what she had learned from the London homes for the dying, and others she had studied at a distance.

The Catholic Ambience

There must have been something rather strange for an earnest evangelical — they called her the 'Protestant heretic'[14] — suddenly moving into this very traditional Catholic environment during the years before the Second Vatican Council in 1962, that sought to reform the church in the face of the modern world. Despite this, two nuns in particular made it easy for her: Mother Mary Paula and Sister Mary Antonia. They could see the value of her contribution and seemed to sense this was about something more than just the direct care of patients at St Joseph's. Cicely also considered herself to have begun a process of spiritual 'loosening up' by this time. The outer shell of her Billy Graham–inspired evangelicalism was beginning to show some hairline cracks and she was open to other perspectives. She was very happy with the nuns, and they were very prepared to let her in, although 'they all prayed like beavers to get me into being a Catholic and I remember a patient saying to me once: "Perhaps I might be the one to bring you in, doctor"'[15]. Her evangelical friends, like Rosetta Burch, worried that she might join the Church of Rome, and had to be placated: 'Don't worry, I know my friends wonder about me and Rome and some take it quite seriously. I am far less likely now that I have seen it near to'[16]. She much later declared:

> I could never become a Catholic. I couldn't take the authority or some of the dogma either . . . . I've always been a reader around this area. I find it absolutely enthralling. I really do. [But,] you can't be with dying people and remain strict within boundaries, because there aren't any boundaries when you're dying[17].

As we are beginning to see, this was not a point about spiritual matters alone.

Cicely became a familiar sight across the whole of St Joseph's, spending time with Sister Mary Antonia in St Michael's ward, Sister Joseph Xavier in Lourdes ward, and Sister John Francis in St Anne's. Sister Joseph Xavier was the oldest. Cicely got on 'terribly well' with all of them. She would have a 'splendid lunch' and tea given to her by Sister Mary Antonia in St Michael's. They kept an eye on Sister John Francis, who was younger, ensuring she didn't go off to the chapel with the drug cupboard keys in her pocket. Quite simply, Cicely had a 'lovely time'. Once again, she was fitting into the routine and fellowship of institutional life, albeit with half of her own life being lived outside the institution. She could enjoy and feel comforted by the daily routines, the sights, the smells, and the ringing of the Angelus bell at noon. Until after 'Vatican II', the nuns still wore white hooded habits, that cloaked them from head to foot. Cicely could see things were changing at St Joseph's, but she was also aware of a bigger goal and the need to bring about change elsewhere. This kind of community was 'one foot in Eden'[18], but there was much to be done in the harsher world beyond. Her orientation to both institutional life and to the wider context would continue for the rest of her days, even when she had established St Christopher's as a force for influence and herself as its doyen.

Medical Routines

Looking back in later years, Cicely and others continued to have particularly fond memories of her medical companion at St Joseph's, Dr John Browne. He was remembered for his 'caring concern for both the patients and staff', for generosity with his time, and for making each patient feel 'they were the only one that mattered'[19]. Perhaps it was his colleague, Dr Ross, who was more concerned than he that Cicely shouldn't sign the cremation forms and thereby deprive them of the income that thereby accrued[20]. More generally, money issues were never far away from St Joseph's. On one occasion she was in front of a committee about the large quantities of drugs they were ordering. She took a look at the prescribing patterns and the death rates of the patients. It seemed that both had gone up after she got there. She speculated that people were dying sooner as a result of having their pain better controlled. As she much later remarked, slightly abashed:

> I never pushed anybody off, but I think it must have shown that there were people who just weren't getting the drugs they ought to have had, because morphine doesn't hasten death if you use it properly. But not having it, you may drag on in pain. I mean some of the ones I gave the Brompton Cocktail to no doubt got pneumonia, but that was, you know, 'double effect'. I remember some reason for looking at two or three years of death rates. I've never told anybody else that, and I'd completely forgotten it; but, yes, I think it's so, but don't go chasing it up[21].

She quickly fell into a settled routine at St Joseph's. Three times a week she drove in her green and rather sporty Triumph Herald to Hackney[22]. She took a northerly route through Cannonbury to get to the east of the city. It was a massive contrast in social worlds, from the wealth and poise of the West End to the poverty, diversity, and bustle of working-class Hackney. Driving home one evening, she was waiting to cross Harley Street. The red light seemed to take forever without changing, so she slid across the junction, only to be stopped immediately by the police. 'What's the number of this car?' the officer asked. She replied correctly. 'We always ask that because sliding over a light is so often a stolen car.' She told them she was just on her way back from St Joseph's. 'Are you going to visit the dying?' he asked. 'No, I have just been with them', she replied, relieved at her good fortune in not getting booked[23].

Patients who required terminal care usually arrived at St Joseph's through the Emergency Bed Service:

> They used to come in with a very little chit from a G.P., no notes or anything. It really was veterinary medicine: You started out with a very ill patient, hardly able to give a history and really nothing else — carcinomatosis, carcinoma of breast, and that was it[24]. They were referred from hospitals around London. Patients who lived near St Joseph's would often refuse to go there, and would be sent right across London to St Luke's, and vice-versa. You couldn't, as I discovered later on, when you discharged a patient, have the possibility of re-admitting them other than going back on the Emergency Bed Service waiting list[25].

They were often poor people, with advanced disease that had been diagnosed late. Cicely sensed that St Joseph's had some inspiring aspects, but there was much room for improvement. It was battling against a tide of indifference to the needs of terminally ill people which existed in the care system. In time, this would need reform on a major scale. For the moment, Cicely had to concentrate on her individual endeavours and build up the wherewithal to tackle bigger problems later. She would arrive at the hospice around 9:30 each morning and stay until 5 pm, and she was given free rein to move about as she wished (Figure 4.1). She encouraged the nurses to start writing ward reports and was guided by her conversations with them about which patients to see.

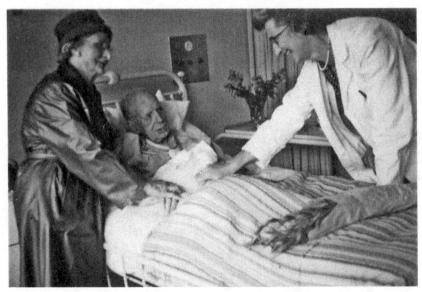

FIGURE 4.1 Cicely with a husband and wife at St Joseph's Hospice. *Source: Cicely Saunders.*

Pain Relief and the 'Brompton Cocktail'

They used the services of the pharmacist at Hackney Hospital. The main approach to pain control in 1958 was injections of morphine using a formulation called Nepenthe — the drug to drive away sorrows and induce forgetfulness — along with pethidine by mouth. Cicely gradually reduced the amount of sometimes painful and awkward injections and started up a liquid formulation which would be easier for the patients to take. Soon she favoured the use of diamorphine over morphine in the mixture because, anecdotally, the former was thought to have fewer side effects. They called this 'St Joseph's mixture'. She was eager to build on her earlier learning, as she explains in detail here many years later:

> The 'Brompton Cocktail' was oral morphine and quite a mixture, with gin and honey . . . that had been put together by the pharmacist at Brompton Hospital for patients who were dying of tuberculosis and had desperately sore throats and so on. At St Luke's, I saw they had a slightly different version, but it was basically morphine by mouth that was given on a four-hourly basis, and sometimes they did move over to injections. They never went up to more than sixty milligrammes. Of course we were talking grains in those days. But it was very effective. It was before the psychotropic drugs came in, so we were able to use an anti-seasick pill that I suppose must have been Dramamine, and phenobarbitone as a sedative, and Soneryl as another barbiturate at night for sleeping. So we had a very limited armamentarium. And what was so fascinating was that during the 1950s, when I was a medical student, and I went on for about four years volunteering until I really was so busy with revising and things, but all the psychotropic drugs, the antidepressants, the antispasmodics, the anxiolytics, all come in in 1951. The [phenothiazine] . . . Largactyl [was] introduced in the 1950s and the non-steroidal anti-inflammatory drugs, apart from aspirin, started to come in then. The pain clinics were working, just began to publish, and there was a chap, Dr Maher up in the north somewhere, who was one of the first to write. And Bonica in America was coming along and beginning to write, all about the same time, and some of the earlier research on experimental pain and the earlier research on clinical pain, which was done by Beecher in Boston, was done on post-operative patients, and so there was a group in Memorial Sloan Kettering in New York. So there were a whole lot of tools waiting to be used when I arrived at St Joseph's[26].

Cicely observed that, in Hackney, pain relief was being administered on demand and not regularly. She seems to have found it easy to persuade Sister Mary Antonia (Figure 4.2), first that she could get a patient onto the regular giving of analgesia and also to begin keeping a 'pain diary'. This would give insight into what pain meant for the person and could be further explored by listening and talking. The Catholic Sisters quickly saw that this tall, evangelical

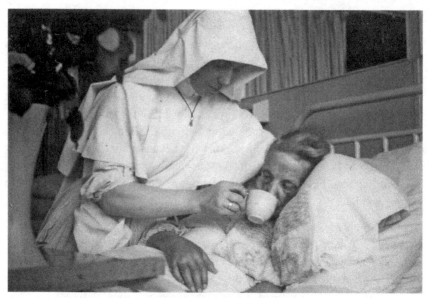

FIGURE 4.2 Sister Mary Antonia with a patient, St Joseph's Hospice. *Source: Cicely Saunders.*

Protestant with a rather patrician bearing, and to them the apparently private means to work in the hospice, was getting palpable results. Whilst in the past the nuns had felt helpless in the face of pain, now their attitude became more positive and they saw they could have patients free of pain and alert. Cicely was bringing this about, effectively as a senior house officer or registrar to the hospice, looking after the forty-five beds for terminally ill cancer patients in Our Lady's Wing, as well as offering assistance with some of the long-stay patients in other parts of St Joseph's. Now the tender loving care of the nuns and their religious composure were being harnessed to a quite specific clinical purpose. The combination was transformational. When Cicely took her supervisor, Dr Stewart, around the hospice to show him the work she was doing, he was immediately impressed. Sensing the change she was bringing about, he encouraged her endeavours and told her not to worry too much about the drug studies they had planned, advising her: 'Do them if you can'[27].

As we shall see, a huge amount of research work *was* achieved, though it did not result in the completion of her M.D. thesis. In late 1965, Cicely said to a colleague in Australia: 'I hope your thesis goes faster than mine does'[28]. By the early months of 1966, her work existed in a very full typed and referenced draft, heavily annotated with handwritten comments and corrections, and numerous notes and tags. She hoped that a period of sabbatical for writing would be the final push to its completion. At one point, it seemed to need only a few more weekends of concentrated effort and tidying up, but it was not to be. She was simply too busy with the more immediate pressures, demands, and opportunities, and she prioritised them over academic achievement. Instead, and among other things, she accepted a growing number of speaking engagements, extended the range of her travel, and, in particular, took on a large number of writing commissions for a variety of journals.

New Connections

As her early publications began to find an audience, they stimulated requests for visits to St Joseph's and, in time, as her networks expanded, Cicely actively encouraged visits from people she was keen to influence. Most typical were medical students from the London Hospital and St Bartholomew's, to whom she offered ward-rounds. Their reactions were often ones of amazement. Cicely would encourage them to talk to the patients, to whom she would say: 'You're doing the teaching. If you don't feel like teaching this afternoon when the students come, just shut your eyes and pretend you're asleep and we'll just go by'[29]. Afterwards, she would gather up the visitors for a discussion and questions. A trainee doctor in a London teaching hospital in 1961 was familiar with referring patients to St Joseph's but had never visited. Cicely invited him to come on a ward-round. She introduced a patient with inoperable cancer of the stomach who was contentedly reading a book, sitting up in bed. As they came away from the bay, the self-confessed 'bright-eyed, bushy-tailed houseman' enquired how they would deal with the patient in the event of a massive haematemesis; he had seen no fridges or drip sacks to give blood. Cicely replied: 'Well, it's unlikely, but if he did, he'd have an injection of morphine and he would either die of his haemorrhage comfortably and unaware of what was happening or, if he didn't die from it, then we would think about and consider transfusion the next day.' The houseman was astonished by the humanity and common sense of it all. The experience stayed with him. Twenty-five years later, he was medical director of a hospice in the north of England[30].

Arthur Norman (A.N.) Exton Smith, a physician at London's Whittington Hospital, had visited Cicely at St Joseph's in 1959 and knew of her interests. He was also acquainted with Dr Leonard Colebrook, of the Euthanasia Society. Exton Smith suggested they all three should meet. Colebrook was a physician and bacteriologist who, like Cicely, had held a fellowship at St Mary's. He had made his name as a champion of sterile procedures and for his investigations into *Streptococcus*. The trio had lunch together at the Royal Society of Medicine. She and Colebrook then corresponded about her recent series of articles in *Nursing Times*, in one of which she had noted that his Society had failed to produce data in support of its cause. She told him: 'I do feel strongly that yours is not the answer. We can relieve suffering if we will put our minds to it. It is just because so few people do, that pathetic cases exist'[31]. She felt he must visit the hospice if he was really to understand her approach. He said he would believe it when he saw it and eventually came to look around in February 1960. At the end of his time there he seemed convinced and told her: 'Well, you know, if everybody could have this sort of care I could disband the Society'[32]. Cicely remarked shortly afterwards that she might have paid her patients to say what they did to him, so convincing were they on the benefits of the approach at St. Joseph's: 'A little while, and I shall have the Society working to produce Terminal Homes rather than to produce a Bill which will obviously never get through Parliament anyway'[33]. In a subsequent letter to her, Colebrook was less positive but did acknowledge that this kind of hospice care was solving a lot of the problems, though it would be a long time before the idea and the practice were widely spread. Despite their implacable differences on euthanasia, the two of them became good friends. She stayed at his home in Guildford on several occasions and they remained in touch until his death, in September 1967, just a few months after St Christopher's had opened.

Based at the Maudsley Hospital in London, psychiatrist Dr John Hinton had published his first paper on the physical and mental distress of the dying in 1963[34]. Cicely read it with interest and wrote to him, inviting him to visit her at St Joseph's. He had been reading her early work too, and although he recognised their very different standpoints, they agreed on some fundamentals. Cicely had a sense of vocation, and was a 'doer' and an organiser. He, by contrast, was a non-interventionist observer in the care of dying people. She was a believer in a religious hospice; he was an agnostic at the Maudsley. What they had in common was an interest in listening to patients' stories — a narrative orientation. Here their ideas meshed; they were in sympathy with each other and kept in touch. Later, he would join the research committee at the new hospice[35].

Patient Inspirations

Not surprisingly, Cicely also found constant inspiration in those for whom she cared, and was particularly drawn to the long-stay patients in St Joseph's. They could be located mostly in the day centre, off St Michael's ward. The most established patients had their own territory in the bay window. 'They were there with bows in their hair and sort of nappies and so on. It was good old custodial care'[36]. She got to be very close to them. The ones she knew best were Louie, Alice, and Terry[37]. She looked after their medical requirements. Terry had multiple sclerosis, collapsed at one point, and had a near-death experience which Cicely recorded. Louie had fragile bones and suffered prolonged pain which required a series of Omnopon injections over a long period before she died in 1965. Alice had spent forty years, two thirds of her life, in and out of hospital with tuberculous arthritis. With these three, Cicely began to discuss in detail her ideas about a hospice she would start herself. She did the same on a visit to Mrs G. in the autumn of 1959. Mrs G. was immediately curious and asked: 'What are you going to call it? Are you going to call it after David?' Cicely replied: 'Well, I don't think so because David has no connection with medicine in any way, but I'm going to call it "hospice"'. 'What does "hospice" mean?' asked Mrs G. Cicely said: 'Well it's come to mean "a stopping place for travellers"'. Mrs G. was quick to respond: 'Travelling. You'll have to have St Christopher won't you?'[38] By 26 November 1959, therefore, Cicely was writing to a friend and referring — for the first time in correspondence — to 'St Christopher's Hospice'[39], and so it was to remain, despite the subsequent irritation caused by those who wrongly added 'for the dying' to it. Early in the process (there was no committee wrangling about this or 'market testing'), the home she was seeking to create had been given a name by one of her patients. It was one that would come to be known in time all around the world of hospice.

Tensions at St Joseph's

But Cicely's influence was not always so welcome. Surprisingly, given her well-established relationship with St Luke's, her association there came to an abrupt end in 1959. Unlike at St Joseph's, where she was a fully engaged doctor, Cicely's status at St Luke's, after the research fellowship began with St Mary's, was that of an observer, not a clinician. It may well have been difficult to stay on the right side of this boundary. As we have seen, and will see again, boundaries were problematic for Cicely. In this context, she had been a volunteer nurse at St Luke's, had completed two hospital house jobs as a newly qualified doctor elsewhere, and was also seeing terminally ill patients in Hackney. Dr Patricia Graham was a registrar from St Mary's, that now had responsibility for St Luke's, and had taken over the medical management role. It may also have been that she was not properly consulted about allowing Cicely in on this basis. To compound the concern, Cicely was clearly very much at home there. It was not to last.

> I had done seven years as a volunteer nurse at St Luke's, so I was used to going over and having coffee with the Sisters and relating with the Sisters rather than the doctors, which probably got up their noses a bit. But what happened was that, I don't think I'd been there very long, and one day I was asked by a patient a very direct question, 'Am I really dying?' and foolishly, as a researcher, I didn't say, 'I'm only a researcher; I don't know', I'd obviously said something — 'I'm afraid it doesn't look very good' — or something like that. The patient said to her mother: 'The doctor told me that I wasn't getting better' and the daughter complained to Patricia Graham that 'a doctor' had told her mother she was dying and she didn't want her to know. And so the axe fell, and I was written a letter, which was sent to Dr Stewart and to me that my presence was no longer welcome because I had overstepped my brief as a researcher in talking to a patient. At which the nurses were very upset and I saw the chaplain

to say, you know, 'I'm terribly sorry but I had a feel for St Luke's because I'd done volunteering there, and I was very upset but I didn't suppose we could repair the damage'. And certainly one of the doctors — Dr Brinton, I think — wrote me quite a nice letter saying that he was sorry this had happened. That's right, but that was it. I mean, there was no chance of going back and Patricia Graham I think . . . felt I was making a great fuss about terminal care, that was perfectly simple and regular giving [of analgesia] wasn't all that special, and I was getting some limelight by the *Nursing Times* articles and things like that. Quite a long time later, I was lecturing at St Mary's and I think she came and listened, and I mean she felt less strongly than I did that communication was important and that, if honesty seemed to be right, then that was a path to pursue, even gently. I think we eventually parted on reasonable terms, but she might have a different view of it[40].

In 1965, six years after the departure from St. Luke's, the time also came to leave St Joseph's. Now she jumped before she was pushed. Again it was a clash with the hierarchy, though this time with Reverend Mother rather than one of the doctors. From the start at Hackney, Cicely had got on well with Mother Mary Paula, who enjoyed the enthusiastic presence of the evangelical champion of terminal care. This provided a solid platform for Cicely's work there. Mother Mary Walter followed, but was soon moved elsewhere. Her successor, ironically named Mother Dolores (meaning 'pain'), was less sympathetic. From Northern Ireland, she seemed to dislike the idea of a Protestant doctor in the house. She may also have caught some word about a special relationship that had developed between Cicely and one of her patients in 1960. Nor did Mother Dolores care for Cicely's friendly colleagueship with the younger Sisters. Most overtly, she didn't like Cicely's clinical methods and the unconventional approach she was adopting in some instances — discharging patients home when symptoms were under control or referring them for radiotherapy to ease their symptoms. Later, it would become clear that these were examples of a 'modern' approach to hospice and to what would come to be called 'palliative' care, but they did not impress Mother Dolores, who told Cicely: 'When I'm dying, I want to grow fat in the bed'[41]. The implication was that patients 'shouldn't be got up and got going by an eager doctor'[42]. Cicely sensed that her time was nigh. Sister Joseph and Sister Mary Antonia were bewildered and supportive, but no one would go against Reverend Mother. Chuckling as she said it many years later, but not wishing to cause offence even then, she recalled: 'I gave in my notice just before I got thrown out in '65, in the summer. Oh yes, Mother Dolores was going to get rid of me . . .[43]'.

There was no sense that this was deeply problematic, however. In September 1965, Cicely wrote to a colleague in the United States:

My time at St Joseph's is coming to an end at the beginning of October when I am due to have some holidays anyway . . . . I will miss very much being

with patients, but I feel that I do need a sabbatical after such a long time . . . .
Certainly the end of my time at St Joseph's was shown very clearly, not least
in the fact that for the first time since I have been there, the first time in this
whole seven years, I find that there is not one single patient about whom I feel
the kind of responsibility that makes me unhappy about going away for a holiday. They will manage alright without me and this is entirely as it should be[44].

Antoni Michniewicz, Mrs. G., and Gordon Saunders (1960 – 1961)

But earlier, as the work at St Joseph's began to pick up momentum at the start
of the 1960s, Cicely could hardly have been prepared for the events that were
to unfold. It was to be an intensely formative time, as we shall see — one of
deep reflection and consultation with others on the precise nature of her vision
for her own hospice. It was also a period of keening loss associated with one
particular patient, Antoni Michniewicz, that created in her such a powerful
and abiding sense of sorrow for a relationship which, as with David Tasma,
never came to fruition. Yet, this time, it made her feel that she had experienced something far deeper and consequential, something capable of giving a
true authenticity that was imperative to the work she was undertaking. Within
months of the new decade starting, the energy and resolve she would need to
push forward her ideas for a hospice of her own were being challenged by
other things that bore in on her. She was on the brink of a trilogy of hammer
blows, encountered in a period of twelve months, and the like of which she
could scarcely have countenanced:

> You see, after Antoni died, Mrs. G died the following January, and my father
> the following June, and I really got my bereavements muddled up[45].

Antoni Michniewicz

On 2 January 1960, Cicely admitted the fifty-nine-year-old widowed Polish
patient Antoni Michniewicz (Figure 4.3) to the ward in St Joseph's[46]. He
had a rare liposarcoma, or bone cancer of the right shoulder, and had been
operated on in October 1958. An electrical engineer, he could no longer
work, had developed multiple symptoms, and was described in the notes
as 'semi-bedridden'. He had dry, scaly skin and eczema on his hands and
feet; was experiencing pain creeping down his right arm; and had lost mobility in that hand. He had clearly shed a great deal of weight from his tall
frame. Cicely quickly established him on the Brompton mixture and this
seemed to help. In his early days at the hospice, she found him cheerful and
calm, asking for a Polish priest, but also quizzical about his worsening condition. His only daughter, Anna, was in her final year of study for a degree

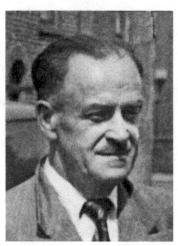

FIGURE 4.3 Antoni Michniewicz, probably in London. *Source: kept by Cicely Saunders.*

in Chemistry, and he told Cicely on 20 January that he would so much like to survive until the summer, when her results would be known. Anna seems to have had only one other relative, a cousin, in London, but she visited her father 'devotedly'. Sensing her needs, Sister Antonia gave her an evening meal each time she came to the hospice.

At the end of January, Cicely referred Mr Michniewicz to the Medical Research Council Radiotherapeutic Research Unit at Hammersmith Hospital, where he was commenced on a weekly palliative dose of X-ray therapy to the right neck to ease his symptoms. But by the beginning of March, he was no longer well enough to travel to the hospital and the sessions were discontinued. Despite his problems, he became in some ways a model patient. Speaking eight languages in total (English apparently his worst), he helped with translation for a patient in an adjacent bed. He liked, and was given, his shaving water really hot, and took pride in maintaining his smart appearance. Intelligent and insightful, he gave every indication that he was aware of his worsening condition, but was desperate to stay alive until after Anna had completed her finals and gained her results.

Cicely explains:

> He was just an interesting and challenging patient — an ex-Eight Army, very patrician Pole. He was an electronics engineer. He was a widower. And after Easter, I'd been on holiday, and I remember coming back and saying, 'We had a marvellous time and we had this wonderful weather'. And Antoni said, 'Oh, I prayed for your weather'. So he was on quite sort of friendly terms, which all my patients were for that matter. But it was when his daughter passed her exams in July and I went to congratulate her [that] she said, 'Oh my father has so much fallen in love with you, Doctor'. And he said, 'I

don't know how to express it. Please don't be offended.' I said, 'Well, no, I'm grateful'. And I left them. But my world was suddenly unmade without warning.

And then we had just a few weeks of becoming incredibly close, with the rigorous discipline of being his doctor, and so I never pulled the curtains 'round more than I would have done anyway for any other patient, and yet we managed. I did allow myself to sit and talk with him at five o'clock in the evening, and sometimes I just couldn't help taking an hour. And that very intense and totally, I suppose I would say, 'spiritual relationship', that people find difficult to believe could be quite so . . . unfulfilled, and in a way it was fulfilled. When he died I was absolutely devastated.

But before he died, I was able to get across to him that he was a giver as well as me, because he was saying, 'I can give you nothing — nothing but sorrow.' We couldn't just sit in silence, which we would love to have done, because that would have been much stranger in a ward, so it was always in a six-bed bay, never, ever anywhere else. But just before he died, just before he lost consciousness, he gave me the most incredible smile . . . and I was writing a prayer down every morning at that time and I wrote a detailed diary every day for the three and a half weeks that we were together. So I wrote that evening: 'I'm not sure what was in it, not sorrow at all, strong somehow and even a gleam of amusement'. It was just the look of love, and it was a moment of suddenly finding all the answers, and it was all right.

And that again was like the feeling about David; he was alright. Antoni was a very mature person, and I had to stretch up to meet him at the level at which we had to function. And it took me months and even years to grow up to that, and to come to terms . . . . My goodness it was bleak. But not a word of complaint, because we couldn't have met any other place or time[47].

It was an intense and private relationship conducted in a public space. Once again, Cicely was playing with dynamite, as this time, now in the role of a fully qualified physician, she formed a deep, personal relationship with a terminally ill patient in a Roman Catholic hospice. She was forty-four and he was fifteen years her senior. Mature adults, they entered into something which would have been seen as deeply inappropriate — even reprehensible — at the time, were it to have been revealed. Blind to any institutional consequences that might result, in late July and August 1960, Cicely recorded on a daily basis, and quite separately from her patients' clinical notes, each of the unfolding aspects of their final weeks together, including a great deal of personal information. Later, she typed up these notes and then went on to edit them further by hand until a complete version was achieved. They amounted to twenty-seven quarto pages, with an additional ten pages of material written in the days following his death, and were to remain extant[48].

Now she wrote in far greater detail than had been the case with David Tasma. Her daily account covered the period 20 July to 15 August. She thought he might die at any time. She records the minutiae of their conversations, the details of his care, his medications and routines. He told her that Monday, Wednesday, and Friday had become his best days — those when she was at the hospice. He was tall, thin, confined to bed, and limited in his movements. He would kiss her hand, which she would then surreptitiously hold to his cheek. He had pain and needed frequent injections. He slept a great deal. He admired her watch, which had been left to her by David Tasma. He had lived on an estate which was then in eastern Poland, but mainly spent his winters in a flat in Wilno, that later became Vilnius, the capital of Lithuania. She learned of his interest in wireless making, in music (Schubert and Strauss), and in birds. He told her he had lost the art of conversation, so long was it since he had talked to anyone. He spoke of the 'happiest time of his life' at the University of Wilno, of his two-storey partly wooden home, with servants, a big garden, water nearby, and his Doberman Pinscher. They shared brief words about his wartime deportation by the Germans to Siberia; his escape by train to Persia, where he joined the British Eight Army; and his eventual arrival in London, where he decided to stay after demobilisation and was eventually reunited with his wife.

On 1 August 1960, the diary records:

> And I said that I was a doctor and he was my patient and we couldn't ever be alone and I couldn't come as often as I wanted and he said, 'For me, it is enough'. And I said, 'There has not been anyone like you'. And I tried to say, 'There won't be very long', but it was so hard to quench his dawning hope. He said, 'I do not understand. I have never done anything for you'. I said, 'I love you just because you are you'. He said, 'Thank you'.

In the following days, she told him more about her own life and continued her fitful and intense visits. At 3 pm on 14 August, the sun was shining. He looked out of the window and said, 'It is getting darker'. She knew his time was near. The Viaticum was called for. He lay watching the crucifix, before his eyes looked over her face and back again. 'He was at peace. I think it was our best moment of all and really timeless . . . . I do not know how long'. Next day, the Feast of the Assumption of the Virgin Mary, there was a greater urgency. He took communion but was restless, and terribly emaciated and breathless. He was offered a further injection. The ominous sense of the diary is that this would be his last. Cicely slipped in to give him a drink. His daughter arrived, the curtains were drawn, and the prayers began. Seeking against all odds to maintain a complete sense of normality, in the midst of all this, Cicely was elsewhere in the hospice at the time, taking tea with a colleague. Antoni died shortly before her return, towards four o'clock in the afternoon.

As she recalled more than forty years later, the experience had so many dimensions:

[I felt] tremendous satisfaction that such a special person should love me. Also, very much a depth of spiritual things. I remember him looking across the ward through the glass partition to the crucifix and saying, 'I can see my Saviour' and saying to him that he's my Saviour too, so wherever we are, we shall be together. Then another time [me] saying, 'He'll be here when you're gone'. But the day after he died, I went back and there was another patient in his bed and I remember standing at the door and thinking, 'I can't go in; it hurts too much', then looking at the crucifix and letting it hold me, and getting around. But I couldn't really think for the next few days, so I went away for just a few days before I came back to work[49].

Cicely went to see her father, spent time talking with Madge Drake, and then threw herself back into her duties. As she later explained: 'It was the only resource, apart from prayer — and singing'[50]. She was also 'endlessly on the phone', talking to those few friends with whom she could share her experience, especially Rosetta Burch and Betty West (Tom's mother), with whom she also exchanged many letters. By this time, Tom West had joined the Church Missionary Society and, on 28 April 1960, sailed for a posting in Nigeria. She had been there to see him off, with the ever-supportive Gillian Ford waiting at the flat afterwards with a smoked salmon supper to cheer her up. West and Cicely had been corresponding regularly since his departure for Africa, and she was the chief source of his reading matter there. But when she wrote him about Antoni, he failed (or refused) to understand the magnitude of it all 'and he wrote me a rather silly letter and I wrote back *scorpions*, ticking him off and he came back rather hang-dog . . .'[51]. It was an emotional ebb and flow in the currents between Cicely and West that would continue for at least another decade.

Months later, on Wednesday, 2 November 1960 — All Souls' Day — Cicely trudged through the wet London streets to attend communion in Langham Place. Despite the day and the name of her church, she was disappointed in the service. There were two options for post-communion prayers that day. One spoke of the communion of saints and the other did not. The priest had chosen the latter. Still raw from the death of Antoni, Cicely felt hurt and let down. She quickly made a resolution: 'That's it. I'm not going here anymore. I can't. I must go somewhere else'[52].

After Antoni's death she began keeping a prayer diary. For the next four years, she wrote down her devotions each day. Relentless outpourings couched in the language of prayer and addressed directly to her Lord, they are almost, without exception, about Antoni. They make for painful reading that might also induce irritation or impatience, such is the degree of personal introspection. Day after day, year after year, they recall Antoni on his deathbed, their brief moments together, his suffering more at their parting more than at the prospect of his death, and her longing to meet him in heaven. There were dreams about Antoni, many of them disturbing. The first one to give comfort was on the night of 2 – 3 April 1961, when she encountered him alive and strong, kissing her 'with deep sure loving, but not with physical passion' and then reading to her a passage from Genesis 120:4 about God speaking in deep silence[53]. She recorded more dreams of Antoni in 1961, 1963, and 1964. She came to inhabit a world of profound self-absorption, carapaced with spiritual exploration. The emotional labour this required of Cicely and the time she devoted to it cannot be under-estimated. Yet when she might have slipped into uncontrolled morbid grief and psychiatric illness, she never, ever lost sight of her goals for a new hospice, and also the wider world and its issues.

One aspect of this was the intense interest she now developed in Poland, its history and culture, finally getting to visit for the first time in March 1963. She took extracts from Christine Hotchkiss's *Home to Poland* based on an extended visit made by an émigré in 1956, and had them typed[54]. She accumulated many, many articles about Poland from the Sunday newspapers and elsewhere. She donated to the Polish Airforce Association in Great Britain and made contact with St Andrew's Bobola Polish Church in London. She wrote out Polish phrases for use in letters. She started subscribing to the illustrated magazine *Poland* and acquired all the back issues for 1960. She was especially intrigued by the journal's competition asking readers to write on the theme 'My encounter with a Pole' and submitted an entry in February 1962. Although never published, it comprised a seven-page account of her time with Antoni[55]. His name and other details altered, it dwells less on their relationship and much more on his personality and manners, and the Polish culture that must have shaped them. It is something too of a manifesto for special places devoted to the care of the dying, and is the only source in which Cicely pays homage to a Polish doctor she had when she was a child and 'whose courtesy and friendliness had helped me to lose my shyness and begin to meet people more easily'. Following her patient's death, she describes how she became fascinated with Poland, even proud of its people, and 'also ashamed that I had known so little before'. She had seen how someone who had been deprived of so much by war, forced migration, the death of his wife, and then his own terminal illness could maintain a sense of integrity and faith, and remain rich in his interest and friendship for others. This dying Pole could so much focus on the present moment as to forget other troubles and foster an independence of circumstances which she believed may be characteristic of a nation which had lost so much and lived under — and eventually outlasted — its oppression. Drawing on a metaphor which she would use many times in the future when speaking of hospice care, she concluded: 'Perhaps this position in geography and history which has brought them so much suffering has now given them the unique opportunity to be a *bridge* instead of a battlefield'. Meanwhile, her own battles would continue, as she too faced further losses.

The Death of Mrs G.

As we have seen, by the end of 1960, Mrs G.'s condition was also worsening rapidly, and the final weeks of her life were painful for those around her, when dark moods and suspicions threatened to under-mine long-established relationships. It was made worse when Mrs G. sensed that the Ward Sister, to whom she was devoted, was going to be moving elsewhere. She became very distressed; her old anxieties of abandonment and being sent away were once more re-kindled. The hospital matron was brought in and promptly did two things. First, she ordered Mrs G.'s favourite lunch from the kitchen. Second, she called for Cicely to come as quickly as possible. Things calmed down. Christmas came and went with Mrs G. in slightly better spirits, but soon she drifted into unconscious and left the world, just as the new year was beginning.

> And when she died, she had made an incredible impression on an enormous number of people and I still, from time to time, meet people who were nursing at that time and never forgot her. And she said one very important thing to a student, three or four weeks before she died: 'Some people can go to church and get their help there, some people can read their bibles and get their help there, but He deals with me differently: He sends me people'. And that is one of the things about hospice: It is quietly meeting as people[56].

The links with Mrs G. would not be severed. Cicely stayed in touch with her husband and mother-in-law, whom she later described as 'two of my best friends'[57]. When Cicely opened her own hospice in 1967, Mrs G.'s Ward Sister (Joan Steel) was its Senior Sister and Mrs G.'s husband took on the duties of head porter. It was further evidence of Cicely's boundary-hopping and close intertwining of the personal and the professional — an orientation that would continue when St Christopher's became operational.

For now, in early 1961, two absolutely special patients had died in fewer than six months. Cicely was on her knees, but one more blow was still to descend.

The Visit to Grandchamp and the Death of Her Father

The previous year, when Cicely visited her father on regular occasions in his home at Hadley Chase, he was still showing an interest in property deals and getting around the garden for walks. Despite cardiac problems, as Cicely put it to her brother Christopher, he would 'probably surprise his doctors yet'[58]. But in the spring of 1961, Gordon Saunders's health had deteriorated significantly as he succumbed to the distressing signs and symptoms of heart failure. Cicely began spending more time with him to give a break to Mrs Diamant. But at the same time she had a plan to go to the Communauté de Grandchamp in Neuchatel, Switzerland, and to complete a visit which had been put off the previous year. Her father encouraged her to go ahead. He would travel down to Hythe on the Kent coast and stay at the Hotel Imperial for a few days for a change of scene and air.

The visit to Grandchamp marked a profound shift in Cicely's spiritual orientation. Since early spring 1960, and following the advice of her theological confidant, Olive Wyon, she had been in correspondence with Sister Genieviéve at Grandchamp, the sister community to Taizé, in Burgundy, France[59]. She had received information about life and work there, with an invitation to attend a retreat in the summer, but had so far been thwarted in her efforts to go. In July 1960, a visit was postponed as she felt unable to leave Antoni just as they had shared their feelings for each other. Now, almost a year later, and despite worrying about her father, she was on her way. She quickly felt at home in the community. In the quiet contemplation of Grandchamp, she made a confession to Gibberd, one of the visiting Fathers. This was a striking new departure in her spiritual life, revealing in dramatic fashion how her move away from the evangelical world was gathering momentum.

> [It was] a load that needed to be got rid of. Snapping at people and not getting on, fighting like anything with my father at various times, and all the business of my father and my mother . . . and finding her just so difficult. I can't tell you how difficult[60].

The confession was a profound experience that brought to a head several years of ill feeling and tension in Cicely's family life. It ended in bathos. As she left the confessional, on the brink of relief at what she had shared, she reached for the light and pulled on a great rope which, to her huge embarrassment, sounded an enormous bell across the community. Perhaps unconsciously, it was a wider announcement that something very profound was happening to the 'Protestant heretic'.

On the morning afterwards, she spent time in the chapel, going through Psalm 95, the *Venite*, just as she had done with David Tasma. Then she was by a riverbank, deep in prayer and reverie, again just as she had been in the Highlands after the death of David. Running water and the natural world drew her towards them in some of her most profound moments of reflection. She found solace in the hills and mountains, in the rippling light of sunshine on watery pebbles, and in the purity of the country air. Some of her deepest moments of insight were in these places, far away from the city backdrop to her quotidian life. Now, the great tree behind her appeared to transform into a huge cross — the Cross of the World. She felt the words 'Come; for all things are now ready', said before the communion at Grandchamp. On returning to her room, there was a message waiting for her with the request to make a call to England. She received the news that Gordon Saunders had just died in his hotel, while she was at the riverbank[61]. It was 13 June 1961.

Sensing her growing pain and disorientation, Father Gibberd took time to give advice on her spiritual path. He considered her to be in the wrong sort of fellowship and advised that she begin worshipping at the St Marylebone Parish Church, in a more Anglo-Catholic environment. When she returned to London, she did as suggested and at first warmed to the 'high church' orientation. But when a new vicar was installed who greeted her by name at the door, she felt her anonymity had been compromised. She wanted to be able to worship alone in a metropolitan setting, without the need for social contact with others. She realised later it was an aspect of her complicated grief reaction, when she was 'euphoric' at times but angry and resentful at others.

Daily Light seemed to help, and reading the Psalms every day.

> And then I got myself a rosary and using the Jesus Prayer, I used to say it in the car driving over to St Joseph's to stop telling myself how miserable I was. And I was always dropping it on my lap and then getting out of the car and losing it. Sister Mary Antonia had one left and she said, 'You won't lose that now'. And I used that for a long time[62].

Cicely drifted towards Westminster Abbey as a place of worship and then to Christ Church at Lancaster Gate in Paddington, where she couldn't get on with the modern approach of the Rev Antony Bridge. As she put it much later:

> I was just too raw to be too close . . . . I wasn't feeling less sure of God, but I just didn't want people fretting me about it. I wanted to go and worship quietly and not be bothered with other people — tellingly, I suppose — because I had a pretty bleak three years after Antoni died. We simply had no past. We'd no common memories. We'd no common anything except that one intense time[63].

Complicated Grief

These were only some of the contradictions in her life. At the same time, she could live without financial worry, leading a busy social life and entertaining in her rooms in Connaught Square. As the idea for her own hospice developed, she began wooing members of the establishment and working her way through the foundations, trusts, and livery companies which made up part of the fabric of London life and which might be willing to lend support. Moreover, as we shall see, when in 1963 a new man and potential lover came into her life, she seized the moment and threw considerable energy into pursuing him. There was complexity in her existence, but also a sense of completeness and purpose that could be the envy of others, despite her sorrows and searching.

But when the terms of her father's will became known in the midst of all this, her distress increased[64]. The will had been made in January 1955, when Cicely was still a medical student. Probate was given in London on 13 November 1961 to her younger brothers John and Christopher, along with Ronald Walker, a retired bank manager. Cicely was completely excluded from the executorial process. The gross value of the will was £188,873. After death duties of £50,343 had been paid, there were various small cash allocations to specific individuals. A trust fund of £20,000 was formed to provide income to Gordon's wife Chrissie, and a similar arrangement for £2,000 was provided for his sister Daisy. The residuary value of the estate was then split into fifths. Cicely received one fifth, interest only. Her brothers received two fifths each and a controlling interest in her share. She panicked that she might not have enough money to live on. She was outraged too at the way Mrs Diamant had been treated — being left with just £15,000 after all the support she had given to Gordon:

> She'd given up her home. She was living with him. And as she said to me, 'I feel as if all my clothes have been blown off'. So I said to the boys, 'She's got to have the coach house and she's got to have all the furniture in her room . . . .' And she got it, but then I took myself off to another lawyer, just saying, 'I really want to be sure that I'm going to be alright'. He said, 'That's a very Victorian will'. And it was at that time that I thought, 'Really, I'm in a mess'[65].

She went to see her G.P., Dame Annis Gillie, at the Connaught Square practice and told her: 'I'm really getting depressed and angry and in a muddle'. Dr Gillie referred her to psychiatrist and psychotherapist Anthony Storr, whose book *The Integrity of the Personality*[66] had appeared the previous year and who had a special interest in aggression[67]. In the two sessions they had together, he told her to express her anger and 'let it out'. She seemed temperamentally disinclined to do this and told him she had a calling to serve the dying but felt unworthy to follow it. He replied that she had to get on and do it. It wasn't possible to be 'worthy first'; she must act. Cicely took this as good advice, but didn't continue the sessions and 'went on battling'[68]. Instead, she heeded the advice of a Catholic Sister with whom she was corresponding, who told her: 'Listen to God. Don't express your anger. You should listen to your God, not your psychiatrist'[69].

Over time she realised that her father was at the centre of her grief, sometimes clouding her thoughts about Antoni[70]. She was relieved that Gordon had finally understood what her work was all about, but despite the terms of the will, she felt guilty she had taken so much money from him during his life and never properly thanked him for it. Nevertheless, they had parted well. His boasting was over, along with his criticisms of her chosen path. He had been confident in her and rationalised that his moneymaking had found a purpose. Even before she made her confession at Grandchamps, she knew that God had forgiven her. But there was something deeper still that troubled her and which, only years later, she came to understand when she read a passage in a book by Henri Nouwen, Dutch Catholic priest, writer, and theologian. Published in January 1999, she had Nouwen's *The Inner Voice of Love*[71] on her lap when, in an interview, on 15 December of that same year, she said:

> There's something I absolutely battled with at the time. I mean a feeling that you love somebody more than God. When you try to die to that love in order to find God's love, you are doing something God does not want. The task is not to die to life-giving relationships, but to realise that the love you received in them is part of a greater love. And I had a great battle to discover that[72].

Paradoxically, her prayer diaries spoke not of anger and confusion, but of gratitude.

> We will rejoice in Thy Salvation O Lord. Whenever we rejoice and we rejoice in Thee, then we are together. A.M., my father, Mrs G., all my patients. O Lord, here is home and safety, here is strength and redemption, here is love. All in Thee and from Thee[73].

Perhaps it is the last group on her list that is the key here — 'all my patients'. Whilst attention has focussed on the three named persons, it might well be that every one of her patients that had died — now running into the hundreds — had laid in each case a feather of grief on her shoulder. The accumulation, further inflamed by personal losses, had simply become too much to bear.

Total Pain

In these years at St Joseph's, and woven from the threads of her clinical and personal experiences at that time, Cicely created a radically new approach to the conceptualisation of pain. We have seen that she was already tuning in to the close relationship between physical and mental suffering, but she could see that suffering had other dimensions. It included physical symptoms, spiritual distress, social problems, and emotional difficulties. She began to grapple with this and searched for inspiration to make sense of it, drinking deep from many sources. She prepared an extensive typed extract of a work by Jesuit priest and modernist George Tyrrell titled *Water and Wine*[74]. She was assiduous in collecting clippings and holding on to handwritten notes about distress, illness, loss. She read Laurens van de Post's *A Bar of Shadow*[75] and Evan Hopkin's *The Mystery of Suffering*[76]. She extracted passages from Kahil Gilbran's *The Prophet*[77] and took detailed notes from Kierkegaard's *The Gospel of Suffering*[78].

Helped by these diverse influences and interwoven with what she was feeling, what she was hearing from her patients, and what she knew of the clinical literature, she forged the notion of 'total pain'. In so doing, she bequeathed to medicine and health care a concept of enduring clinical and conceptual interest which was still attracting commentary and analysis fifty years later. The concept emerged from her unique experience as nurse, almoner, and physician. It reflected a willingness to acknowledge the spiritual suffering of the patient and to see this in relation to physical problems. Crucially, it was tied to a sense of narrative and biography, emphasising the importance of listening to the story and of understanding the experience of suffering in a multi-facetted way. This was an approach that saw pain as the key to unlocking other problems, and as something requiring multiple interventions for its resolution. Her way into it was through close attention to what patients were saying, aided by tape recordings and subsequent transcriptions. She describes it here:

> Well I knew from what patients were saying that this wasn't just a physical problem and I knew from my previous nursing and social work that anxiety and depression were major components. I was certainly alert to the fact that family problems were difficult, very often adding to distress and I also felt that a search for feeling that they were wanted and still important people was a spiritual pain and so, out of what one patient said, very neatly describing her pain to me, developed the idea of 'total pain' with those four components. And that seemed to me to be a structure that, although it was a whole package as far as the patient is concerned, it was almost an internal checklist for you when you were listening to them to spot the main problems of their suffering[79]. The person who really sparked me into looking really widely, apart from the patients themselves, was a chap called Buytendijk, who wrote a book on pain and he was absolutely fascinating[80].

F.J.J. Buytendijk was a Dutch doctor and phenomenological scholar whose 1943 book *Over de Pijn*[81] was published in English in 1961, as well as translated into German, French, and Italian. He had completed his medical studies in 1909 and later wrote widely on philosophical anthropology. Cicely was inspired by his work, telling him in a letter that his book was 'one of the most exciting things I have read since I started five years ago trying to do research on the control of pain among patients with terminal cancer'[82]. On that basis she planned a holiday to the Netherlands with her mother in October 1963 and asked if she could meet him at the University of Utrecht. They stayed in the Hotel Poort von Cleve in Amsterdam, during which time she was able to slip away for her meeting with him. The much anticipated encounter seems to have fallen a little flat however. Buytendijk 'was a bit disappointed when he found I wasn't a psychologist or a psychiatrist, and was just a basic doctor'[83]. Nevertheless, she responded to his interest in the history of the terminal care homes in London, sending him various notes and articles and later inviting him to St Christopher's, though there is no evidence he was able to make the trip. The 1963 holiday with her mother, however, who had now emerged from the shellshock of separation from her husband, was deemed a huge success.

The inseparability of physical pain from mental processes is alluded to by Cicely in some of her earliest publications. Even then she was on her way to a completely new conceptualisation of pain as a multi-faceted and complex phenomenon[84]. In 1959, she could note: 'Much of our total pain experience is composed of our mental reaction . . .'[85]. At this stage we have the idea of total pain in a weaker, more preliminary sense than was to emerge within a few years. Here it is a general descriptor, indicating there may be several layers which have to be understood to have a full grasp of the problem of pain in the terminally ill. The specific context of this understanding is the stage of illness 'when all curative and palliative measures have been exhausted'[86]. This moment, at which modern medicine typically states 'there is nothing more to be done'[87], thus becomes the starting point for an emergent medicine of terminal care, central to which is a multi-faceted understanding of pain. This is a medicine concerned also with the meaning of pain. A cry simply to be rid of pain is not worthy of humans, who must question the pain which is endured and seek meaning in it. Seen this way, pain somehow breaks the yoke of material values and allows the finest human sentiments to shine through.

In this sense, Cicely began to realise pain is something indivisible from both the body and the wider personality. So she observed that 'the body has a wisdom of its own and will help the strong instinct to fight for life to change into an active kind of acceptance that may never be expressed in words'[88]. In the following narrative, from a 1964 article in *Nursing Mirror*, Cicely describes for the first time the key elements of what came to be viewed as 'total pain'. It is about Mrs Hinson, a patient cared for at St Joseph's Hospice, Hackney. It was later quoted extensively within the palliative care literature, becoming emblematic of the whole principle of care within the emerging specialty.

> One person gave me more or less the following answer when I asked her a question about her pain, and in her answer she brings out the four main needs that we are trying to care for in this situation. She said, 'Well doctor, the pain began in my back, but now it seems that all of me is wrong'. She gave a description of various symptoms and ills and then went on to say, 'My husband and son were marvellous but they were at work and they would have had to stay off and lose their money. I could have cried for the pills and injections, although I knew I shouldn't. Everything seemed to be against me and nobody seemed to understand'. And then she paused before she said, 'But it's so wonderful to begin to feel safe again'. Without any further questioning she had talked of her mental as well as physical distress, of her social problems, and of her spiritual need for security[89].

That same year, 1964, in an article for *The Prescribers' Journal*, Cicely used the phrase 'all of me is wrong' more formally to introduce the concept of total pain in its stronger and definitional sense — to include physical symptoms, mental distress, social problems, and emotional torment. Although often over-looked by subsequent commentators, this is the foundational piece in which total pain is fully described for the first time[90]. In a 1965 article, a patient at St Joseph's used the phrase, 'it was all pain and now it's gone, and I am free'. Cicely had understood that 'total pain' calls for analysis, assessment, and an-ticipation[91]. As early as 1959, she had acknowledged that pain in this multi-facetted sense could not be relieved solely through analgesics[92]. Likewise, it posed greater challenges than could be overcome by the technologies of reg-ular administration for pain relief. By 1967, a new conceptualisation of pain had emerged: 'Pain demands the same analysis and consideration as an illness itself. It is the syndromes of pain rather than the syndromes of disease with which we are concerned'[93].

Clinical Studies

Part of Cicely's remit on being given the fellowship at St Mary's was to find out what was going on in the field of clinical pain. She became increasingly energetic in writing to clinicians and researchers, making contacts, requesting offprints of articles, and sharing what she had of her own. In those days, offprints were a scarce commodity, sent by post and often backed up with extra copies laboriously (and inkily) printed from a hand-turned duplicator machine. She sought out anything on which she could lay her hands. By the time she went to the United States in 1963, she had acquired enough credi-bility to gain entrée to the worlds of noted pain researchers such as Stanley Wallenstein and Ray Houde at Memorial Hospital, New York, and Henry Beecher at Massachusetts General Hospital. But they were on parallel lines to her, working with post-operative pain and conducting 'single-dose' studies. As she was coming to understand, morphine in a single-dose study is far less satisfactory than morphine given regularly, and morphine in a single dose by injection is different from morphine by mouth. She couldn't accept their findings that morphine is no more effective than aspirin or that by injection it is six times stronger than by mouth — all things that clashed with her growing clinical insights. She also saw that this body of work, that focussed on post-operative or post-trauma pain, was addressing something quite different, both clinically and at the level of meaning.

> Chronic pain and the pain of end-stage cancer is a situation in which you're ab-
> solutely held. Whereas the first kind of pain has got a nice built-in meaning —
> 'Of course I've got a pain; I've had an operation' — for the second one, the
> only meaning is really one of threat. 'This is undermining me'. So you're

absolutely bound, I think, once you start looking at that kind of pain, to say it's quite ridiculous to do a one-dose study here. What we've got to look at is coping with it all the time. Then you obviously have to look at what else is happening and then you're into the field of total pain[94].

The British and American approaches were radically different. Quite soon, Cicely would witness first-hand the scepticism of her American pain research counterparts when she visited them in the United States: 'I think they thought I was a bit of a nutter when I went over the first time.' In due course, there would also be a standoff between them at the world's first cancer pain congress, in Florence. 'But it got picked up later'[95].

The Influence of New Studies

This momentum around the study of pain was expanded during the early 1960s with research by other British clinicians who began to show an interest in terminal care and with whom Cicely developed contact. Coming both before and after her chronologically, they also became her contemporaries and fellow travellers as enthusiasm for this new aspect of medicine began to gain momentum, not only concerning pain, but also in relation to caring for the dying more generally.

In this context, A.N. Exton Smith had asked Cicely to comment on the draft of an article he was preparing for *The Lancet* and that was published in 1961[96]. It reported observations on a series of 220 patients, age sixty to 101 years. Although the numbers were modest by the scale of those Cicely was amassing, the findings were important. He reported that twenty-five per cent died within the first week of admission to hospital and eighty-two per cent within three months. Exton Smith's purpose was to assess the pain and distress experienced by this group of patients, who had a range of malignant and non-malignant diseases, including conditions of the cardiovascular, locomotor, and central nervous systems. Interestingly, he suggested that cancer was less likely to be a cause of pain and suffering in the elderly than in younger patients and that 'processes which lead indirectly to death are associated with most pain and suffering' — in other words, the chronic conditions. Nevertheless, effective analgesia in the form of narcotics was usually denied to them because of fear of habit formation. Exton Smith noted that 'the suffering of this group of patients was aggravated by the fact that they were all mentally alert and recognised their helplessness'[97]. He argued that a 'natural death' in old age is experienced by but a few and called for more comprehensive inpatient facilities, allied to hospitals, for terminally ill patients who could not be cared for at home. Although Cicely did not follow Exton Smith's focus on the dying aged, and fastened her attention instead on those, often younger, patients in the final stages of cancer, especially those with the most complex problems, nevertheless, she had an ally in him. He was one of the few clinicians at that time gathering empirical evidence about the care of the elderly and the dying. It meant that she was not alone. Moreover, an editorial in *The Lancet* endorsed the work of Exton Smith, and took a swing at those supporting euthanasia:

> [I]f the known means to make death, when it comes, easy and happy were applied by individual and collective effort with intelligence and energy, could not all but a few deaths be made at least easy and, in our ageing population, even happy? And should we not avoid this pressure to assume the right — even the duty — to take life, with all the implications and consequences that assumption carries?[98]

John Hinton's 1963 paper was written in 1962 and based on research conducted at a teaching hospital in 1959 through to 1961[99]. He pointed out that, before Exton Smith, only Osler, more than fifty years earlier, had described the incidence, severity, and relief of distress among the hospitalised dying. As we have seen, like Cicely, Hinton was inclined to a conversational approach to data collection and his 1963 paper is based on interviews with 102 patients thought unlikely to live for more than six months, with control subjects. The dying group were more commonly depressed and anxious, and half of them were aware their illness might be fatal. Physical distress was more prevalent in those with heart or renal failure (fifty-seven per cent) than those with malignancies (thirty-seven per cent) and was, in general, more severe and unrelieved for longer within the dying group.

Just as the Exton Smith paper had stimulated comment in *The Lancet*, now the *British Medical Journal* took notice. A leading article in August 1963 acknowledged the absence of 'objective inquiries into this matter' and praised Hinton for building on the contribution of Exton Smith[100]. It focused in particular on mental distress and the need for doctors, described as 'at a disadvantage in this respect compared with nurses and patients' relatives', to pay attention to the problem of such distress in their dying patients. By so doing, 'we should re-examine the comfortable supposition that the majority of our dying patients are not suffering overmuch, or they are not pondering the outcome just because they do not ask the most dreadful question of all'.

Pressing the Case Against Euthanasia

Cicely then took up her pen, and the following month wrote a letter in response which underscored the importance (so much a feature of her methodology and of Hinton's approach) of giving patients opportunities to talk, seeing this as the pathway to the relief of both mental and physical suffering. More generally, however, this was an opportunity for her, building on a leading article in one of the world's most eminent medical journals, to press the wider case for terminal care homes:

> In spite of what is already being done in this field there remains a need for more units planned for those patients who do not need the resources of a large hospital and who cannot be at home. There is also a need for more research and still more teaching in this unusually neglected subject. It is hoped that a hospice being planned by a recently founded charity will be able to stimulate further interest and skill in this important part of medical care[101].

The countervailing argument, however, was also in evidence. A letter published on the same page from euthanasia supporter Dr Maurice Millard, likewise welcomed the work of Exton Smith and Hinton, but in what looks like a particular swipe at Cicely, proposed that those 'not inhibited by dogmatic religious views' should use these papers as an opportunity to 'think again about our "Hippocratic" ethical opposition to permissive euthanasia — that is at the request of the sufferer — when all the resources of physical, mental and spiritual help have been exhausted'[102].

In fact, Hinton did not offer objections to euthanasia on religious grounds (though Cicely certainly did). In his important paperback published in 1967, Hinton included a lengthy and balanced discussion of the subject[103]. Acknowledging powerful arguments in favour of euthanasia, he also pointed to the need for a bulwark against the erosion of human values which prohibit the deliberate taking of life. At the individual level, judgements would become too complex, particularly in relation to the question of whose interests were being served by the euthanasia — patient, friends, relatives, professional carers? Acknowledging the difficulties, Hinton concluded his discussion on the subject by introducing the question of improving care for the dying:

> As long as we can truly say that for the patient merciful death has been too long in coming, there is some justification for euthanasia. It seems a terrible indictment that the main argument for euthanasia is that many suffer unduly because there is a lack of preparation and provision for the total care of the dying[104].

Other Enthusiasts

In late summer 1963, Cicely received a letter from Dr Eric Wilkes, a G.P. in Derbyshire, explaining that he was interested in establishing some form of hospice along the lines that interested her. This was a telling and early example of the enthusiasm that was later to develop in Britain, leading to what came to be known as the 'Hospice Movement'. Indeed, Wilkes would be closely associated with that wider development. She was full of enthusiasm in her response to him ('bursting with ideas about beginning such institutions!'[105]) and went on to read his two important papers in *The Lancet* in the following years[106]. Wilkes had qualified in medicine from St Thomas's in 1952, but eventually opted for the life of a country G.P. in Baslow, just outside Sheffield in the Derbyshire Peak District. His entry into the field was not insignificant. Fond of straight talking, and a masterful speaker and writer, he could see no reason why hospital provision for the terminally ill should be so inadequate or why the National Health Service was not taking a more active interest[107]. It was not without justification that he would later be referred to by some as 'the Cicely Saunders of the North'.

There were other points of contact within London itself. Cicely first wrote to British psychiatrist Colin Murray Parkes in March 1965[108], requesting a re-print of an article he had written on the pastoral care of the bereaved, for the journal *Contact*[109]. She explained that she was interested in knowing more about how relatives could be helped at an earlier stage of the care for their relative, and also more of what could be done after a death — something that was completely ignored at St Joseph's. He rang her up and they arranged to meet in London for lunch with his mentor John Bowlby. Quite soon Murray Parkes was drawn into the ambit of Cicely's plans and was giving advice on the role of liaison psychiatry in the new hospice. The growing body of published works began to raise interest in the problems of care for the dying, though it was still the case, as John Hinton noted, that 'the large number of articles in which remembered experience is distilled into advice on the management of dying awesomely overshadows the few papers attempting to measure the degree of success or failure of treatment'[110]. Over time, however, a research-based approach to improving care at the end of life began to be more visible and Cicely did a great deal to foster it[111].

By the mid 1960s, there was also sociological interest in these issues, found in ethnographic studies of the care of the dying in American hospitals[112] and later in surveys of bereaved relatives who were asked about the experiences of the deceased person in the last year of life[113]. Cicely wrote to their authors, praising and critiquing in turn. For example, to America sociologist Anselm Strauss, whom she had met a month earlier when he was in London, she wrote an extraordinarily long and detailed letter[114], explaining that she was in her sickbed ('I happen to have perfectly fearful cold') when his eagerly awaited book, written with Barney Glaser, had arrived. It was based on observations in six San Francisco hospitals and placed a heavy emphasis on the 'awareness contexts' that surrounded the dying patient, where knowledge of the situation might be concealed from the person or restricted only to certain people. It became a sociological classic in the field. From cover to cover, she read it in one day and quickly dictated her reactions. She disliked the use of 'terminal patients' in the text. She did not accept the notion of 'pretence' among patients who were close to death but who behaved otherwise.

> I do not think it is necessarily a contradiction to live life, as it were, on two levels at once. Both can be true, in a sense, without necessarily contradicting

each other as so often I think truth is something that does not entail reconciling two opposites, but in holding them in some kind of tension so, as it were, sparks fly between them.

Likewise she was disappointed to hear of the book's poor assessment of the quality of pain management in the hospitals studied, but she liked everything said about families, and the remarks about encouraging patients to manage their own dying. In a typical example of confident forward planning, she asked him to make a visit to St Christopher's when next in London 'to tell us what we are doing and what we ought to be doing better'[115].

M.D. Thesis and a Growing Knowledge Base

In these years we can see Cicely becoming instrumental in defining a new knowledge base about the care of those dying from malignant disease. In 1960, her chapter on the management of patients in the terminal stage, published in Ronald Raven's six-volume set *Cancer*[116], contained reference to forty published works; by 1967, her pamphlet titled *The Management of Terminal Illness*[117] included 184 references. By such means, a new field of healthcare practice—*terminal care*—began to be defined. It would be a multi-disciplinary endeavour combining many skills and aptitudes. Cicely's background in nursing and social work meant she was not loathe to draw on influences from other caring professions. Her early papers drew on other contributions, less well known, but important in shaping the new discourse of terminal care. There was Margaret Bailey's survey of patients with incurable lung cancer, conducted at the Brompton and Royal Marsden Hospitals[118] as well as a survey of public opinion on cancer[119] and a study of delayed help-seeking among cancer patients, that noted 'the fact of palliative treatment is not understood, and hospitals appear to be trying to cure all their patients and failing in a high proportion of cases'[120]. She gathered evidence from a study of one hundred patients in Boston[121] and from another helpful paper on social casework with cancer patients[122]. It was from the United States in particular that concerns emerged on more psychosocial issues, such as truth-telling[123], anxiety and depression[124], and anticipatory grief[125].

Against this widening background, it is perhaps not surprising that the rather narrowly conceived study which had been the basis for Cicely's move to St Joseph's was never concluded. The uncompleted draft of Cicely's M.D. thesis gives careful consideration to the study design, albeit buried away in an appendix[126]. She begins by pointing to the value of reporting on unsuccessful clinical trials, and the learning that might be derived from them. Her own study was set up to compare (1) Nepenthe with a placebo tablet, (2) Nepenthe with soluble aspirin, and (3) Nepenthe with soluble codeine. The second and third of these had been in regular use at St Luke's, where the Ward

Sisters were convinced they could detect a difference in their analgesic effects. The trial was designed to test this conviction, along with the strong belief in the regular giving of such analgesia. It was therefore originally trialled in St Luke's before being transferred to St Joseph's — probably because of Cicely's rather peremptory departure from the home in Bayswater. At St Joseph's, other problems emerged. The number of patients considered suitable for the trial was much smaller than expected. Many were too ill and there was the inexorably changing 'baseline' of their condition to consider. The patients were also on other drug regimes, for other symptoms, and these also were subject to change. The trial was too complex, with its emphasis on both the regime and the different medications. The small differences in effect were further complicated by the patients' generalized illness. Moreover, the staff quickly decided they could distinguish the placebo tablets by their greater effervescence, and this introduced a prejudicial bias. To make things worse, the nurses were often loathe to enter patients into the study at all — too concerned were they for the vulnerability of those for whom they were caring. Nor did they respond well to the extra work of planned observations and record-keeping. After a huge effort and considerable time, therefore, just fifty patients had been entered into the trial — and no difference was found amongst the three tablets. It was decided to call a halt, leaving Cicely to ruminate on whether a difference would have been observed with a larger number of patients. She had also learned why it was that Beecher and colleagues in the United States preferred single-dose studies; they were much more straightforward to carry out.

Nevertheless, the research potential at St Joseph's was obvious and she capitalised on this through the punctilious keeping of patient records. In the days before the computer, this involved the use of a Copeland-Chatterson ('Cope-Chat') punch-card sorting system which required holes to be punched in oblong cards against a pre-defined set of codes. The combined columns and rows allowed a large number of variables to be stored on a single card, one for each patient. Using a mechanical technique to select any chosen combination of variables, it was possible to count associations and grouping in the data — in the manner of simple cross-tabulations which could be expressed as tables. The method was in wide use for social surveys, and epidemiological and clinical studies at the time. Variables were separated out by inserting long needles into the requisite holes, allowing particular categories to be removed and identified — for example, all female patients, older than sixty years, who were receiving morphine. By such means, Cicely was able to build an unprecedented database of information about patients being cared for at St Joseph's. In total, during her time at the hospice, eighteen hundred patients were treated there. Of these, an astonishing eleven hundred were described in detail in various publications.

In a substantial early paper, published in July 1960[127], Cicely defines the terminal stage being reached 'when all curative and palliative measures have been exhausted'. Addressed to G.P.s, the article was based on Cicely's experience to date with 340 patients in a 'terminal-care hospital' (St Joseph's). Amongst these, one hundred had severe pain; 105, moderate pain; and 135, mild or no pain; less than ten continued to complain of pain once a course of analgesia was established or were only relieved by drugs which rendered them sleepy all the time. This might seem 'a counsel of perfection to a busy general practitioner or district nurse', but the article suggests that the methods could be adapted for use elsewhere. A section on the treatment of pain invokes her mantra about the constant control of pain, and that severe pain 'is a potent antagonist to the effect of any analgesic'. Recommended analgesics for mild and moderate pain are listed as aspirin and codeine, Nepenthe, pethidine, and the Brompton mixture (of morphine hydrochloride, cocaine, gin, aqua chloroform, and syrup of chlorpromazine). Severe pain calls for drugs by injection and the properties of Omnopon, morphine, and diamorphine are discussed. The question of addiction is raised, but dismissed as an insignificant clinical problem. A brief section looks forward to the benefits of longer acting drugs. There is a discussion of mental distress: 'Our experience is that as they draw near to death, fear fades away and acceptance brings peace'. There are suggestions for improving the sleep of patients at home, and a call is made for better casework and planning between G.P.s and almoners. The article concludes by emphasising how the doctor who visits the dying patient and family may 'potentiate the action of the drugs used and the treatment provided, and transform the illness into something for the relatives to remember with pride in spite of their loss'. It was a telling observation from Cicely that the research, the drugs, the techniques must never obscure the importance of the intangible inter-actions which can take place between the physician, the patient, and the family.

Into the Lion's Den

By March 1963, Cicely was reporting on problems and treatments in a series of patients that had grown to nine hundred in number, and whose care she had now documented[128]. Presented to an intimidating audience at the Royal Society of Medicine Section of Surgery in early December of the previous year, the focus of that day had been on the management of intractable pain. For the occasion, London was enveloped in a 'pea-souper' fog that had delayed several participants, and to add to her stress, Cicely had only just managed to get back to Heathrow following a short visit to Warsaw. Now, just four years after she had begun at St Joseph's, and with the experience of her own studies to report, she acknowledged that 'we have not found that controlled clinical trials are suitable either in this setting or with this particular group of patients'. The article concentrates, therefore, not on the drugs used with these patients, but rather the methods of their use. Cicely sets out her 'cardinal rules' in this respect: careful assessment of the symptoms that trouble the patient, assessment of the nature and severity of pain, and the regular giving of drugs. Diamorphine still finds particular favour: 'In the doses we use, it does not cause changes in personality, frank euphoria, or a "could not care less" attitude'. It may, however, be short-lived in effect and require more frequent administration. The article concludes with a discussion of mental distress ('perhaps the most intractable pain of all') and the appropriate drug treatments which may be used, as well as the importance of listening. The presentation was a triumph at the event itself, and a milestone in Cicely's growing confidence.

The still newly qualified Cicely was working at this time in a hospice setting which was probably unknown to most of the audience, she was tackling a clinical issue which most preferred to ignore, and she was doing so from an undisguised religious motivation. Christina Faull and Alexander Nicholson point out in a detailed reflection on the meeting and the article[129] that, as a physician, she would have been nervous of her surgical colleagues and also her fellow speakers. Cicely later recalled a degree of anxiety about the event, but felt that 'I had done a lot of solo singing in my time and that stood me in good stead'[130]. In any event, she seems to have eclipsed the talks by Joseph Burford Pennebacker, a neurosurgeon from the Radcliffe Infirmary in Oxford, and John W. Dundee, a professor of anaesthetics at Queens's University, Belfast, with whom Cicely had corresponded previously. Her message was confident and clear: Pain was very common in patients with advanced cancer, but it could be relieved in the large majority of cases given an assured approach to the regular giving of opiates and, to boot, the patients could be kept 'alert and cheerful', with no hint of tolerance or addiction. She must have gone back to Connaught Square after the meeting feeling a sense of relief, but also success. She had knocked over some profound and deeply entrenched assumptions held by her senior colleagues.

In the summer of 1967, Cicely was able to conclude her reporting on research undertaken at St Joseph's[131]. An article in the *Annals of the Royal College of Surgeons* signifies the growing esteem in which her work was held and reflects back on her experience of working in Hackney. She details the referral patterns, diseases, clinical problems, and methods of treatment in a series that had now amounted to the full eleven hundred patients. Although the article concentrates on the role of the doctor, the work of the whole team, including the patients, is also emphasised. As with most of Cicely's works of this time, she picks up on a particular illustrative example. Special attention is given to the moment of admission to the hospice, at a time when '[p]atients watch us as we watch them'. Half of the patients had openly discussed the fact that they were not getting better, but '[w]e must not forget the human capacity to hold two incompatible truths at the same time'. On looking back to her years at St Joseph's, Cicely concluded with the memorable observation: '[W] e remember not what death has done to them, but what they have done to our thoughts about it'.

From the start of 1960, Cicely had begun making recordings of conversations with patients on a newly acquired tape recorder. These were then carefully transcribed by her secretary. Over time, she gathered detailed narratives of patient stories, to which she could turn again and again for inspiration and for teaching purposes. These narratives were also a constant feature of her papers and articles, some of which were almost entirely given over to individual stories, like that of a patient called Mrs Hindmarch, which was published in 1961[132] and based on one of the early recorded interviews from the previous year. So in addition to the quantifiable material she held on the St Joseph's patients, she now had extensive accounts of personal experiences, stories, case illustrations — captured in the words of her beloved hospice patients. It was possibly the most powerful combination on which she could build and elucidate the architecture of 'total pain'.

Put in this context, it is impossible to say that Cicely 'failed' to complete her M.D. thesis. She simply gave priority to other things, using what she had learned from her studies and observations to construct a compelling argument for modern hospice care, before going on to create the setting in which it could be fully practised. But it was not all work, and out of the ashes of grief following the death of Antoni Michniewicz, a new flame was about to erupt. Her personal life was to remain on a roller coaster.

Marian Bohusz-Szyszko

One Saturday in December 1963, to fight off the continuing feelings of sorrow and loss which still besieged her more than three years after the death of Antoni, Cicely forced herself to go out to the public library to get some new classical music records and find something different to think about[133]. She had no idea what the day held in store. Driving past the Drian Galleries in Porchester Place, Bayswater, she glanced at the window and was suddenly struck dumb by what she saw. 'I thought, "Gosh! I must go in"'. Parking the car around the corner, she entered the gallery and spoke to its owner, Lithuanian born Halima Nalecz, who had fled war-torn Europe for the Middle East before settling in London in 1947. A trained artist herself, she had opened the Drian Galleries in 1957 and given the first big exhibitions in England to John Bellany, William Crozier, Michael Sandle, Yaacov Agam, Douglas Portway, and other emerging artists of the period[134].

The picture that enthralled Cicely was *Crucifixion*. It was a 'wonderful blue, very blue[135]', painted in oil in a modern, expressionist style. The artist was Marian Bohusz-Szyszko, an émigré Pole. The exhibition was closing that day. There were pictures still for sale. Untutored in art acquisition, Cicely bought her first painting — at half the listed price. It was called *Christ Calming the Waters*. She had somehow experienced an 'instant alignment'[136] with the work of Bohusz-Szyszko, that would eventually go far beyond the purchase of one of his paintings.

Marian Bohusz-Szyszko was born in 1901 in Trokienniki near Wilno, then in Russian Poland. His family was said to be wealthy and aristocratic. He served with the Polish Army during the First World War and as it resisted the Soviet invasion of Poland in 1919. Subsequently, he trained in fine art at Stefan Batory University (1921 – 1923) and the Academy of Fine Art in Krakow (1923 – 1927). He then became a teacher of art and mathematics. His first exhibition was held in Gdansk in 1934. At the start of the Second World War, Bohusz-Szyszko joined the Polish Army again and was captured at an early point in the hostilities. He was held prisoner for more than five years, during which time he made some four hundred paintings and pencil drawings, mostly on scraps of paper, that he managed to hold on to despite the constant moves from one camp to another. During his internment, he lectured on both his specialist subjects. When released from imprisonment, he travelled to Rome, where he became a teacher of Polish art students. In 1946, he settled in London and founded the Polish School of Art[137]. 'On the opening of his first London show in 1959 at Grabowski Gallery, the *Manchester Guardian's* art critic, Eric Newton, described Bohusz-Szyszko as "one of the great artists" of his generation'[138]. Redolent with Christian imagery, expressive and colourist, with bold use of the palette knife and, at times, richly textured surfaces, his 1963 exhibition at the Drian was a retrospective, signifying the body of work he had accumulated at that time, when he was in his early sixties.

Driving back to Connaught Square, Cicely was in a daze. What she had briefly learned about the artist had stunned her as much as his paintings. He was around the same age as Antoni and from the same region of Poland. She had time to ruminate over the weekend before she went back to collect the painting on the Monday. The gallery gave her Bohusz-Szyszko's address. She would write and thank him for painting such a picture. It would go, from the very beginning, into the chapel of the new hospice she was planning.

Meeting the Artist

Cicely's next step was characteristic. She wrote him a letter on the following Sunday, explaining how she had found his work and the immediate impact it had on her. By this time, she had become quite knowledgeable about Poland and things Polish. She was keeping up to date with current Polish affairs, literature, and films, and had become interested in the story of Our Lady of Cztestochwa, the revered icon of the Black Madonna housed at the Jasna Góra Monastery. She gave him details of her hospice plans and explained:

> The message of your picture is so fundamental to what we are going to try and do that I am certain that it was no mere chance that made me attracted by your pictures and drew me to the gallery, the last evening before it closed[139].

His reply came three days later, flowery and hyperbolic. He considered her letter to be the most important thing he had experienced in his forty-year career as an artist. He invited her to his studio to select a large painting suitable for the chapel, explaining that: 'The right of giving it as a present I shall consider as my greatest privilege'[140]. As she later observed: '[I]f you are going to fall in love with an artist eventually, it's a good thing to fall in love with his pictures first. That's how we met'[141].

When they did meet in person, it was just before Christmas. He proved to be a 'splendid, wild, mad artist, eighteen years older than I was'[142]. He was also married, though he had not seen his wife since 1939, and had a son in Poland and, as Cicely would learn in due course, a daughter in Italy. Cicely was immediately drawn to him, but not comfortable with his situation. Nor did his treatment of her inspire confidence. 'He was much more absent than present for the first eighteen months or so . . . being available, not available, and not too available'[143]. Far from his origins, experienced, and moving in an artistic if not exactly bohemian world, he was, as du Boulay puts it, 'enjoying his freedom and in no hurry to see it end'[144]. So strong in her resolve professionally, now Cicely became submissive, putting up with his poor treatment of her as he would disappear off the radar for long periods, only to turn up again, always charming, romantic, and fulsome in his words, before vanishing once more to a world unbeknownst to her. He could embarrass her thoughtlessly in front of others, such as in an example described by du Boulay when, in 1966, Cicely stopped off in Paris when returning from the United States, especially to meet him and attend the opening of an exhibition of his paintings[145]. When she reached the airport in Paris, there was no word, no details from him. By chance, she was able to find out the venue. Still, he failed to appear. She even assisted with the setting up of the show. The next day, he breezed into the gallery with his admirers and then unapologetically took Cicely out to dinner when the opening was over.

His was a chivalry that lacked consideration. He was patrician but impoverished. Religiously opposed to divorce, he seemed to be untroubled by adultery. Such attributes combined unpleasantly. They unsettled Cicely, but she remained available to him, not confronting his unkindness, desperately hoping to reel him in at some point. When she eventually purchased *Crucifixion*, and another painting with money from her father's legacy, Marian's response seems to have been predictable and clichéd: '*Now* I can tell you that I love you. If I were younger and if I were free, I would offer you my hand'[146]. As she noted later, of course he was not free to marry, 'so he was quite safe to say that'[147]. She had truly fallen for him and seemed prepared to wait for events to unfold.

Writing, Writing, Writing

In later years, Cicely's curriculum vitae (C.V.) recorded the publications from her time spent at St Joseph's and in preparation for St Christopher's. The listing belies the reality. On the C.V., there are half a dozen citations from 1958 to 1967. In fact, almost sixty works were published during this period, covering medical and nursing journals; Christian periodicals and magazines; items published in America, Norway, and India; and contributions to textbooks and edited collections. The publications include detailed descriptions of clinical practice, case studies, research reports, opinion pieces, book reviews, and lengthy summaries of the clinical literature. It is an astonishing output for one who, at the beginning of the period, was still a newly qualified doctor, who in the same years experienced major personal and family stresses, and who simultaneously was working towards the challenging goal of establishing a new kind of terminal-care home. Her careless recording of her publications and lack of interest in cataloguing them speaks of someone focussed on acting in the world, getting on, and making a contribution. Hers was not the orientation of the academic, quietly cultivating a resumé and building a reputation for scholarship through published works. Rather, she was busily doing things, accepting invitations, turning talks and lectures into published articles which could be more widely read, and, in the process, starting to build what would later be known as an 'evidence base' for the clinical approach she was advocating.

The Craft of Writing

Cicely had learned to write at Roedean, then honed her skills as an Oxford undergraduate, and, as a medical student, quickly came to grips with the genre of clinical reporting. It would be incorrect to say she was a natural and easy writer. As she once remarked: 'I'm a natural speaker; I'm not so easily a natural writer'[148]. But from the outset, she wrote with confidence, with knowledge of grammar and syntax, and a measure of authority which, in the early years, masked her relative inexperience. Cicely's writings present dilemmas, challenges, and paradoxes. Her readers are drawn into them and are invited to explore them. But, they are always guided out of the ambiguities and uncertainties to a place of assurance, where things are, in a phrase she was very fond of, 'gathered up' and resolved.

She worked hard for her results, dictating, drafting by hand with many revisions, and sometimes feeling under pressure from editors' deadlines. The early writings were hard won. Her first major commitment was the series of articles she wrote for *Nursing Times* in 1959. They had been commissioned by the editor, Peggy Nuttall, whom Cicely had known from her nursing days. Initially committed to four pieces for *Nursing Times*, she eventually expanded the number to six. On 26 May 1959, she wrote to her editor with four pieces, already heavily revised but still in need of further correction. Another was being actively 'beaten into shape'. At the same time, she had an eye on the future. Enquiring about copyright, she closed the letter by remarking that one day she might try to write a book on the subject[149]. The series proved to be a remarkable statement about Cicely's interest and a key landmark not only in her thinking, but also in the development of others who became drawn to her ideas. Published in *Nursing Times* in consecutive weeks, it quickly built up an excited and committed following. She began in controversy and chose to commence with the subject of euthanasia[150].

The *Nursing Times* Series of 1959

The first article took its cue from a recent public discussion of 'mercy killing' and asked two key questions: 'Is euthanasia morally right?' and 'Is there really no other way of relieving the distress of patients in the terminal stages of cancer?' The argument drew on an explicitly Christian theodicy which claims that 'disease and all our other ills were caused in the first instance by the sin of man'[151]. But in this context, the relief of suffering can also be seen as a Christian duty. The first question is refuted on both theological and empirical grounds, and case illustrations are used to show how dying patients may continue to grow 'in patience and courage right up to their last moments'. For those unmoved by 'transcendental values', there is a second argument that euthanasia can and should be unnecessary. Cicely's experience in two 'terminal homes' is drawn on to suggest that 'we can relieve the suffering of 90 per cent of the patients and bring it within their diminishing compass where we cannot relieve it entirely'. It was an astonishingly bold claim.

From there, in the second article, she moved on to tackle the dogmatism and general rules concerning the question of whether patients should know they are dying[152]. A detailed account of a forty-four-year-old female patient with carcinoma of the stomach is used to illustrate 'how the lies which are intended to shield from fear may in fact add to distress, and that a patient must be allowed to take the initiative because she may well know her real need much better than we do'. Patients should not be deceived deliberately, but not all need to know they are dying. Above all this is 'pre-eminently the time for doctor, nurse and chaplain to co-operate'.

The third article describes the case of a woman of fifty-four years with advanced carcinoma of the cervix[153]. Pain control began with 'Mist. aspirin, gr. 10, with Nepenthe, 30 minims four times a day'. Later, an injection of 'Omnopon, gr. 1/3' was given at night and, on waking, with the aspirin and

Nepenthe continuing during the day. When the Omnopon was increased to gr. 2/3, the patient complained of feeling 'dopey'; the Omnopon and the mixture were both stopped in favour of injections of 'morphine, gr. 1/2, with amiphenazole, 30 mg, four times a day at routine times'. The amiphenazole was discontinued during the last few days before death. Regular giving of drugs is described here as 'the cardinal rule in the treatment of pain in this type of patient'. Despite the detailed description of the drug regimen for this patient, the article makes the point, consistent with Cicely's developing and wider orientation, that '[a]nalgesics are not the only means we have of relieving pain'; physical nursing care, antibiotics, and the understanding of mental and spiritual worries may all have a part to play.

It was this latter theme that was picked up more strongly in the next offering, that focussed on the case of 'Miss R.', a patient of fifty-four years, who proved 'difficult to help'[154]. Miss R.'s mental suffering was all too apparent, but there were language and communication difficulties (she was Prussian), and her irregular behaviour was a 'continual worry' to the staff. A German–speaking visitor, a trained mental nurse, was found who was able to listen to Miss R.'s story of loneliness, exile, her love of art and music — and her lack of personal relationships. At Miss R.'s request, letters were written to her relations in Europe. Eventually, 'Miss R. seemed comforted and peaceful at last'. The article again highlights the problems of 'mental pain' and argues for the value of the 'real listener' as well as opiates, barbiturates, and alcohol in these cases. 'Suffering', it is suggested, 'is only intolerable when nobody cares'. The article demonstrated the detailed lengths to which caring could go in the hospice setting.

For the fifth article[155], Cicely chose to eschew the individual case-study format of its predecessors, in favour of a discussion of each of the nursing problems encountered in the care of the dying patient, together with suggestions for how they might be overcome. The material is 'culled from several sisters who have cared for these patients for years and from my own observations in terminal homes'. Cicely dealt with a dizzying array of problems, including intractable vomiting; dysphagia, fungating growths; the mouth; pathological fractures; fits; urinary complications, bowels; sleep; bedsores, hiccoughs; persistent coughs; asphyxia; and dyspnoea. Again, it was a proving ground for Cicely's knowledge of the many physical problems, other than pain, which could be encountered amongst dying patients.

'It is not so much death itself as the actual process of dying that most men fear . . . .' Thus opens the final article in the *Nursing Times* series[156]. Here is presented the case of 'Mr B.', a patient who had received cancer treatment for twenty years before admission to a terminal-care home. He had an advanced rodent ulcer of the face, was blind, and was very deaf. His pain was treated with Omnopon and morphine. One episode of climbing out of bed was controlled with an injection of hyoscine. He died peacefully a few days later. 'Observant care' can contribute to such an outcome, for example through frequent and gentle moving, sponging and rubbing, cleansing the mouth, and talking (for hearing is often the last sense to go). The role of relatives in this process is discussed, together with advice on how they should be cared for immediately after the death.

These articles sent reverberations through the nursing world, and beyond. The following year they were brought together in a pamphlet of thirty-three pages[157]. This found favourable reviews in the Left–leaning broadsheet newspaper, *The Manchester Guardian*, as well as in *The Lancet*. The latter could find occasion to comment on the place of religious thinking within her argument:

> She early makes it clear that she writes also as an Anglican Christian, believing that 'by Man came death', but any medical reader who quits at this point because he cannot accept this doctrine will lose a very great deal of practical instruction in devices for the relief of pain and distress and the skilful use of drugs[158].

Other Successes

This was praise indeed from one of the world's leading medical journals. It was underscored by the invitation she had received from Ronald Raven to contribute the last chapter to his major six-volume series of books on cancer[159]. Opening with a plea for 'the art rather than the science of medicine', the chapter can be seen as a consolidation, more fully referenced, of the ideas expressed in her preceding publications. It begins with a discussion of home care, taking in the work of the social worker, home nurse, doctor, and the relations. ('If the family is united, the relatives are often the best nurses, but they will need understanding and support in these demanding situations'.) A section on symptomatic treatment includes an extended discussion on analgesia for mild, moderate, and severe pain. As in earlier articles, problems of addiction are dismissed and the emphasis is upon the regular giving of pain relief and the avoidance of over-sedation. Further attention is given to vomiting, dysphagia, asphyxia, fungating tumours, oral involvement, pathological fractures, malignant effusions, pleural effusions, persistent cough, fits, urinary complications, the bowels, sleep, bed sores, anorexia, and hiccough. It is an extended and detailed treatment of the physical problems that can occur in the face of terminal illness, born of sustained clinical observation. Of course, a section on mental distress highlights the limitations of drugs and the value of the 'real listener'. The section on 'How much should the patient know?' again advocates an individualised approach and the avoidance of deceit. The absence of pain is highlighted as an important feature of the dying process, and there is guidance on physical nursing procedures. Euthanasia is opposed, but she puts her finger right on the clumsiness of then-current clinical practice, noting that: 'With the means we have at present, although the motive is different, it is not always easy in practice to distinguish between proper relief and the hastening of death'.

In February 1964, Cicely received an invitation from the Episcopal Church Center in New York to write for *The Living Church*, an American journal, on the topic of 'Facing Death'[160]. The theme of the article was the denial of death and, in it, she suggested that acceptance of one's mortality was a route to finding meaning in life itself. She described the case of a young woman, about to die, who wanted to assist her children and husband through the process, and the reaction of the staff. The article rejected the apparently 'swift and easy' solution of euthanasia in these cases and suggested that religious peace may come to dying people in such circumstances, even those who seem most indifferent and recalcitrant before the end.

Inspired by this article, Dorothy Nayer, associate editor of the *American Journal of Nursing*, wrote to Cicely requesting an article which would help her readers come to grips with their attitudes about death and which would assist them in their service to dying patients and their families. Characteristically, a detailed correspondence ensued. Cicely checked on various themes that might be explored in the article, discussed the use of illustrations, and also asked for advance copies of two papers by American sociologist Anselm Strauss which were to appear in the journal at a later date. After the back-and-forth of discussions, the editor was delighted with the result. Illustrated with impressive line drawings, the article took as its theme the idea that the last stages of life should not be seen as defeat, but rather as life's fulfilment. Using case illustrations from St Joseph's Hospice (although the name appeared incorrectly in the text), there was a focus on the nursing aspects of care, especially the responsibility of telling or not telling the prognosis. Readers were as enthusiastic as the editor, and nurses from around the country wrote in with their endorsement. Typically, each received an individual and detailed reply from Cicely. Some of those who read the original article in 1965 were still writing with requests to visit St Christopher's Hospice many years later.

The third American publication for which Cicely wrote in the decade before her own hospice opened was the journal *Geriatrics*, in 1966, and this took the form of an extended letter, produced by invitation[161]. In it she gave details of the developing plans for St Christopher's and the goal of making an impact on the lack of interest in research, teaching, and care relating to the dying. It emphasised the concept of a 'hospice' as a resting place for travellers and pilgrims, something between a home and a hospital, and also noted that the project already had established international links, particularly with the United States.

American Connections

By now Cicely's reputation in the United States was growing rapidly. Media attention followed, along with requests for her help and guidance, as well as for her to speak at meetings and write for other publications. In 1965 and 1966, she got involved in correspondence with Professor Willis W. Harman of Stanford University, concerning his research into the use of lysergic acid diethylamide (aka L.S.D.) for pain relief in cancer patients (she decided not to take the idea forward). In May 1966, Cicely took part in a series of lectures at Western Reserve University in Cleveland, Ohio (later published[162]), titling her talk 'The Moment of Truth: Care of the Dying Person'. She had found a niche with so-cial scientists, therapists, and thanatologists in the United States who were struck by her direct clinical and practical knowledge, whilst at the same time they were to broaden her own perspectives far beyond the clinical world. By the autumn of 1966, there was a sense of an emerging critical mass of interest not only in her work, but also in the wider field to which she was contributing. These early publications and the many talks and lectures to which they were linked in the United States spanned several key disciplines and audiences: the church, nursing, medicine, and psychiatry. America was learning about the work of Cicely Saunders and she was learning from America as she 'picked up thoughts and ideas from all around, like a kind of a sponge'[163].

Adding in the new cadre of pain specialists, from whom she received en-couragement and inspiration, it was indeed a rich mixture of influences and skills that she was encountering, and one that was later to become such an im-portant aspect of the modern multi-disciplinary specialty of hospice and palli-ative care. There was a sense of forces coming together, of new possibilities. A special relationship was forged between Cicely Saunders and her American friends and colleagues during the middle years of the 1960s, and this con-tinued for the rest of her life. The relationship was part of an extraordinary groundswell of interest in the care of the dying and the bereaved out of which new social movements and professional specialisms were quick to emerge, not only in Britain and the United States, but worldwide.

Religious Considerations and the Ambition for St Christopher's

It was while writing the six articles for *Nursing Times* that Cicely had one of her moments of spiritual revelation and epiphany. She often described these as 'God tapping me on the shoulder'. In this instance, on 24 June 1959, she sensed he was saying: 'Now you've got to get on with it.' It stemmed from *Daily Light*. The reading that day was from Psalm 37: 'Commit thy way unto the Lord; trust also in him; and he shall bring it to pass'. Why this passage appears to have moved her more deeply than innumerable others she would have read in the previous fourteen years of Christian belief is not clear. The wider context may help to explain.

At this point she was almost one year into her time at St Joseph's. She had just celebrated her forty-first birthday. She was neither wife nor mother. Her busy social calendar of concerts, singing, Highland holidays, and church-related activities could not disguise a drifting lack of direction to her life. David Tasma had inspired her to work with the dying. Now she was caring for dying people every day and could see the enormous challenges and opportunities that it presented. She had sensed that more could be done. There was more to this work than could be encompassed by homes like St Luke's and St Joseph's. Although she had never held any kind of managerial role, she ruminated that some strategy was needed. Conversations with her brother Christopher, who was immersing himself in the business world and the management ethos he had learned at Harvard, were telling her she must make plans and gather the wherewithal to support them. It is also clear from her correspondence that she was turning her thoughts more and more to organisational matters. Just twelve days before God's 'tap', she was writing to Dr J.R. Heller of the National Cancer Institutes in Maryland, United States, and noting: 'I am becoming more and more convinced that institutions of this kind are the best places for a very large number of these patients'[164]. By now she had also put in a huge effort to write the requested chapter on terminal care for Ronald Raven. It was in this that she observed: 'Nearly half of the patients in the terminal stage need institutional care' and had gone on to discuss the role of hospitals, geriatric units, nursing homes, and 'terminal hospitals or homes'. These latter, she considered to offer two things: 'skilled and specialized nursing and an atmosphere of individual love and care, stemming in most cases from the strong sense of vocation of the staff'[165].

Seeking Spiritual Guidance: Sister Penelope at Wantage

But if the context was heavily circumscribed by institutional issues, Cicely nevertheless sought a spiritual path through them. She was aware of Sister Penelope Lawson at the Mother House of the Church of England order of St Mary the Virgin, at Wantage, Berkshire, in southern England. Beginning in the late 1930s, C.S. Lewis had been a friend and active correspondent with Sister Penelope, who helped him to slough off some of his earlier misgivings about High-Church religious practices — in particular, the confession of sins. As their friendship grew, they shared notes on wartime broadcasts for the B.B.C., that she too was asked to undertake, and Lewis would read her books in manuscript and offer in-depth comments[166]. So there was an interesting link here with events and circumstances that had shaped Cicely's own religious thinking as a student nurse during the 1940s. Moreover, by 1957, when Lewis wrote his last known letter to Sister Penelope, he had married a woman dying of cancer. He told her, 'As you can imagine, new beauty and tragedy have entered my life. You would be surprised . . . how much of a strange sort of happiness and even gaiety there is between us'[167]. As we have already seen, it was not long until, in 1961, Lewis published, at first pseudonymously, his memoir of loss, *A Grief Observed*[168], a work which Cicely would also read in the depths of her own sorrows.

Sister Ruth Penelope Lawson was now retired, having spent much of her time as the librarian to St Mary's[169]. She was a translator of early and medieval Christian writings and an author of works like *God Persists: A Short Survey of World History in the Light of Christian Faith*[170] and *Light in the Night: A Book for Those in Bed*[171]. Cicely had read some of these and was confident enough to approach her. So, in July 1959, Cicely found herself motoring west from London to Reading, then to Newbury before turning north over the Downs to Wantage. Established in 1848 by the local vicar, William John Butler, it is one of the earliest Church of England religious communities. Cicely found Sister Penelope receptive to her story and to her nascent idea for a new kind of hospice. Sister Penelope could also see that Cicely was taken with the idea that this should be some form of 'community', but was unsure whether it should be religious or secular in character. She immediately suggested a source of help and expertise, and advised Cicely to approach theologian Olive Wyon, who had a special interest in these matters. Cicely also talked to the Reverend Mother and asked if perhaps the hospice idea should be nested within an established religious order. The reply was negative: 'What you're doing is a new thing. You're not going to, by any means, want to use an old Order like ours. You're going to set out on your own'[172]. The advice had been given. Cicely then recused herself and spent the remainder of her time at Wantage in private contemplation and prayer. Sitting in the chapel in front of a carved wooden crucifix, she reflected on verses from St John's gospel and asked: 'Lord, what do I have to do?' By evening, 'it seemed to be sorted out'[173]. She now felt confident to tackle the balance between the religious and the medical in her vision for the hospice.

'The Scheme'

The day after returning from Wantage, Cicely committed a ten-page document to paper. Pouring out her ideas in writing which demonstrated more confidence than she felt, she was suddenly equipped with 'The Scheme'[174]. It was her plan so far, her distillation of hopes and ambitions. It was a manifesto, something she would share with others and use as a basis to convince, to cajole, and to advocate. du Boulay saw an eleven-year gestation to the document, to the extent that 'the child, like the goddess Athene, was born fully fledged'[175]. Just as her first medical paper had laid out the whole challenge of caring for people at the end of life, so this more strategic document set out in broad but precise terms what the hospice would be for and how it would function. The template was clearly St Joseph's. There would be sixty beds for terminally ill people, as well as long-term accommodation for the elderly and chronic sick, that would include former staff and relatives. There were detailed descriptions of ward layout, decoration, and organisation, along with estimates of capital and revenue costs, and of anticipated contractual arrangements with the National Health Service. Notwithstanding such links to the public health system, the hospice would safeguard its independence and thereby maintain freedom of thought and action. It would reflect the values and beliefs of a religious community.

First to receive a copy of 'The Scheme' was Brigadier Glyn Hughes, who — as we shall see — was busily preparing his own report on the state of terminal care in Britain at this time. Cicely sent her draft to him with a long letter on 22 July 1959, explaining that 'this problem has been on my mind for a long time and somehow it seems to me that the time has come to try and do some practical planning and to find the people who would want to help'[176]. In the months that followed, Cicely built on the first version of 'The Scheme', clarifying her ideas, striving to create a programme for action, and worrying away at practical first steps. For a while — and it was something she felt compelled to work through — the over-arching and dominant question concerned the religious and spiritual foundation of her ambition. This was the key problem she had taken to Wantage. So as she pulled around her, at first, an informal group of friends and associates who might help in her quest to found a new home for dying people, she tackled them in turn on the question of its religious priorities and orientation.

Religious Emphasis and the Question of 'Community'

Throughout the early part of 1960, there were numerous meetings and extended correspondence with a clutch of evangelically inclined Anglican friends: John Stott (her vicar at All Souls, Langham Place), Rosetta Burch (her friend and confidante since the almoner days), Madge Drake (a friend since the visits to Devon in the late 1940s), and, in particular, solicitor Jack Wallace. The process was characteristically 'Cicely' in the way it wove together her emotions and personal pre-occupations, together with matters of her professional judgement, along with highly specific questions of religious belief and how that might shape the ethos and practice of the new home. By the end of 1960, a certain clarity had emerged which was sufficient to take St Christopher's forward. Though the protagonists were likely unaware of it at the time, their deliberations were also to have a profound influence upon the later development of what became known as the 'Hospice Movement'.

A good deal of initial thinking centred around the involvement in the hospice of those of different 'churchmanship', and Stott in particular advised her against bringing in those inclined towards the 'higher' (more Anglo-Catholic) wing of the Anglican church. It was Wallace with whom she shared her practical and theological struggles over the following months. Wallace, and his wife Lucie, had met Cicely at a Christian weekend house meeting during the early 1950s. When she began to articulate her ideas to them after her arrival at St Joseph's, they were taken aback by the scale of her ambition. But Wallace was impressed by Cicely and was fond of her[177]. He saw that her vision was important and he made it his business to support her both professionally and spiritually. He was an important sounding board for her as she thrashed out her ideas and strategy. In a letter written to Wallace on 20 January 1960, her lack of agreement with Stott is apparent. There is a strong sense of courage here. As we have seen, Stott had become a figure of great influence in the evangelical world to which Cicely belonged, yet here she was openly arguing against him:

> I am not sure what John Stott is going to think about final control being in the hands of a rather diverse body of people. I feel more and more definitely that this is what I want and if he doesn't feel that Evangelicals are having enough control I'm afraid I can't agree with him. What about you? Do you feel I'm getting too broad?[178]

Perhaps unsurprisingly, Wallace replied by return in cautionary tones, agreeing with Stott and taking the view that 'ultimate control' must be in the hands of the 'convinced minority'[179]. In Wallace's view, there were two main tasks: 'To build up firstly a Medical Unit, and secondly a Christian Community'[180]. He felt these tasks should be organised by the same people, and was concerned the two might become separated. On the second, he noted, however:

> What in effect you are doing (though perhaps not in name) is to establish a dedicated Spiritual Order, and this must inevitably mean Spiritual Discipline and Rule, with a recognisable basis. I am sure you will find Anglo-Catholics more amenable to these ideas than Evangelicals . . . [181].

It was the question of community which was to prove so taxing. So energized was Cicely by it that she wrote back to Wallace's hand-delivered letter on the day of its receipt, 10 February 1960. The frustration was clearly showing:

> You need not tell me what a difficult part this is! I quite agree that what I am in effect being led to do is to establish a dedicated Spiritual Order, and what I have been trying to find out is whether this does inevitably mean spiritual discipline and rule with a recognisable basis. I don't know if I can make more comments on that. I am just trying to find out. And I will bring with me a letter from a nun at Wantage — an ex-evangelical. This is not exclusively the province of the Anglo-Catholic, she refers to Calvinist nuns. There are

also the Lutheran deaconesses; there are also the Iona Community and St Julian's . . . one of the works of the Spirit in the Church of England today is this idea of forming communities. I do not believe that I am in the van of a new spiritual movement. I know that this is away outside my own spiritual capacity. All I know is the way the spirit has been leading me so far. If it is His way, it will be all right if we follow Him slowly. I do not feel that we need hurry over this; it need not hold us up now. We may not know till we begin[182].

There is a suggestion in this letter, with its quasi-prophetic language, that the 'medical unit' could be more easily conceived than the notion of a religious community and, over time, Cicely's sense of caution about the latter was to grow. A meeting, at Wallace's suggestion, with church consultant Bruce Reed saw the same themes raised again. The Rev Reed had come up through the Billy Graham crusades, and had major responsibility for following up the converts and collating their commitment cards. Seeing the prosperous and influential backgrounds of some of those coming forward, he developed a strong interest in assisting them to bring their Christian beliefs to their secular involvements. Now he was devoting much of his Church of England ministry to fostering a bridge between Christian theology and the insights of the behavioural sciences[183]. He quickly spotted some of the tensions in Cicely's ideas, but she could not agree with his analysis:

During the course of our discussion you asked me more than once what I thought I was really aiming at. You were not certain whether my vision was a spiritual or medical one. Whether my interest in the medical side — the control of pain and so on, and my desire to spread the knowledge of how to do that — was really more important to me than my desire that every patient in our Home and in many similar Homes elsewhere in England should come to know the Lord . . . [but] in this work the medical and spiritual are inextricably mingled. I long to bring patients to know the Lord and to do something towards helping many of them to hear of Him before they die, but I also long to raise standards of terminal care throughout the country from a medical point of view at least, even where I can do nothing about the spiritual part of the work[184].

Olive Wyon

This dual longing was a heady mixture. It risked tangling up an enthusiasm for death-bed conversion with a broader move to reform medical care at the end of life. Cicely would have to tread carefully in seeking to prosecute both interests. Sensing the difficulties, she finally took the advice first given by Sister Penelope the previous July and reinforced in subsequent correspondence, and on 4 March 1960 wrote to Dr Olive Wyon, then a retired theologian living in Cambridge. Among Wyon's interests were the new religious movements and communities that had developed in the post-war era across Western Europe and about which she was writing a book[185]. It was her knowledge of these which was to prove so helpful. Cicely's letter sets out the background in detail:

> The problem . . . is the question of the 'Community' which some people seem to see envisaged in my plan. I am tremendously impressed by the love and care with which the Irish Sisters give to our patients — something more than an ordinary group of professional women could ever give, I think. But I was not really thinking of anything nearly so definite as a real new Community. I think I was using the term in a much less technical way. I asked Sister Penelope if I was attempting the impossible to hope that a secular group of people without any kind of rule would be able to hold together and give the feeling of security, which I want so much to help our patients . . . . So I am really faced with two problems. On the spiritual side, I know that the spiritual work is of paramount importance and, while it goes hand in hand all the time with our medical work, it is the only lasting help that we can give to our people . . . I feel that the work should be a definitely Church of England one rather than interdenominational and that it must be widely based in the Church, and not just in one wing. Then the other problem is this question of a Community of those who work there. I think myself that this matter should be held in abeyance; I may have adumbrated it in my scheme, but I had not been thinking of going any further than pray for the right people to come, and wait for the leading of the Spirit should He want us to draw together more definitely[186].

In just over a week, Cicely had visited Olive Wyon and came away feeling helped: 'I feel that I have been floundering around in rather a fog for quite a long time, and you showed me one of the first really strong beams of light . . .'[187]. Wyon could see that this extraordinarily earnest and driven woman that had turned up at her door was in a difficult and transitional stage of her spiritual journey. For Wyon, Cicely was 'bursting out of her chrysalis', not wanting to lose what she had been given but searching simultaneously for much more[188]. It was an extraordinary insight about Cicely made several months before the death of Antoni and its aftermath.

For now, Cicely could see that two issues required resolution. The first was dealt with straightforwardly. The second remained unclear, and continued to be so, even as the hospice moved towards its opening day.

First was the question of the precise religious character of the hospice. The debate was initially about in which wing of the Church of England it should be located, but quickly ecumenical ideas and the influence of discussions about Christian unity became apparent. This was the extent of inter-faith considerations; Britain in these years was still some way from addressing multi-faith issues, and the question of non-Christian religions was not given any acknowledgement. That would come much later. To a considerable extent, the issue was resolved pragmatically. A major source of charitable funds, the City Parochial Foundation, was showing an interest in the project, but the Foundation was unable, under its terms of trust, to give to a purely Anglican venture. As Cicely therefore noted in a letter to her brother on 30 August 1960: 'I very much prefer something that is "inter" rather than "un-"'. In this clunky language, she was referring to the question of the denominational character of the hospice[189]. Betty West had reassuringly captured this months earlier in a letter encouraging Cicely not to be too dismayed by the apparent diversity of Christian influences which were helping to form St Christopher's: '[C]ould it be, do you think, that in heaven our ways don't seem quite so different as they appear to us — and who knows that the edges might well melt away or not matter so much?'[190]

On the second question, however, that of the hospice as some form of community, no such categorical statement appeared. Indeed, there was a sense that this issue remained something to be explored and encountered, even as the work of the hospice got underway. Cicely would return to it from time to time, not least when she engaged with ideas of 'therapeutic community', and explored them with others. Whereas on the question of denominational identity, Cicely had felt that her supporters and collaborators were taking a broader view than her own, on this second issue it was as if some held her back from the possibility of a more strongly communal orientation. Her dear friend Rosetta Burch expressed this clearly:

> To the outside world you must be first and foremost a medical concern . . . . You are a Christian doctor, not a spiritual leader with a medical vision. You have lots of experience of working with others on a professional basis, but God has never given you the experience of being a member of a Community. Don't you think He would if that were to loom large in His plan?[191]

So it was that Cicely was able to write to Olive Wyon at the end of 1960:

> We have decided that it shall be an inter-denominational foundation, although we will have something in the documents stating as firmly as possible that it must be carried out as a Christian work as well as a medical one . . . . I found that I just couldn't think it was right to be exclusive. First of all, I could not be exclusively evangelical and thought that perhaps it would therefore have to be Anglican to keep it safe from heresy or secularisation. But then it didn't seem right to be that either, and in our legal Memorandum stands the statement: 'there shall be a chapel available for Christian worship', and I do not think that really we could be much broader than that! . . . It does not seem to have been right to think much more along the lines of a Community for this Home at the moment. I think that if we are to be drawn together in this work, that it will happen when we get there[192].

A New Authenticity

It is clear that this had been an intensely formative year for Cicely. It was one of deep reflection and consultation with others on the precise nature of her vision for the new hospice, St Christopher's. Cutting through it like a knife in the summer months of 1960 was Cicely's sudden and deep affection for Antoni Michniewicz, triggered within the jaws of death. The issues which she had explored at such length with her friends and associates during that year would continue to tax her imagination and energy, but a clear turn had occurred which enabled her purposes to be explained succinctly to the wider public and to those whose financial support she would need. It was on the latter that her energies began to focus, as in the following months she actively engaged in the communication of her ideas to those who had the material wherewithal to turn them into reality. Despite, her sorrow, she felt able to do this with a new authenticity based on her time with Antoni. It was a complex mixture of terrible longing and loss, matched to a strengthening resolve about how she should proceed with her plans. Antoni was not the catalyst to her actions, but he was the musical *continuo* to everything she did at this time — one which would fill out the harmonic structure of her work and go on resonating throughout her life. In that sense, and not until much later when she was able to accept love between persons as no barrier to the love of God, he also became woven into the narrative of her entire spiritual biography.

In 1962, the supporters of St Christopher's began meeting under the guidance of the Bishop of Stepney for discussions in which they sought to clarify and set down in a statement the basic principles of their work. It was at one of these meetings in June 1964 that Olive Wyon, in Cicely's words, 'made an excellent digest of my woolly thoughts'[193]. The result was a document which was to have currency at the hospice for many years into the future, titled *Aim and Basis*[194]. Within it, St Christopher's Hospice is defined as a religious foundation based on the full Christian faith in God. Five underlying convictions are listed: (1) all persons who serve in the hospice will give their own contribution in their own way; (2) dying people must find peace and be found by God, without being subjected to special pressures; (3) 'love is the way through', given in care, thoughtfulness, prayer, and silence; (4) such service must be group work, led by the Holy Spirit, perhaps in unexpected ways; and (5) the Foundation must give patients a sense of security and support, that will come through a faith radiating out from the chapel into every aspect of the corporate life. The *Aim and Basis* therefore provided St Christopher's with a statement of under-pinning motivation, and was reviewed from time to time in subsequent years, even in the years preceding Cicely's death. The discussions which preceded it, however, were to shape the work of the hospice for many years to come. They reveal a profound sense of purpose coupled with a rigorous approach to debate and discussion, that were essential in establishing the dominant themes in the life and work of the world's first modern hospice, defined as a place which would undertake the tripartite duties of care, education, and research.

The real importance of the early thinking which led to St Christopher's, however, was as much in what was decided against. The ideas which were not pursued or which were allowed to recede are themselves significant. In particular, it was decided that this would not be an endeavour located in a narrow evangelical wing of the Church of England, and in which the primary purpose would be to proselytise. Nor was it to be a new religious community in which a dedicated few, operating outside of the secular world, would care for the dying in their own special way. Instead, it became a foundation underpinned by the Christian religion, where the contributions of various disciplines were also fostered, where research and teaching could take place, and where others came to develop their own ideas and skills. Without such omissions and commissions, it is difficult to see the subsequent development of the international Hospice Movement being possible in quite the same way. The success of the vision, as defined, was that it could be emulated or elaborated, and this made possible its global spread in the following years

Making It Happen

Peace at the Last — H.L. Glyn Hughes

The new decade of the 1960s had also got going with some intense practical thinking on Cicely's part. Central to this was the report by Brigadier Glyn Hughes on the state of terminal-care provision in Britain. It was titled *Peace at the Last*[195]. Like the Joint Cancer Survey Committee almost ten years before, Glyn Hughes, himself a former army doctor, gave considerable attention to the social conditions of the terminally ill, but his report was more wide ranging in character and gave greater prominence to matters of policy and service organisation. His focus was upon the terminal care of those with an expectation of life of no longer than twelve months, and particularly upon the very last stages of life. He began by highlighting the fact that, whilst numerous enquiries and reports existed on the medical and social problems of the aged and the chronic sick, none had given adequate attention to the problem of terminal care. A particular aspect of his enquiry concerned 'the extent to which the Welfare State has made adequate provision to deal with this problem both now and in the future'[196]. In this context he criticised both the Philips Committee[197] and the Boucher report[198] for failing to deal with terminal care in their considerations of old age and chronic illness. However, a 1957 Ministry of Health circular[199] had sought to clarify the separate responsibilities of local authorities and hospital services in this regard. The former were responsible for elderly persons in welfare homes who were not expected to live more than a few weeks and who could not benefit from treatment or nursing care beyond what could be given there. The latter were deemed responsible for the chronic bed-fast who required little medical treatment, but who were in need of prolonged nursing care.

On this basis, Glyn Hughes identified 'a serious gap in the National Health Service'[200], for the circular made it clear that it was not the responsibility of the hospital authority to give all the medical or nursing care needed by an old person, nor to admit all who needed nursing care as they entered upon the last stages of their lives. Against the background of the Joint Committee's findings, this left unanswered the question of where and by whom the elderly terminally ill would be cared for.

The Glyn Hughes survey sought information from every medical officer of health in the United Kingdom. In addition, the senior administrative medical officers, who were responsible for the hospital services throughout the regional hospital boards, provided a range of statistical data on the use of hospitals for terminal care. Many voluntary organisations, religious orders, and other groups were also consulted, and three hundred site visits were made. The National Council of Social Service provided information on 150 of its local groupings. Finally, a survey of more than six hundred family doctors was conducted. Hearing of this work, Cicely had been in touch with Glyn Hughes since 1959 and he had even invited her to comment on a draft of his report.

He showed that two fifths of all deaths occurred in National Health Service hospitals, with less than a half taking place in the home. Almost forty-six thousand cancer deaths (approximately one third of the total) took place at home, and it was considered that many of these would have required continuous medical and nursing care. Similar needs were thought to be in evidence amongst some of the 121,000 who died at home from diseases of the circulatory system. Overall, Glyn Hughes estimated that about 270,000 people in need of 'skilled terminal care' died each year outside of National Health Service hospitals.

The conclusions to the report began by acknowledging that 'for a long time to come there will remain a need to make use of accommodation outside the National Health Service, both in voluntary and profit-making establishments'[201]. By the former, Glyn Hughes referred to homes for the dying run by charitable organisations and religious orders, of which only a small number existed — such as St Joseph's. By the latter, he made reference to the much larger number of nursing homes. Neither could be given a clean bill of health in his opinion. In the homes for the dying, although 'love and devotion'[202] were in evidence from the staff, there were poor staff – patient ratios, a paucity of fully trained nurses, austerity, a lack of comfort, and an air of financial constraint. Amongst the nursing homes, a large proportion were deemed quite unsuited to provide the terminal care of patients who, in their last stages, require the most skilled nursing attention; in fact in many of them the conditions were bad, in some cases amounting to actual neglect when measured by standards that could reasonably be expected[203]. It was a damning judgement all round.

Whilst dying at home was seen as the preferred alternative for most patients, Glyn Hughes stressed the importance of calculating the total number of inpatient beds which would be needed for terminal care. He was eager to stress the value of special terminal care beds 'within the curtilage of hospitals for the acute sick'[204]. At the same time, the independent homes for the dying should develop closer links with hospital services to reduce their isolation. As a review of the report in *The Lancet* put it:

> We must attack the problem on every side: hospital services must be improved and extended, staff in residential homes increased, and voluntary as well as profit-making institutions helped in return for an approved standard of care[205].

At the same time, the review recognised some of the impediments to this — the limits to hospital expansion, the inadequate supply of trained district nurses, and the paucity of home helps. *The Lancet* did, however, endorse Glyn Hughes's radical policy suggestion that payment be made to women for the full-time care of their dependent relatives. But Glyn Hughes had revealed the absence of a serious policy commitment to terminal-care provision and his recommendations highlighted the need for voluntary and for-profit organisations to work in conjunction with the National Health Service to achieve the necessary results.

Crafting a Response

For Cicely, the report was both a wake-up call and a mandate.

As we have seen, she had written to Glyn Hughes the previous summer with a newly minted copy of 'The Scheme'. Then, on 28 January 1960, she elaborated a long letter with extended thoughts about his draft report which he had shared with her some months before and on which she had been 'brooding' for some time[206]. She summarised her then-current findings at St Joseph's, explaining that he might be particularly interested in the patients who were admitted too late and pondered on the value of a home-based study to find out why that should have been. Inviting Glyn Hughes and his wife to dinner, should they feel strong enough to tackle the stairs up to her flat, she also touched again on her own plans for a new hospice and explained her search for people to be trustees and the process of drawing up Terms of Trust for discussion among them. She was already a couple of months into this and, in the summer of 1959, she had been getting advice from Jack Wallace and John Stott, as well as Betty Read, Head Almoner at St Thomas's[207]. She was also seeking out other possible candidates for the group, such as Dr Dennis Brinton, a neurologist and former dean at St Mary's who had served in the mid 1950s on the Archbishop of Canterbury's Commission on Divine Healing. In February 1960, she wrote to Evered Lunt, the Bishop of Stepney, again enclosing 'The Scheme' and copies of her *Nursing Times* articles[208]. They had met when Lunt, the local bishop, came into St Joseph's to conduct a confirmation service for a patient. Now she explained to him her sense of being led by God to found a work similar to St Joseph's, but located within the Church of England. She set out her experience as an established member at All Souls, Langham Place, as one helped by 'evangelical churchmen', but also impressed by the work of others differently motivated. The letter is open about her need for help. She feels the whole thing may be beyond her capacity — 'both spiritually and practically' — but makes it clear to Lunt that this is work in which the church should be engaging.

These deliberate and rather formalised approaches, always made through well-crafted letters of introduction and explanation, each one tending to build on an earlier personal link of some kind, marked the beginning of a loose circle of supporters which soon expanded and consolidated. It included influential figures in the Anglican world, such as Sir Kenneth Grubb, President of the Church Missionary Society and Founder with Bruce Reed of the Christian Teamwork Trust, and widely regarded as the Church of England's leading layman. There were also prominent individuals from nursing and, in time, from medicine. It may not have been surprising that Cicely was able to bring into the fold her long-standing supporter Peggy Nuttall, editor of *Nursing Times*. There was also Muriel Edwards at the King's Fund Nursing Division, who offered help. Capturing the interest of the civil servant, Dr Albertine Winner was another matter, however. When Winner visited St Joseph's in 1961, she could see that good medicine was on offer, as well as tender loving care. She also saw something that could be replicated elsewhere. As deputy chief medical officer, and thus inspired, she could open up a whole world of politics, policy, planning, and finance which would then be so crucial to the success of the St Christopher's initiative:

> Albertine was brilliant because, you know, I was really rather a maverick and had really no experience in administration at all, whereas she had been a very good administrator in the Department of Health, then Ministry, and she was 'establishment' and respectable, whereas I was wild, and we made a very good pair[209].

In March 1960, Cicely was again flat on her 'beastly back' with a return of her problems. The pace of work was perhaps taking its toll. Her days were full of clinical activity, research, and teaching. Her evenings were more and more taken up with writing, making plans for the new hospice, and giving dinner to the many contacts she felt might be able to help her. Being laid up didn't stop her from writing to her brother Christopher, with further comments on the 'The Scheme' and ideas about an organisational structure, a topic on which she had also received helpful advice from the King's Fund Nursing Division[210]. She wrote again to Christopher on 5 April, feeling ready to finalise the arrangements about the trustees, who would be the legal owners of the new hospice. She ignored her father's advice that she should concentrate on 'big names' and asked her brother to be in a small group in which she could have 'complete confidence'. In addition to Cicely and Christopher, the list comprised Jack Wallace, Madge Drake, Rosetta Burch, Betty Read, and, probably, Miss Edwards at the King's Fund[211]. There was starting to be a degree of urgency about it all. Now someone had offered to leave money to Cicely's cause, but in the absence of any organisation, it would have to go to St Mary's. It was time to make things more formal. Two days later, Cicely wrote to Betty Read:

> [I]t really is time to get ahead with the terms of trust and attacking the Inland Revenue about becoming a charity. I have decided the actual drawing up of the terms should be done by a small group, and that we should not bother with the 'big names' at this stage (even if we knew which ones we were going to have anyway)[212].

Beginning to Organise

In the summer of 1960, Cicely had been sleep-walking her way into a love affair with her patient Antoni Michniewicz. In July, she coyly noted to Christopher Saunders that 'I continue to enjoy the work over at St Joseph's immensely and have had some particularly rewarding patients lately'[213]. It was not surprising that, until recently, she had not noticed Antoni's growing affection for her. She had just begun the clinical trial that was central to her studies, she was becoming more and more immersed in planning for St Christopher's, and, on this, momentum was gathering. Talks with friends like Rosetta and Martin Burch reinforced her thinking about the spiritual components of the work and, in particular, the support that could come from Evered Lunt. They also began to provide the first leads on a charitable trust that might be approached for financial support with St Christopher's. Betty Read was the link to Sir Donald Allen, of the City Parochial Foundation and described by Shirley du Boulay as 'the spider in the middle of the web — he knew everybody in the world of fund-raising'[214]. For Cicely, he was 'an exceedingly important person with whom to get on well!'[215] Now the organizing committee for St Christopher's was taking shape and Jack Wallace had taken on the role of interim chair. By late June 1960, in a clear statement of intent, she arranged to meet the architect of Our Lady's Wing at St Joseph's.

Justin Smith (usually known as Peter) was a partner in the London architectural practice of Stewart, Hendry and Smith. He had designed the new wing at St Joseph's and first met Cicely in 1958, when working on a ward extension at the hospice. She could see the effectiveness of his approach — widely in vogue at the time — that 'form should follow function'. Perhaps surprisingly, she was drawn to his modernist orientation, that somehow fitted perfectly into the otherwise traditional ambience of St Joseph's. His design brought light, practicality, and a sense of opening to the outside world, coupled with clinical efficiency and ease of movement. Devoid of ornamentation, the main characteristics of this style were 'straight lines, geometric forms, metalwork and extensive use of glass and cantilevered elements'[216]. Cicely seems to have looked no further for architectural inspiration. Smith jumped at the chance to create what he subsequently called 'a new English hospice'. Cicely was not asking for a converted building, nor in-fill or an extension to existing facilities. Her vision was for something on its own site and, crucially, independent from though linked to National Health Service facilities. Avnita Amin acknowledges the detail of Cicely's proposed design, that expanded on that of Our Lady's Wing:

[It] envisioned three terminal wards, a mixture of six and four-beds, providing a total of sixteen to twenty beds. In addition, there ought to be three single rooms to provide privacy and intimacy for those in the final stages of dying[217].

Saunders was even more specific — beds were to be placed sideways to maximise space and she emphasised the need for 'a feeling of space on entering the ward'. A day room was important to encourage patient interaction, which should be 'cosy', perhaps with a fireplace. With her experience as a nurse, Saunders was aware of the practical needs — cupboards along the passage would be useful and that the bathrooms needed to be bigger to 'bring in beds', as well as a shower. Emphasis was also on hygiene and cleanliness — hallmarks of modern medicine but also providing a direct contrast to the squalid conditions described in home death reports — there was to be a sluice at each end of the ward for waste disposal . . . . Lighting was also considered; practical needs dictated the use of fluorescent lighting in main areas, but attention was given to creating a more welcoming atmosphere — tungsten, that provided a warmer, incandescent light, was used for bedheads, in the Chapel, and entrance hall. Natural light filled the patient areas through the incorporation of a cantilevered space running the length of the building, providing a 'projecting day space to the wards, angled to catch the early sun[218]' — a modernist architectural twist to Saunders's request for a balcony. For privacy, the 'balcony' spaces could be curtained off from the ward[219].

Quite quickly, Smith produced some designs which could be used for briefing others and for fund-raising. The estimated cost of the build at this point was £376,000, though in the inflationary environment of the times, the architect warned that prices were rising on a daily basis. But nothing could proceed without a site, and as yet nothing had been identified. Cicely knew only that she preferred a location south of the Thames, where she would not have to compete with St Joseph's either for funds or for patients. The working relationship between Cicely and Smith was to prove fruitful and collaborative. Over time, it was not always clear where the ideas of each of them began and ended. It was a remarkable partnership not always found between architect and client. The result of their efforts became a source of inspiration to others and a strong influence on hospice design in Britain into the 1970s, for example at St Luke's Sheffield, where Smith was again the architect.

The drafting of the Trust document for St Christopher's was undertaken by the legally qualified Wallace during the autumn of 1960, and in November Sir Kenneth Grubb gave advice on the memorandum and articles of association. Importantly, '[h]e talked at some length about the various people and Trusts who might be interested, most of whom he seemed to know personally'[220]. Together with advice from Sir Donald Allen, this fuelled an intricate and in-creasingly elaborate mosaic of approaches to various charitable organisations, in the search of funding for St Christopher's. Typically, the pattern would in-volve an initial, informal approach, after which Cicely would meet up with the relevant official of the organisation in question, often taking in a visit to St Joseph's, where favourite patients were on hand to assist. After this, a formal written application would be submitted, by which time the ground had been well prepared. It was a roller coaster of successes and disappointments that lasted for five years and continued right up to the months before opening.

Throughout 1960 and into the early part of the following year, Cicely was also scouring the House of Lords in search of a medical peer who would take on a role within the organising committee for St Christopher's. Geriatrician Lord Amulree seemed suitable; he had been on a committee at St Columba's, but was unable to make a commitment. The pool of eligibles seemed small[221]. Cicely remarked to Evered Lunt, 'I only wish it were as easy to find important people in the medical world as it is to find such Christians'[222]. She maintained her efforts, writing to Jack Wallace in February 1961: 'I am lobbying the Peers at the moment!'[223]

Late April 1961 saw Cicely in the northwest of England in the unlikely lo-cation of the Blackpool seaside resort. The occasion was the Health Congress of the Royal Society of Health[224], and there she had a chance to get across some of her ideas to officials in the Ministry of Health. In a symposium on teaching, she outlined the salient idea that: 'Before making any attempt to consider what to teach others about the care of terminal illness, one must begin by looking at some of the things we must try and teach ourselves'. Cicely's starting point was facing our own attitudes, emotions, fears, and faith relating to death. On this basis, the caseworker could then involve families in the pro-cess of care and also prepare them for the impending death. She then went on to explore the issues of physical deterioration and the sense of personal deg-radation in the patients themselves. 'Weariness of the mind may be harder to bear than that of the body', but pain should not be a source of defeat. She laid out a set of ideas for teaching patients how to find a key to the problems being faced, engaging with spiritual advice, and the importance of an individualised approach. The whole thing was rounded off with a case illustration from St Joseph's in which all these issues were inter-twined. In the audience was Dame Enid Russell-Smith, Deputy Secretary to the Minster of Health, who was none other than Enoch Powell at the time serving in the Conservative government led by Harold Macmillan. Cicely had dinner with Dame Enid, who subsequently wrote: 'I think you know how much I, in common with everyone else who heard it, admired and appreciated you address at Blackpool'[225]. It did not bring the sought-after senior medic, but it was instrumental in cementing the link with Deputy Chief Medical Officer Albertine Winner, who was soon involved with Cicely in the selection of a site for St Christopher's.

Options and Developments

Through this route, an option was put forward for a location on the Denmark Hill campus of King's College Hospital, in Camberwell, south London. The discussions with King's got underway in early 1962. Cicely then met with Dr Frank Cooksey, Director of Rheumatology and Rehabilitation at King's and a leading pioneer of rehabilitation medicine along with Oswald Phipps (Lord Normanby), who was chairman of the hospital. The conversation was cordial and, in March, Cicely met with Mr Banks, the house governor at Camberwell, to discuss possible locations. Even before approval in principle was given by the Development Committee in April, however, Cicely had her doubts about the arrangement. She wrote to Albertine Winner:

> I am not quite certain whether there is a suitable site available a bit further away from the hospital but I must admit if there were I think I would choose that rather than the one just below their own planned extension on Denmark Hill. With the new long term road planning there is obviously going to be a great deal of traffic along there, there would be no room at all for any kind of extension, and also although I know the present committee only want a friendly kind of liaison and quite understand our feelings about being independent yet one does have the feeling that, say in twenty years' time, our nearness to the hospital might make us feel a little like Naboth[226].

Despite her reservations, when a specific site was offered, she asked Peter Smith to draw up some plans and he produced a preliminary layout in June 1962. As Amin points out[227], the cheaper site — with its ability to share other resource burdens with the main hospital — would have offered a shorter building time and less financial challenges. Cicely could see the attraction and considered it at length. But, the site was smaller than she wished for. She felt that being in the shadow of the hospital would only limit the flexibility and freedom which she envisioned for the hospice and as an independent charity with a religious ethos. It was delicate. She had no wish to offend Albertine Winner or the people at King's, but in the end she declined the offer, despite having no viable alternative with which to proceed.

Meanwhile, other developments were advancing steadily, if more slowly than Cicely would have wanted. She had written to Evered Lunt in January 1961 explaining they were in the process of forming a company limited by guarantee and of being recognised as a charity by the Inland Revenue. An 'appeal' document was in preparation for printing and would be sent first to the City Parochial Foundation[228]. The search for a chairman was also proving to be protracted. If it were to succeed, Cicely and her associates were convinced their venture needed the involvement of a high-profile and respected figurehead. Until such a person could be found, the humble and unassuming Jack Wallace was in the chair, a role he would demit with the greatest of modesty when a replacement was eventually identified some years into the process. With help from Lord Taylor, views were canvassed from Lord Hailsham, former Leader of the House of Lords and Chair of the Conservative Party. A short-list was produced: Lord Limerick, Lord Amery, the Earl of Arran, Lady Ravendale, and Lord Hawke[229]. None of these materialised, and Lord Limerick (Hailsham's preference as he had recently been Chairman of the Medical Research Council) appeared to mistake the project for one in support of euthanasia, a matter on which Cicely quickly corrected him[230].

By late autumn 1963, the matter had still not been resolved and Cicely proposed to Wallace that they should expand the list of eminent vice-presidents they had been signing up[231]. Although this was an impressive roster which included, as we shall see, distinguished colleagues from the United States, it lacked a well-placed individual who would also be able to give significant time and energy to the project. The breakthrough came the following year, with the suggestion of St Christopher's Treasurer, Captain T.L. Lonsdale, that Lord Thurlow might be approached. Cicely met with him in the House of Lords and was given a 'delightful lunch'. They immediately hit it off. Thurlow seemed eminently suitable. He had just retired from the army. His father had founded the Missions to Seamen, and Lord Thurlow himself had been a member of its Council for some years. He agreed readily, being duly elected by telephone, such was the haste and enthusiasm for his appointment, at the end of July[232]. He chaired his first meeting on 17 September 1964.

Fund-raising and the Acquisition of a Site for the Hospice

Between 1961 and 1964, more than £330,000 was accumulated through vigorous fund-raising. It came from such London–based groups as the King Edward's Hospital Fund, the City Parochial Foundation, the Draper's Company, the Nuffield Foundation, the Sembal Trust, the Max Rayne Foundation, the Kleinwort Benson Charitable Foundation and Settlement, and the Goldsmith's

Company. The hospice was not only going to be located in the capital city, it would also be suffused with London's cultures and traditions, exemplified in the support of such benevolent and charitable organisations. But it was a roller coaster of suspense that at times brought the project, and those supporting it, to the point of collapse and despair. The initiative prevailed and the goal was realised, in fact within a brisk time span, though it may not have seemed that way at the time. The first breakthrough arrived in October 1961 with a pledge of £50,000 from the City Parochial Foundation. It was conditional on evidence that the whole project could be shown to be moving forward, so it proved a spur to greater efforts. Sadly, Jack Wallace was not around to celebrate this first success. He was ill in hospital, and Dr Harold Stewart had stepped in to cover for him[233].

When it eventually came, the acquisition of the site was assured by the involvement of Cicely's brother John. She describes what happened after the King Edward's Hospital Fund had made a visit to St Joseph's in the autumn of 1962 and suggested in passing that she might make an application to them for the cost of the land she required:

What happened then was I was talking to a group of students on a round one day and they said, 'Where are you going to start?' And I said, 'Well I'm going to have to start with having some land and getting going with it'. And that afternoon my brother John, estate agent and chartered surveyor, rang me up to say, 'We've found a site down in Sydenham which might do for you'. And I went round this site at the weekend and it was really ideal. And so that was when I came back to the King's Fund and rang up Mr Peers who was the secretary then, and who I had seen once or twice, and I said we'd found a site. So he said, 'Well you'd better put a bid in for it. How much is it?' And I said, '£27,000. It's got planning permission for twenty-seven flats'. So he said, 'Well you'd better go ahead.' So with the £500 from David Tasma in the bank we bid that, and the town planners were meeting on the same day as the major part of the King's Fund were meeting to consider my bid for the £27,000. And so they said, 'We will put it through to the big group who can get a grant of that size', And then they got in touch with me and I went and saw Mr Peers and he said, 'What are you going to do next?' And I took some-body with me who I hoped at that time might come in as an administrator, although he didn't in the event. And so it was the big group who were meeting on February 7, 1963, and the town planners, because the architect for the new wing of St Joseph's had taken me on board, and he had produced the outline planning document . . . . When I got up that morning I was reading this little book, *Daily Light*, and I turned over the page and *Daily Light's* top text for the day was 'Thou shall bless the Lord thy God for the good land which he hath given me' . . . so I had several of my patients, Louie and Alice and Mr Pettit, and other people, all praying like beavers. And Mr Edward Halton, the secretary to the original committee, rang me up at about five o'clock to say,

'It's alright Dr Saunders — up to £30,000 to pay for the cost of purchase'. And the first person I told was Mr Pettit because he was quite near the new wing, and then I went over to the old wing and told Alice and the others. And Alice, and particularly Louie, said, 'We knew we'd get it'. And so the town planners, though, deferred us because people on either side said, 'It, it looks awfully big but . . . , can you not come back a bit from the boundary?' But they both sold the pass by saying that 'We would rather have this than a block of flats'. And even the second time they deferred us. And by that time I flew off to America for my first jaunt, and I was over there six or seven weeks. They found there was a restrictive covenant on the land and we had to insure against that. And I just got back from America in time to sign the contract[234].

The site in Lawrie Park Road, Sydenham, south London, appealed enormously. Covering 1.3 acres, it had once contained two houses, now demolished. It was on a bus route, a walk away from the tube station, and had lots of potential for development. Located on a leafy street, with a tennis court opposite, it even had its own mature trees, which were carefully preserved. First, the Bishop of Stepney and Cicely went there together to bless and dedicate the location. Then, more detailed preparations could get underway.

With the City Parochial Fund safely confirmed, other monies began to come in smaller amounts from individual donations, along with the proceeds of a B.B.C. charitable appeal. With a third of their needs catered for by the spring of 1964, Cicely and her committee could start to think about building. The Nuffield Trust (£60,000) and the Sembal Trust (£22,680) had also given support. An unexpected donation from the United States led to a well-judged decision to purchase a second plot of land at 57 Lawrie Park Road. It would eventually house the Study Centre.

Elsewhere, it was clear that Cicely's work was gaining recognition beyond her immediate circle. When in January 1965 the Queen's New Year Honours list was published, there under the category Officer of the Order of the British Empire (O.B.E.) was the name Cicely Mary Strode Saunders. It was a huge encouragement to her ambition and, she felt, a salute to the shared vision that was St Christopher's. Tuesday, 9 March, saw her at Buckingham Palace to receive her honour. She was with Penelope, her niece (the daughter of John), and also her mother. Each with a hat for the occasion, with Mrs Saunders in an elegant fur coat, they cut a dash. Later, even greater honours would come Cicely's way. For now there was a quiet pleasure and a sense that she was on the right track and somehow being watched over.

The Ups and Downs of Building in Faith

Two years after the original acquisition, and with the green light showing, it was time to engage a building company and to get on-site. The preferred option when the tenders came in was a firm of 'Christian' builders called Fairweather and Sons. The name was thought propitious and the proprietor was a friend of Jack Wallace, so that may also have been a factor. He came well recommended for efficiency and budgetary control and, with Cicely's involvement, the workers soon became enthused with the whole project. Peter Smith put forward orders for bricks and steel, and a start date was agreed of 22 March 1965, with a two-year building plan[235]. On that day a band of around fifty enthusiasts, including nuns from St Joseph's and people from the Salvation Army, gathered to see the ceremonial digging of the first spit. Neither Cicely nor Lord Thurlow looked particularly adept at handling a spade, but digging together with a highly polished implement, they accompanied the task to considerable pleasure. Around them were Mrs G.'s mother and mother-in-law, Joan Steel, Jack Wallace, Peter Smith, various Polish friends, and Evered Lunt. As Cicely put it: '[W]e had dogs, children, workmen hammering, birds singing and a general atmosphere of informality and welcome which I hope will always be part of St Christopher's'[236].

Two months later, there was further occasion for celebration when, on 22 July, the foundation stone for the hospice was laid by the previous Archbishop of Canterbury, Lord Fisher. In a month of heavy rain, about 140 people gathered on the muddy site for the occasion. Away from the building works it was a sylvan scene with the grounds resembling a wildflower meadow and the trees in full leaf. Lord Fisher was assisted by the Rev Dr Almon Pepper, one of St Christopher's American Vice-Presidents who Cicely had met on her first visit to the United States in 1963. Cicely herself was just back from her second trip stateside. It was extraordinary how she was beginning to inter-leave extensive and demanding foreign travel with the day-to-day responsibilities which were emerging in south London. With rain the day before, rain the day after, and rain in the surrounding suburbs, a bright sun shone through at Sydenham. The Christians took it as a good omen. In the event, the stone was not laid precisely on its designated spot. Unflustered, Peter Smith and the workmen quietly worked around it afterwards. It would be inappropriate to move it. Everyone was content that 22 July had brought sunshine and a simple service with the theme: 'Except the Lord build the house, they labour in vain that build it'. This was 'building in faith' and it would later be stretched to the limit, not by technicalities, but by cash flow. The work had begun without the full amount required in the bank and, moreover, inflationary times were driving up the cost.

The last of the site ceremonies came on Friday, 26 November 1965. It was the 'topping off', when the highest point of the structure was reached and the roof was completed. Cicely was able to show the men some slides of the progress on the building. The warden said a prayer. They ran up a flag from the roof and the men were left to their generous supply of beer. This was very much their celebration, suggested by the workers, and readily agreed to by Cicely.

By 1966, and with Cicely fully on her sabbatical, the building (Figure 4.4) was well underway and the project budget was in excess of £400,000. Now she needed to give serious attention to how the revenue costs of the hospice would be met, along with details of how it would be staffed, the models of care that would be adopted, and all the minutiae of running a small hospital on a day-to-day basis. These things had to move forward, even when immediate capital fund-raising needs bulked large. In January, she wrote to Lord Thurlow, who was newly returned from a holiday in Nigeria, bringing him up to date on new grant offers from the Halley Stewart Trust and the City Parochial Foundation, along with details of discussions with the Wolfson Foundation. She told him; 'The building looks splendid and seems to be growing at great speed'[237]. But at the same time, dark clouds were gathering which would make 1966 a troubling year.

By July, things were considerably more worrying. Wolfson, after lengthy deliberations, had declined to support the hospice. There was little money in the bank, Fairweather's had written a 'restive' letter, and a cheque had to be produced[238]. It was a perfect storm. Cicely and her group were up to their ears in financial commitments to an expensive building project. Costs were inflating

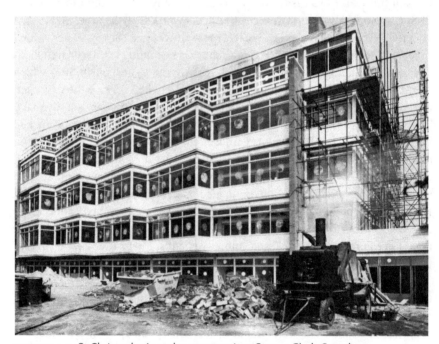

FIGURE 4.4 St Christopher's under construction. *Source: Cicely Saunders.*

monthly. Meanwhile, Britain as a whole was locked in a balance of payments crisis which had led to a credit squeeze and widespread financial jitters. The long-lasting economic post-war boom had come to an end. Thirteen years of Conservative rule had given way to Harold Wilson's Labour government, elected in 1964 and re-elected with an increased majority in March 1966. The country was sitting on an economic crisis. It was a time of low growth and poor industrial relations. The Chancellor's budget of May 1966 was designed to reduce liquidity in all sectors of the economy and was followed by a freeze on wages, dividends, and prices. The devaluation of the pound sterling was not far away. In this hostile economic environment, the St Christopher's group, led by Cicely, had entered into extremely choppy waters. Embarked on their voyage without sufficient supplies to reach home, they were putting in at every available port in search of replenishment. The grant applications were ramped up and every donation — however small — was treasured and put to immediate use. Commercial and non-commercial loans were explored, with no success. Delicate discussions took place with the building contractor and, in turn, with the sub-contractors. At a time when Cicely might have been worried to the point of paralysis, she kept up the effort, continued with her writing and planning, and — perhaps born of her breeding and upbringing — refused to give way to any notion that things would not come right in the end.

On 10 July 1966, Cicely wrote a crucial letter to the treasurer, Captain T.L. Lonsdale[239]. She digested at length the decision by the Wolfson Foundation, on whose support she had informedly been relying. She explained that 'the position is rather acute' but 'it is no good just saying we are unlucky in that giving has been much more tight for the last 18 months and borrowing now very hard indeed'. The builder and architect should have been better informed of the difficulties. Instead, she had — it might seem carelessly — gone off on a visit to Vienna for an international conference of gerontologists and said the builders would simply have to wait. She sent Lonsdale a list of things they must discuss at their next meeting. Five out of seven were about fund-raising, including 'make a bleat to Mr Peers of the King's Fund, Admiral Bingley of the Sembal Trust, and perhaps Mr Young of the Nuffield Foundation'. The last was: 'The good prayers were mobilized some time ago. Perhaps they had best be directed to Kleinwort Benson's?' It shows a combination of her indomitability, humour, and ultimate assurance that 'it will be sorted out somehow'. She could also spare a thought that others might be hurting in the process, such as the builder and sub-contractors: 'I feel rather guilty over them and very much so over Mr Smith, who is not having too easy a time with his own business at present and hangs back from sending us any bills'.

A week later she updated Sir Kenneth Grubb on the situation[240]. He was at home in Wiltshire, suffering with arthritis in his neck. After enquiring after his condition, she used an ornithological analogy to describe herself as 'rather like that small and diligent wader the turnstone, who bustles up the beach turning over every single stone it meets to find out what lies underneath'. She was not letting up on any front. That week, 150 people were expected for the group's annual general meeting, to be held in the unfinished building. On the day itself, she was making an appearance on B.B.C. Radio's long-running magazine programme 'Woman's Hour', and an article about St Christopher's was expected to appear in the *Guardian* newspaper.

At the end of July, Evered Lunt was given a full update[241]. Where it mattered to her, Cicely was the expert communicator, spending hours dictating and typing letters to members of her committee and the wider network of supporters, informing on progress, outlining problems, demonstrating optimism, and, above all, showing them she was fully engaged and tirelessly committed to this project. She wrote to the Bishop, explaining they still needed £212,000 to finish and equip the hospice. Of this, £150,000 was essential to keep building over the next six months. On the previous day there had been a long meeting with the builder. Fairweather's had agreed to wait for their money and be paid as funds became available, so long as the sub-contractors would do the same. Here, Peter Smith did excellent work to smooth the negotiations, and everyone agreed to wait for three months. They had avoided the unpleasant alternative: 'make the building watertight, put in a watchman, and begin again when the money has come in'. There were acts of personal generosity to report. The chairman of one bank that had refused a loan made a personal donation of £5,000 and encouraged a colleague to do the same. Meanwhile, there were many other irons in the fire, with results awaited. She told Lunt: 'Somehow we will get it, and those who have helped us will not let it sink'.

In the autumn, the tide suddenly turned. Money came in from the Ministry of Health for the capital costs of the pain clinic. The Goldsmith's Company gave £25,000.

> This, with the wonderful number of smaller gifts which have come our way since July, enables us to give the 'Go ahead' to an accelerated building programme to the contractors and means that not only have we have paid everything up to date . . . but that everyone is tremendously impressed by the way it has all happened[242].

In the same letter, Cicely hinted at bigger things to come, and this in due course was made official. By February 1967, a donation of £50,000 had been confirmed from the City Parochial Foundation. They were now just £90,000 short of their target of £480,000. Yet by June, the building was commissioned, a team of staff had been appointed to work at the hospice, and the first patients were beginning to arrive. Cicely also felt confident enough to move out of Connaught Square and take up residence from 12 June in a modern flat nearer to Sydenham, at 4 Restmorel House, Chester Way in Lambeth, south London.

By opening day at the hospice, 24 July 1967, the long struggle was over, all debts had been cleared and Cicely was ready to embark on the next set of challenges.

Growing Networks

Any appraisal of the people to whom Cicely was writing in the years since 1959 could not fail to note her capacity to make extensive use of social networks and, in particular, her ability to drill into those elements of the British social class structure that could be helpful to her cause. There is correspondence with bishops, barristers, peers and aristocrats, senior figures in the military and the Foreign Service, together with those prominent in medicine and the world of charitable trusts. There is a systematic quality, a thoroughness about much of this which was operationalised by boundless energy and purpose but which was made possible by an ease and confidence in matters of protocol. It is no small achievement that this was, as we have seen, orchestrated in times of great personal sorrow and huge strain on her mental and physical resources. Nor was Cicely's uncanny knack of charming the elite classes achieved at the expense of ignoring those of many other stripes who showed an interest in her work. She could be just as solicitous to the visiting medical student as to the trust secretary. She could find time for the unannounced visitor just as much as the one whose arrangements had been planned meticulously in advance. She wasted no opportunity to get her message across and to soak up information and insights from elsewhere that might help to improve it.

Always Making Connections

Despite all the pressures upon her, therefore, she was welcoming to those who came to St Joseph's and was just as eager to learn from them as they were from her. One bleak day in November 1960, just months after the death of Antoni, she was called on by Dr K.J. Rustomjee, of Colombo, Ceylon. He arrived at St Joseph's Hospice in Hackney eager to meet the enthusiastic doctor who had been working there for the past two years, improving her understanding of terminal care and also attracting attention for her recent publications. The two bonded immediately and soon 'Rusty' and she were in regular contact by air-mail. A prodigious worker, he had done much to champion the need for cancer care in Ceylon. His interests spanned the entire spectrum from disease prevention to treatment and terminal care. In particular, Dr Rustomjee harboured his own ambition to establish a terminal-care home in Colombo. Some years before, the Ceylon Cancer Society, of which he was president, had pledged to the then-Prime Minister S.W.R.D. Banderanaike that the Society would establish such a home for the shelter, comfort, and peace of terminal cases of cancer. By the time he and Cicely met in 1960, plans were well advanced and, by early 1961, an elephant was deployed to clear the site in preparation for building.

In their correspondence, Cicely and Rusty exchanged news and updates on their parallel projects. Whilst her letters were carefully typed by her secretary, his were handwritten. Hers were quite formal; his, less so. But they did exchange pleasantries about the weather, bouts of illness, and events of the day. Over the years she updated him on the fund-raising work for St Christopher's and the successes and disappointments along the way. She also supplied him with a steady stream of reprints of her publications from the period.

At the same time, he shared with her the details of the home being built in Ceylon, its facilities, and how it was to be staffed. He then sent a full album of photographs depicting the opening ceremony of 19 November 1962, with its ritual lamp-lighting and Buddhist ceremony. Dr Rustomjee had many connections. When he visited St Joseph's in 1960, he was en route to Ceylon from the United States, where he had undertaken a wide-ranging tour of organisations and facilities engaged in cancer care. On this same visit, he had also attended the Fourth National Cancer Conference, that had taken place over three days in September at the University of Minnesota, Minneapolis. He wrote up the whole experience in a report sent to Cicely in February of the following year. When in the summer of 1962 she contemplated making a similar visit to the United States, he was quick to step in and make the necessary introductions. These included a connection to Mildred Allen at the American Cancer Society, as well as to the Home of Our Lady of Good Counsel in Minnesota. The following year, Cicely headed to the States herself, followed in his footsteps for part of the way, and, on concluding her trip, did just like her friend by preparing a detailed report that she could pass on to others. Her connection with the American Cancer Society was to be long-lasting and beneficial.

More Links with the United States

This close acquaintance with developments and people in the United States became a striking feature of Cicely's approach during these formative years. Perhaps unexpectedly, she drew remarkable strength from her connections across the Atlantic, and they from her. There were three key visits during the 1960s that yielded a huge amount in terms of knowledge, insight, and collaboration. The first, in the spring of 1963, was a tour de force, covering the East and West Coasts and making connections with individuals from a spread of disciplines who would become influential in forging modern ideas about 'hospice' across the United States. She soon ran out of copies of her report from the trip, as demand outstripped supply, and she under-estimated the level of interest it would attract[243]. Three of those she had encountered were asked to become vice-presidents of St Christopher's Hospice. Professor Gordon

Allport, a contact through her brother Christopher, was chair of psychology at Harvard University and executive secretary of the Ella Lyman Cabot Trust, that supported the visit to the United States. Theodate Soule was a consultant to the Hospital Social Service Fund in New York. The Rev Dr Almon Pepper was director of the department of Christian Social Relations at the Protestant Episcopal Church in New York and, as we have seen, subsequently attended the laying of the foundation stone for St Christopher's in 1965.

The first visit to the United States, in 1963, came about almost by chance and once again saw personal and family contacts at work.

> Well I was pretty bereaved at that time and working very hard, but being pretty lonely and being sad and an American student — theological, actually — he was a priest but he was working in Canterbury on an overseas fellowship or something, and he was interested in the dying and he asked for a visit at St Joseph's. And he picked up on my grieving for Antoni and the fact that I was pretty stuck, and he said, 'I think you need to go over to America and meet some of these people'. Later I was sitting next to Peggy Nuttall in the Thomas's Old Girls Reunion at the Nightingale Fellowship and they announced that there were these fellowships for nurses and I said to Peggy, 'Oh, I think I'll apply for one. I'm a nurse and I'll try and get over to the States'. So I got it and at the same time my brother Christopher was interviewed for going to work at McKinsey's management team, he'd been a part of the School of Management [at Harvard], and this chap, as part of his interview, said, 'What are your family doing?' He said I was interested in pain and he said, 'Put her in touch with me', so I met up with this chap and I got an Ella Lyman Fellowship from Boston as well, that enabled me to spend a whole eight weeks in the States[244].

For a lone Englishwoman who had never before travelled to the United States — a country at that time in considerable foment over civil rights and international relations issues — it was a remarkable tour. Taking in New York; Yale; Boston; Washington, DC; Los Angeles; San Francisco; and Vancouver, British Columbia; she visited eighteen different hospitals of varying types as well as the National Institutes of Health in Maryland. Along the way she met with doctors, psychiatrists, nurses, social workers, social scientists, and hospital chaplains. As she noted in the introduction to her report of the whole experience, 'I found it a great asset that I was able to go in my threefold capacity of nurse, social worker, and doctor. It made my own approach a broad one and also made me "one of them" when I discussed problems with each of the different professions'[245]. There are sections in the report dealing with pain in terminal cancer, the mental pain and distress of dying patients, relatives and their problems, home-care programmes, nursing homes, and the work of chaplains. It is an assiduous log of travel, meetings, events, and ideas.

Several of those she met on the trip became long-standing colleagues and friends, and over time an elaborate trans-Atlantic network of individuals concerned with the care of the dying began to develop, with Cicely close to its core. During the early 1960s, airmail letter writing was their main means of communication, coupled frequently with an enthusiastic exchange of reprints from recent publications. Her prolific correspondence gives remarkable insight into the energy with which she pursued her links in the United States and the benefits that flowed from them. Her personal papers contain no fewer than fifteen archive boxes of correspondence with U.S. colleagues, much of it covering the period up to 1967.

Regular correspondents on the West Coast included Dr Herman Feifel, chief psychologist at the Veterans Administration in Los Angeles and author of key early work on aspects of death and dying — notably, his book *The Meaning of Death*, an edited collection that came out in 1959[246]. There was also Esther Lucille Brown, a social anthropologist working with the Russell Sage Foundation — a frequent source of letters and ideas, with specific interests in improving the quality of nursing care. On the East Coast, Florence Wald, then dean of nursing at Yale University; Professor Gordon Allport; and Carleton Sweetser, chaplain at Memorial Hospital, New York, all became close colleagues and friends.

The link with Yale was to be particularly significant. Cicely's first visit was at the invitation of Dr Bernard Lytton, a former surgeon at the London Hospital, from where he had attended St Joseph's Hospice once a week. On moving to Yale and learning of her planned visit to the United States, he invited Cicely to lecture at the university, and it was he who met her when she arrived at the airport in New York. At Yale she spoke first to the student council in the school of medicine, and then, by special request as word of what she had done reverberated across the campus, repeated the talk the following day to the faculty of postgraduate nursing. It was at the second lecture that she met Florence Wald, who was completely bowled over by what Cicely had to say[247]. Somehow, and perhaps without intention, Cicely's message about the care of the dying was resonating with the times. In the air was a heightened sense of social conscience. That same month, May 1963, was when the marches of Martin Luther King began in Selma, Alabama. That summer, doctors and nurses also began to join in the fight against segregation. Cicely was not a part of these causes, but her message about another dispossessed and disadvantaged group, those with terminal illnesses and those facing death, struck a related chord. Wald could tell this was something which had been lost from nursing and health care and yet somehow had to be recovered.

As Joy Buck, the historian of American nursing, has noted, Wald was at a critical point in her own life in 1963. She was an advocate for major reforms in nursing education and the clinical role of the nurse and, like Cicely, she believed that professional nurses should eschew non-nursing tasks to give more focus to care at the bedside. She was also deeply sceptical of the drive within medicine to privilege technology and cure over an emphasis on care of the person. Wald believed the hospice concept — as outlined in Cicely's lecture — offered the perfect vehicle by which she and other reformers could achieve a 'brave new world' in health care, with nursing and medicine working together as equals at the helm[248]. In other words, Cicely's ideas were being picked up by others and harnessed to their specific causes, from which they would gain wider power and influence. From a Catholic home for the terminally ill in the impoverished East End of London, to the privileged portals of Yale, was an enormous leap, albeit one which Cicely took in her ample stride and worked to huge advantage.

With building work at St Christopher's now underway, her second visit to the United States began in May 1965, in New York with a lecture at the Postgraduate Center for Mental Health. This was followed by speaking engagements at Yale and meetings at the Massachusetts General Hospital with Professor Lindemann, a psychiatrist and an early bereavement researcher who developed the concept of anticipatory grief. On this occasion, as before, financial assistance from the Ella Lyman Cabot Trust was made available, mediated through the good offices of Gordon Allport. Cicely observed to Esther Lucille Brown, 'I cannot be too grateful to them, for not only did they help me very substantially on my last trip, but they also sent me a most generous gift as "seed money" for St Christopher's. I am most undeservedly fortunate in the people who support us'[249]. In the case of Gordon Allport, there was also an emotional and intellectual debt, for it was he who, in 1963, had first introduced her to the writings of Austrian psychiatrist and concentration camp survivor Viktor Frankl, whose book *Man's Search for Meaning*, published in 1964[250], was to prove very influential upon her thinking in the coming years. From his account of 'tragic optimism', she learned of the human capacity to make the best of adversity and turn life's negative aspects into something positive, and constructive — even in the face of death.

American colleagues also proved to be useful sounding boards about events and developments taking place back in London. After writing to Esther Lucille Brown about leaving St Joseph's in autumn 1965, her friend wrote back, 'It must have been a wrench to leave St Joseph's after seven years there. I believe, however, that this is a most auspicious moment for you to sever ties and prepare yourself psychologically for initiating your new program in your own new hospital'[251]. On another occasion when the finances of St Christopher's had taken an upturn, Brown wrote, 'Isn't it marvellous how financial sustenance at this very trying moment has been coming to your rescue. I do hope that it will continue . . . '[252].

Regular correspondents all received a newsletter, that contained details of the development of St Christopher's and there was a steady exchange of information and words of encouragement in the letters that appeared with such regularity from American colleagues. Perhaps resulting from the cultural disposition of the Americans with whom she made contact, there was a tendency for her to receive greater recognition of the wider import of her work from across the Atlantic than she found at home. In due course, the UK – US traffic became two-way. American visitors arrived with increasing regularity in London to visit St Joseph's and the still-to-be-opened St Christopher's. Anselm Strauss, for example, the sociologist and pioneering researcher on awareness contexts in dying based in San Francisco, visited her in the autumn of 1965, and many others followed.

The third sojourn to North America went ahead as planned, despite the worries back in Sydenham. It began in April 1966 with six weeks at Yale before moving on to Cleveland and then Vancouver, British Columbia. She opened her lecture at the Yale School of Nursing as follows:

> This is the third time I've been at Yale, and like St Thomas's Hospital, I think you must begin to feel that every time you get rid of me, I come back in another capacity. This time I've chosen the title, 'The Moment of Truth', not because I just want to discuss the perennial question, 'Should you tell the dying patient the truth?' (which is not really the right question anyway), but because meeting dying patients and facing the fact of death does concern all of us, whether we're nurses, doctors, social workers, psychologists, or of any other discipline — I think perhaps almost most of all, when we're just members of the family. This moment is, or should be, a moment of truth, not just a matter of words, who says what and when, but something much more deep and far-reaching than that in its implications, implications which, I think, are relevant to the whole of life[253].

Whilst at Yale, she also met up with two major figures in the emerging psychiatry of dying and bereavement: Elisabeth Kübler-Ross was visiting from Chicago and Dr Colin Murray Parkes, with whom she had already become acquainted in London and who was spending a year at Harvard. Their first encounter brought together a remarkable triad of names that were to become synonymous with the modern care of the dying and bereaved. Kübler-Ross was, at that time, working as a psychiatrist at the Billings Hospital and University of Chicago, where she had begun to embark on a series of important and widely acclaimed works on death and dying. Parkes was later to work closely with Cicely at St Christopher's, where he brought his psychiatric perspective not only to the care of patients and families, and to research, but also to the support of the staff.

Cicely continued her frequent visits to Yale and, later, in June 1969, she was awarded the degree of Doctor of Science from the university, her first honorary degree. Her friendship with Florence Wald was also to grow and thrive over many years, particularly as developments got underway which led to the formation of America's first modern hospice in New Haven. She maintained some contact with Kübler-Ross, though much more at a distance. And with Colin Murray Parkes there was to be long-lasting friendship and collaboration. Recalling their first meeting together, she captures their shared but contrasting approaches:

> In '66, Colin Murray Parkes was over, and Elisabeth Kübler-Ross had started, and Florence Wald put on a seminar with the three of us there. And we had a most fascinating dinner one evening, the three of us together, and Colin had been working with widows and doing a sort of two-year study with the group. Elisabeth was working with, almost with a one-off [encounter]. She'd find a dying patient and interview them in front of a one-way glass screen and they would open up and come through to a sort of resolution of some of their anxieties, all in a great hurry, you know, in one hour. Whereas [I had been] working at St Joseph's and was doing things which were taking . . . which were taking two or three weeks. And Colin said, you know, in a way we were doing the same but we were doing it in such a fascinatingly different timescale[254].

The Hospice Opens Its Doors

An article by Cicely published in *The British Hospital Journal and Social Service Review* soon after the opening ceremony on 24 July 1967 amounts to a prospectus for St Christopher's[255]. The hospice 'will try to fill the gap that exists in both research and teaching concerning the care of patients dying of cancer and those needing skilled relief in other long-term illnesses and their relatives'. At this point it contained fifty-four inpatient beds, an outpatient clinic, and also sixteen beds available for the long-term needs of staff and their families. It was a small hospital in scale and complement. There was going to be an emphasis on providing continuity of care for those able to return home, and there were plans for a domiciliary service. The involvement of family members in the care of their loved ones would be encouraged. Research on pain, developed by Cicely at St Joseph's, would be extended. The hospice was to be 'a religious foundation of very open character', and there was a sense that the whole endeavour amounted to an elaborate pilot scheme which could have extremely far-reaching implications.

Indeed, Cicely and others around her, even before the opening of St Christopher's, had developed a sense that this was a project far greater than building a single new hospice, taxing though that had proved. Colleagues wrote from America urging her to realize that she had two obligations: one, to develop the work of her own organisation, and the other, to spread her learning farther afield. So it was that the practical accomplishment was about more than St Christopher's Hospice alone. Links had already been established with a wide range of hospitals and nursing and theological colleges, and there were plans for exchange visits with colleagues at Yale, Harvard, and other centres in the United States. Within a few years, voluntary, independent terminal-care services would proliferate, and the modern hospice 'project' would have a growing influence on policy and practice. A nascent movement was underway, the starting point for which, most marked in the British context, was *outside* rather than *within* the formal healthcare system. For this movement to flourish and grow, it would need Cicely to apply enormous levels of personal energy and commitment to its development.

From that time, the future of her professional life was determined. At this point she had become the first-ever modern doctor to devote her entire professional career to caring for those at the end of life. Building on her nursing experience through the war years and her subsequent role as an almoner, she had then trained in medicine. At St Joseph's in her clinical practice, research, and teaching, she had learned the craft of terminal care and created a vision for how it could develop in future. There, in the East End of London, she honed her understanding of care at the end of life, listened to the stories of her patients, and discovered a new world — of suffering and how it might be overcome. She read deeply the contemporary writings of authors such as C.S. Lewis, Viktor Frankl, and Teilhard de Chardin. She drew on the emerging ideas about religious community, found in the work of theologians like Olive Wyon. She continued to study Scripture and located her daily actions in biblical texts, prayers, and biblical exegesis. She passed though the darkness of multiple losses, and the extended bereavement from a man whose love she knew for only a few weeks. She also met the man she would eventually marry. Now she set out to re-invent older traditions of terminal care based on religious motivations. She would forge these in a new guise within an architecture of modernity, drawing not only on medical innovations in pain and symptom control, but emerging ideas of personhood, suffering, and identity. To emphasise her understanding of these things, she wrote dozens of articles and book chapters, she took on prodigious amounts of teaching and lecturing, and she engaged with wider audiences through fund-raising appeals, public meetings, book reviews, and constant letter writing. Gathering a diverse range of well-wishers and supporters around her, she had set about a process of deep reflection leading, in time, to a clear plan for a new kind of hospice — one with Christian roots, but capable of wider influence and conceived as a beacon of inspiration to others. Now St Christopher's Hospice had become a reality and opened its doors to patients and families in July 1967, when Dr Cicely Saunders, O.B.E., was forty-nine years old.

Notes

1. Cicely Saunders letter to Peggy Nuttall, 26 May 1959; Clark D. *Cicely Saunders: Founder of the Hospice Movement: Selected Letters 1959–1999.* Oxford: Oxford University Press; 2002: 14 (hereafter *Letters*).

2. House jobs were training posts occupied by medical graduates who had just passed their final examinations.

3. Cicely Saunders interview with David Clark, 11 May 2004.

4. Cicely Saunders interview with David Clark, 11 May 2004.

5. Cicely Saunders interview with David Clark, 11 May 2004.

6. Cicely Saunders interview with David Clark, 16 May 2000.

7. Cicely Saunders interview with David Clark, 11 May 2004.

8. Cicely Saunders interview with David Clark, 11 May 2004.

9. Quoted in Warpole K. *Modern Hospice Design: The Architecture of Palliative Care*. London: Routledge; 2009: 12.

10. Saunders C. Working at St Joseph's Hospice, Hackney. *Annual Report of St Vincent's, Dublin*, 1962: 37–39.

11. Reynolds L.A., Tansey E.M. *Innovations in Pain Management: Welcome Witnesses to Twentieth Century Medicine*, Vol. 21. London: Wellcome Trust; 2004: 6.

12. Sister Mary Antonia interview with David Clark, Hospice History Project, 28 November 1995.

13. Cicely Saunders interview with David Clark, Hospice History Project, 29 April 1997.

14. Cicely Saunders interview with David Clark, 11 May 2004.

15. Cicely Saunders interview with David Clark, 11 May 2004.

16. Cicely Saunders letter to Rosetta Burch, n.d. (probably late 1960). King's College London Archives, SAUNDERS, Dame Cicely (1918 – 2005), Correspondence and related papers, 1948 – 2005, K/PP149/3/1-5.

17. Cicely Saunders interview with David Clark, 2 May 2003.

18. Bloor M., McKeganey M.P., Fonkert J.D. *One Foot in Eden: Sociological Study of the Range of Therapeutic Community Practice*. London: Routledge; 1988.

19. Sister Margaret Deegan, quoted in Winslow M., Clark D. *St Joseph's Hospice, Hackney: A Century of Caring in the East End of London*. Lancaster: Observatory Publications; 2005: 44.

20. Cicely Saunders interview with David Clark, 11 May 2004.

21. Cicely Saunders interview with David Clark, 11 May 2004.

22. Later, she had one in red.

23. Cicely Saunders, interview with David Clark, 11 May 2004.

24. Cicely Saunders interview with David Clark, 11 May 2004.

25. Cicely Saunders interview with David Clark, Hospice History Project, 29 April 1997.

26. Cicely Saunders interview with Neil Small, Hospice History Project, 24 October 1995.

27. Cicely Saunders interview with David Clark, 11 May 2004.

28. Cicely Saunders letter to Dr W.J. Moon, 18 November 1965; Clark, *Letters*, 90–91.

29. Cicely Saunders interview with David Clark, 11 May 2004.

30. Quoted in Clark D. *To Comfort Always: A History of Palliative Medicine Since the Nineteenth Century*. Oxford: Oxford University Press; 2016: 120.

31. Cicely Saunders letter to Dr L. Colebrook, 8 December 1959; Clark, *Letters*, 17–18.

32. Cicely Saunders interview with David Clark, 11 May 2004.

33. Cicely Saunders letter to Dr Hugh de Wardener, 1 March 1960; Clark, *Letters*, 22–23.

34. Hinton J. The physical and mental distress of the dying. *Quarterly Journal of Medicine*. 1963; 32(125): 1–20.

35. John Hinton interview with David Clark, Hospice History Project, 25 April 1996.

36. Cicely Saunders interview with David Clark, 11 May 2004.

37. See du Boulay S. *Cicely Saunders: The Founder of the Modern Hospice Movement*, 2nd ed. London: Hodder and Stoughton; 1994: 78 ff.

38. Cicely Saunders interview with Neil Small, Hospice History Project, 31 October 1995.

39. Cicely Saunders letter to Jack Wallace, 26 November 1959; Clark, *Letters*, 17.

40. Cicely Saunders interview with David Clark, 11 May 2004.

41. Cicely Saunders interview with David Clark, 11 May 2004.

42. Cicely Saunders interview with David Clark, 11 May 2004.

43. Cicely Saunders interview with David Clark, 11 May 2004.

44. Cicely Saunders letter to The Reverend Whitney Hale, 7 September 1965; Clark, *Letters*, 89.

45. Cicely Saunders interview with David Clark, 15 December 1999.

46. See also du Boulay, *Cicely Saunders*, 103–116.

47. Cicely Saunders interview with David Clark, 2 May 2003.

48. Typescript document given by Cicely Saunders to the author. This version, that is a carbon copy containing further handwritten amendments and attached addenda, was apparently typed up sixteen months after the events. A slightly different version of the typescript is at King's College London Archives, SAUNDERS, Dame Cicely (1918 – 2005), K/PP149/2/2/20.

49. Cicely Saunders interview with David Clark, 2 May 2003.

50. Cicely Saunders interview with David Clark, 2 May 2003.

51. Cicely Saunders interview with David Clark, 19 December 2000.

52. Cicely Saunders interview with David Clark, 15 December 1999.

53. King's College London Archives, SAUNDERS, Dame Cicely (1918 – 2005), K/PP149/2/2/20.

54. Hotchkiss E. *Home to Poland*. London: Eyre and Spottiswoode; 1958.

55. Saunders C. My encounter with a Pole. Unpublished typescript, 1962: 1–7. King's College London Archives, SAUNDERS, Dame Cicely (1918 – 2005), K/PP149/2/2/20.

56. Cicely Saunders interview with Neil Small, Hospice History Project, 31 October 1995.

57. Cicely Saunders letter to Colin Murray Parkes, 14 June 1966; Clark, *Letters*, 107–108.

58. Cicely Saunders letter to Christopher Saunders, 4 March 1960; Clark, *Letters*, 24–25.

59. Cicely Saunders to Mother Superior, Grandchamps, 30 March 1960; Sister Geneviève to Cicely Saunders, 5 April 1960, King's College London Archives, SAUNDERS, Dame Cicely (1918 – 2005), Correspondence and related papers, 1948 – 2005, K/PP149/4/1-6.

60. Cicely Saunders interview with David Clark, 15 December 1999.

61. du Boulay, *Cicely Saunders*, 117–118.

62. Cicely Saunders interview with David Clark, 15 December 1999.

63. Cicely Saunders interview with David Clark, 15 December 1999.

64. Last Will and Testament of Philip Gordon Saunders, Principal Probate Registry, High Court of Justice, 13 November 1961.

65. Cicely Saunders interview with David Clark, 15 December 1999.

66. Storr A. *The Integrity of the Personality*. London: Heinemann; 1961.

67. Storr A. *Human Aggression*. London: Allen Lane; 1968.

68. Cicely Saunders interview with David Clark, 15 December 1999.

69. Cicely Saunders interview with David Clark, 15 December 1999

70. Diary notes by Cicely Saunders, 12 August 1962, in possession of the author.

71. Nouwen H. *The Inner Voice of Love: A Journey Through Anguish to Freedom*. New York: Image Books; 1999.

72. Cicely Saunders interview with David Clark, 15 December 1999.

73. Quoted in du Boulay, *Cicely Saunders*, 118–119.

74. Tyrell G. *Water and Wine*. London: Longmans, Green and Co; 1911.

75. van der Post L. *A Bar of Shadow*. London: Hogarth Press; 1954.

76. Evan Hopkins H. *The Mystery of Suffering*. London: Ivp; 1961.

77. Gibran K. *The Prophet*. New York: Alfred A. Knopf; 1923.

78. Kierkegaard S. *The Gospel of Suffering*, trans. A.S. Aldworth and W.S. Ferrie. London: James Clarke; 1956.

79. Cicely Saunders interview with David Clark, 16 May 2000.

80. Cicely Saunders interview with David Clark, 6 June 2002.

81. Buytendijk, F.J.J. *Pain: Its Modes and Functions*, trans. Edna O'Sheil. London: Hutchison; 1961.

82. Cicely Saunders letter to F.J.J. Buytendijk, 17 October 1963; Clark, *Letters*, 62–63.

83. Cicely Saunders interview with David Clark, 6 June 2002.

84. Clark D. 'Total pain', disciplinary power, and the body in the work of Cicely Saunders, 1958–1967. *Social Science and Medicine*. 1999; 49: 727–736.

85. Saunders C. Care of the dying 3: Control of pain in terminal cancer. *Nursing Times*. 1959; October 23: 1031–1032.

86. Saunders C. Drug treatment of patients in the terminal stages of cancer. *Current Medicine and Drugs*. 1960; 1: 16–28.

87. Saunders C. The care of the dying. *Guy's Hospital Gazette*. 1966; 80: 136–142.

88. Saunders C. Telling patients. *District Nursing*. 1965; September: 149–154.

89. Saunders C. Care of patients suffering from terminal illness at St Joseph's Hospice, Hackney, London. *Nursing Mirror.* 1964; February 14: vii–x.

90. Saunders C. The symptomatic treatment of incurable malignant disease. *The Prescribers' Journal*. 1964; 4(4): 68–73.

91. Saunders, Telling patients.

92. Saunders, Care of the dying 3.

93. Saunders C. *The Management of Terminal Illness*. London: Hospital Medicine Publications Ltd; 1967.

94. Cicely Saunders interview with David Clark, 6 June 2002.

95. Cicely Saunders interview with David Clark, 6 June 2002.

96. Exton Smith A.N. Terminal illness in the aged. *The Lancet.* 1961; 278(7197): 305–308.

97. Exton Smith, Terminal illness in the aged, 307.

98. Editorial. Euthanasia. *The Lancet*. 1961; 278(7197): 351–352.

99. Hinton, The physical and mental distress of the dying.

100. Exton Smith A.N. Distress in dying. *British Medical Journal*. 1963; II: 400–401.

101. Saunders C. Distress in dying. *British Medical Journal*. 1963; II: 746 [Letter].

102. Millard M. Distress in dying. *British Medical Journal*. 1963; II: 746 [Letter].

103. Hinton J. *Dying*. Harmondsworth: Penguin; 1967.

104. Hinton, *Dying*, 148.

105. Cicely Saunders letter to Eric Wilkes, 12 September 1963; Clark, *Letters*, 59.

106. Wilkes E. Cancer outside hospital. *The Lancet*. 1964; 238(7348): 1379–1381; Wilkes E. Terminal cancer at home. *The Lancet*. 1965; 238(7348): 799–801.

107. Clark, *To Comfort Always*, 74–75.

108. Cicely Saunders letter to Colin Murray Parkes, 23 March 1965; Clark, *Letters*, 81–82.

109. Murray Parkes C. The pastoral care of the bereaved. *Contact*. 1964; 12(1): 3–19.

110. Hinton J. Problems in the care of the dying. *Journal of Chronic Diseases*. 1965; 17: 201–205.

111. Clark D. Cradled to the grave? Pre-conditions for the hospice movement in the UK, 1948–67. *Mortality*. 1999; 4(3): 225–247.

112. Glaser B., Strauss A. *Awareness of Dying*. Chicago: Aldine; 1965.

113. Cartwright A., Hockey J., Anderson J.L. *Life Before Death*. London: Routledge and Kegan Paul; 1973.

114. Cicely Saunders letter to Anselm Strauss, 19 December 1965; Clark, *Letters*, 94–96.

115. Cicely Saunders letter to Anselm Strauss, 19 December 1965; Clark, *Letters*, 94–96.

116. Saunders C. The management of patients in the terminal stage. In Raven R., ed. *Cancer*, Vol. 6. London: Butterworth and Company; 1960: 403–417.

117. Saunders C. The management of terminal illness. Part three: Mental distress in the dying patient. *British Journal of Hospital Medicine*. 1967; February: 433–436.

118. Bailey M. A survey of the social needs of patients with incurable lung cancer. *The Almoner*. 1959; 11(10): 379–397.

119. Paterson R., Aitken-Swan J. Public opinion on cancer. *The Lancet*. 1954; 267: 857–861.

120. Aitken-Swan J., Paterson R. The cancer patient: Delay in seeking advice. *British Medical Journal*. 1955; 1: 623–627.

121. Abrams R., Jameson G., Poehlman M., Snyder S. Terminal care in cancer. *New England Journal of Medicine*. 1945; 232(25): 719–724.

122. Abrams R.D. Social casework with cancer patients. *Social Casework*. 1951; 32(1): 425–431.

123. Brauer P.H. Should the patient be told the truth? *Nursing Outlook*. 1960; 8: 328–333.

124. Bard M. The psychologic impact of cancer. *Illinois Medical Journal*. 1960; 118(3): 9–14.

125. Lindemann E. Symptomatology and the management of acute grief. *American Journal of Psychiatry*. 1944; 101: 141–148; Aldrich C.K. The dying patient's grief. *Journal of the American Medical Association*. 1963; 184: 329–331.

126. Saunders C. The control of pain in terminal cancer. Uncompleted M.D. thesis, n.d. (probably 1965). In possession of the author.

127. Saunders C. Drug treatment of patients in the terminal stages of cancer. *Current Medicine and Drugs.* 1960; 1(1): 16–28.

128. Saunders C. The treatment of intractable pain in terminal cancer. *Proceedings of the Royal Society of Medicine.* 1963; 56(3): 195–197 [Section of Surgery, 5–7].

129. Faull C., Nicholson A. Taking the myths out of the magic: Establishing the use of opioids in the management of cancer pain. In Meldrum M.L., ed. *Opioids and Pain Relief: A Historical Perspective. Progress in Pain Research and Management*, Vol. 25. Seattle: IASP Press; 2003: 111–129.

130. Cicely Saunders interview with Christina Faull, May 2002, quoted in Faull and Nicholson, Taking the myths out of the magic.

131. Saunders C. The care of the terminal stages of cancer. *Annals of the Royal College of Surgeons.* 1967; 41(Suppl.): 162–169.

132. Saunders, Working at St Joseph's Hospice, 37–39.

133. Cicely Saunders interview with David Clark, 2 May 2003.

134. Nalecz H. Artists Biographies, http://www.artbiogs.co.uk/2/galleries/drian-galleries, accessed 3 November 2016.

135. Saunders, The care of the terminal stages of cancer, 162–169.

136. Evens J. Marian Bohusz-Szyszko. Artway, http://www.artway.eu/content.php?id=1395&action=show&lang=en, accessed 3 November 2016.

137. Marian Bohusz-Szyszko. St Christopher's Hospice, http://www.stchristophers.org.uk/about/damecicelysaunders/marianbohuszszyszko, accessed 3 November 2016.

138. Marian Bohusz-Szyszko (1901–1995). The Gallery, http://www.thegallery.uk.com/artists/bohusz-szyszko-marian-1, accessed 3 November 2016.

139. Quoted in du Boulay, *Cicely Saunders*, 212.

140. Quoted in du Boulay, *Cicely Saunders*, 213.

141. Cicely Saunders interview with David Clark, 2 May 2003.

142. Cicely Saunders interview with David Clark, 2 May 2003.

143. Cicely Saunders interview with David Clark, 2 May 2003.

144. du Boulay, *Cicely Saunders*, 215.

145. du Boulay, *Cicely Saunders*, 215.

146. du Boulay, *Cicely Saunders*, 215.

147. Cicely Saunders interview with David Clark, 16 May 2000.

148. Cicely Saunders interview with Neil Small, Hospice History Project, 10 July 1996.

149. Cicely Saunders letter to Peggy Nuttall, 26 May 1959; Clark, *Letters*, 14.

150. Saunders C. Care of the dying 1: The problem of euthanasia. *Nursing Times.* 1959; October 9: 960–961.

151. Saunders, Care of the dying 1, 960–961.

152. Saunders C. Care of the dying 2: Should a patient know . . . ? *Nursing Times.* 1959; October 16: 994–995.

153. Saunders, Care of the dying 3.

154. Saunders C. Care of the dying 4: Mental distress in the dying. *Nursing Times.* 1959; October 30: 1067–1069.

155. Saunders C. Care of the dying 5: The nursing of patients dying of cancer. *Nursing Times*. 1959; November 6: 1091–1092.

156. Saunders C. Care of the dying 6: When a patient is dying. *Nursing Times*. 1959; November 19: 1129–1130.

157. Saunders C. *Care of the Dying*. London: *Nursing Times* reprint; 1960.

158. Review of *Care of the Dying*. *The Lancet*. 1960; 275(7128): 735.

159. Saunders, The management of patients in the terminal stage.

160. Saunders C. Death. *The Living Church*. 1964; July 26: 8–9.

161. Saunders C. Terminal patient care. *Geriatrics*. 1966; 21(12): 70–74.

162. Saunders C. The moment of truth: Care of the dying person. In Pearson L., ed. *Death and Dying: Current Issues in the Treatment of the Dying Person*. Cleveland: The Press of Case Western Reserve University; 1969: 49–78.

163. Cicely Saunders interview with Neil Small, Hospice History Project, 14 November 1995.

164. Cicely Saunders letter to J.R. Heller, 12 June 1959; Clark, *Letters*, 14–15.

165. Saunders. The management of patients in the terminal stage.

166. Van Leeuwen M.S. *A Sword between the Sexes? C. S. Lewis and the Gender Debates*. Ada, MI: Brazos Press; 2010.

167. Quoted in Van Leeuwen, *A Sword between the Sexes*, 124.

168. Clerk N.W. *A Grief Observed*. London: Faber and Faber; 1961. Later, Lewis C.S. *A Grief Observed*. London: Faber and Faber; 1964.

169. Menzies J. Thank you, I think. 2015, http://catchingacupwithlewis.com/thank-you-i-think/, accessed 10 November 2016.

170. Penelope Sr. *God Persists: A Short Survey of World History in the Light of Christian Faith*. Oxford: Mowbrays; 1939.

171. Penelope Sr. *Light in the Night: A Book for Those in Bed*. Oxford: Mowbrays; 1938.

172. Cicely Saunders interview with David Clark, 12 December 2001.

173. Quoted in du Boulay, *Cicely Saunders*, 86, who notes the laconic phrasing.

174. Saunders, C. *The Scheme*. Typescript. n.d [probably 1959]; 1–10. King's College London Archives, SAUNDERS, Dame Cicely (1918–2005), Papers relating to St Christopher's Hospice, 1943 – 2003, K/PP149/3/1-5.

175. du Boulay, *Cicely Saunders*, 87.

176. Cicely Saunders letter to Brigadier H.L. Glyn Hughes, 22 July 1959; Clark, *Letters*, 15–16.

177. Neil Small interview with Lucie Wallace, Hospice History Project, 13 December 1995.

178. Cicely Saunders letter to Jack Wallace, 20 January 1960. King's College London Archives, SAUNDERS, Dame Cicely (1918 – 2005), Correspondence and related papers, 1948 – 2005, K/PP149/3/1-5.

179. Jack Wallace letter to Cicely Saunders, 22 January 1960. King's College London Archives, SAUNDERS, Dame Cicely (1918 – 2005), Correspondence and related papers, 1948 – 2005, K/PP149/3/1-5.

180. Jack Wallace letter to Cicely Saunders, 10 February 1960. King's College London Archives, SAUNDERS, Dame Cicely (1918 – 2005), Correspondence and related papers, 1948 – 2005, K/PP149/3/1-5.

181. Jack Wallace letter to Cicely Saunders, 10 February 1960.

182. Cicely Saunders letter to Jack Wallace, 10 February 1960. King's College London Archives, SAUNDERS, Dame Cicely (1918 – 2005), Correspondence and related papers, 1948 – 2005, K/PP149/3/1-5.

183. The Reverend Bruce Reed, 25 November 2003, http://www.telegraph.co.uk/news/obituaries/1447609/The-Reverend-Bruce-Reed.html, accessed 2 November 2016.

184. Cicely Saunders letter to Bruce Reed, 14 March 1960. King's College London Archives, SAUNDERS, Dame Cicely (1918 – 2005), Correspondence and related papers, 1948 – 2005, K/PP149/3/1-5.

185. Wyon O. *Living Springs: New Religious Movements in Western Europe*. London: SCM Press; 1964.

186. Cicely Saunders letter to Olive Wyon, 4 March 1960. King's College London Archives, SAUNDERS, Dame Cicely (1918 – 2005), Correspondence and related papers, 1948 – 2005, K/PP149/3/1-5.

187. Cicely Saunders letter to Olive Wyon, 16 March 1960. King's College London Archives, SAUNDERS, Dame Cicely (1918 – 2005), Correspondence and related papers, 1948 – 2005, K/PP149/3/1-5.

188. Cicely Saunders letter to Jack Wallace, 16 March 1960; Clark, *Letters*, 26–27.

189. Cicely Saunders letter to Christopher Saunders, 30 August 1960. King's College London Archives, SAUNDERS, Dame Cicely (1918 – 2005), Correspondence and related papers, 1948 – 2005, K/PP149/3/1-5.

190. Betty West letter to Cicely Saunders, 11 February 1960. King's College London Archives, SAUNDERS, Dame Cicely (1918 – 2005), Correspondence and related papers, 1948 – 2005, K/PP149/3/1-5.

191. Rosetta Burch letter to Cicely Saunders 16 June 1960. King's College London Archives, SAUNDERS, Dame Cicely (1918 – 2005), Correspondence and related papers, 1948 – 2005, K/PP149/3/1-5.

192. Cicely Saunders letter to Olive Wyon, 6 December 1960. King's College London Archives, SAUNDERS, Dame Cicely (1918 – 2005), Correspondence and related papers, 1948 – 2005, K/PP149/3/1-5.

193. Cicely Saunders letter to Olive Wyon, 11 June 1964. King's College London Archives, SAUNDERS, Dame Cicely (1918 – 2005), Correspondence and related papers, 1948 – 2005, K/PP149/3/1-5.

194. King's College London Archives, SAUNDERS, Dame Cicely (1918–2005), Papers relating to St Christopher's Hospice, 1943 – 2003, K/PP149/3/1-5.

195. Glyn Hughes H.L. *Peace at the Last: A Survey of Terminal Care in the United Kingdom*. London: The Calouste Gulbenkian Foundation; 1960.

196. Glyn Hughes, *Peace at the Last*, 10.

197. Her Majesty's Stationery Office. *Report of the Committee on the Economic and Financial Problems of the Provision for Old Age*. Cmd 9333. London: Her Majesty's Stationery Office; 1954.

198. Her Majesty's Stationery Office. *Survey of Services Available to the Chronic Sick and Elderly 1954–1955*. Ministry of Health Reports on Public Health and Medical Subjects No. 98. London: Her Majesty's Stationery Office; 1957.

199. Ministry of Health. *Geriatric Services and the Care of the Chronic Sick*. Circular HM(57)86. London: Ministry of Health; 1957.

200. Glyn Hughes, *Peace at the Last*, 12.

201. Glyn Hughes, *Peace at the Last*, 48–49.

202. Glyn Hughes, *Peace at the Last*, 22–23.

203. Glyn Hughes, *Peace at the Last*, 24.

204. Glyn Hughes, *Peace at the Last*, 49.

205. Review of *Peace at the Last. The Lancet.* 1960; 275: 195.

206. Cicely Saunders letter to Brigadier Glyn Hughes, 28 January 1960; Clark, *Letters*, 18–20.

207. Cicely Saunders letter to Betty Read, 6 August 1959. King's College London Archives, SAUNDERS, Dame Cicely (1918 – 2005), Correspondence and related papers, 1948 – 2005, K/PP149/3/1-5.

208. Cicely Saunders letter to The Right Reverend the Lord Bishop of Stepney, 9 February 1960; Clark, *Letters*, 20–21.

209. Cicely Saunders interview with Neil Small, Hospice History Project, 7 November 1995.

210. Cicely Saunders letter to Christopher Saunders, 4 March 1960; Clark, *Letters*, 24–25.

211. Cicely Saunders letter to Christopher Saunders, 5 April 1960; Clark, *Letters*, 29–30.

212. Cicely Saunders letter to Betty Read, 7 April 1960, quoted in Clark D. Originating a movement: Cicely Saunders and the development of St Christopher's Hospice, 1957–67. *Mortality.* 1998; 3(1): 43–63.

213. Cicely Saunders letter to Christopher Saunders, 19 July 1960; Clark, *Letters*, 31–33.

214. du Boulay, *Cicely Saunders*, 122.

215. Cicely Saunders letter to Christopher Saunders, 19 July 1960; Clark, *Letters*, 31–33.

216. Amin A. St Christopher's Hospice: A space for dying. 2015, https://cicelysaundersarchive.wordpress.com/2015/12/14/st-christophers-hospice-a-space-for-dying/, accessed 2 November 2016.

217. Saunders C., Summers D., Teller N., eds. *Hospice: The Living Idea.* London: Edward Arnold; 1981: 45.

218. Smith P. A new English hospice [report], Box 7. Progress reports: 1963–66. 1/2/10. King's College London Archives, SAUNDERS, Dame Cicely (1918–2005), K/PP149/3/1-5.

219. Amin, St Christopher's Hospice.

220. Cicely Saunders letter to Jack Wallace, 7 November 1960. King's College London Archives, SAUNDERS, Dame Cicely (1918 – 2005), Correspondence and related papers, 1948 – 2005 K/PP149/3/1-5.

221. Cicely Saunders letter to Jack Wallace, 28 June 1960; Clark, *Letters*, 30–31.

222. Cicely Saunders letter to The Right Reverend the Lord Bishop of Stepney, 13 January 1961; Clark, *Letters*, 41–42.

223. Cicely Saunders letter to Jack Wallace, 2 February 1961. King's College London Archives, SAUNDERS, Dame Cicely (1918 – 2005), Correspondence and related papers, 1948 – 2005, K/PP149/3/1-5.

224. Saunders C. Terminal illness. In *Proceedings of Health Congress, Royal Society of Health: Symposium on 'Teaching, an Aspect of Home Care'.* London: Royal Society of Health; 1961: 112–114.

225. Dame Enid Russell-Smith letter to Cicely Saunders, 12 May 1961.

226. Cicely Saunders letter to Dr Albertine Winner, 22 March 1962; Clark, *Letters*, 50–51.

227. Amin, St Christopher's Hospice.

228. Cicely Saunders letter to The Right Reverend the Lord Bishop of Stepney, 13 January 1961; Clark, *Letters*, 41–42.

229. Cicely Saunders letter to Sir Kenneth Grubb, 2 February 1961. King's College London Archives, SAUNDERS, Dame Cicely (1918 – 2005), Correspondence and related papers, 1948 – 2005, K/PP149/3/1-5.

230. Cicely Saunders letter to Jack Wallace, 28 February 1961. King's College London Archives, SAUNDERS, Dame Cicely (1918 – 2005), Correspondence and related papers, 1948 – 2005, K/PP149/3/1-5.

231. Cicely Saunders letter to Jack Wallace, 12 September 1963. King's College London Archives, SAUNDERS, Dame Cicely (1918 – 2005), Correspondence and related papers, 1948 – 2005, K/PP149/3/1-5.

232. Cicely Saunders to Lord Thurlow, 28 July 1964. King's College London Archives, SAUNDERS, Dame Cicely (1918 – 2005), Correspondence and related papers, 1948 – 2005 K/PP149/3/1-5.

233. Cicely Saunders letter to Sir Kenneth Grubb, 17 October 1961; Clark, *Letters*, 47.

234. Cicely Saunders interview with Neil Small, Hospice History Project, 24 October 1995.

235. Cicely Saunders letter to Olive Wyon, 2 March 1965; Clark, *Letters*, 80.

236. Cicely Saunders letter to Sister Anne-Beatrice (Grandchamp), 25 March 1965; Clark, *Letters*, 82.

237. Cicely Saunders letter to Lord Thurlow, 3 February 1966; Clark, *Letters*, 100–101.

238. Cicely Saunders letter to Captain T.L. Lonsdale, 19 July 1966; Clark, *Letters*, 109–110.

239. Cicely Saunders letter to Captain T.L. Lonsdale, 19 July 1966; Clark, *Letters*, 109–110.

240. Cicely Saunders letter to Sir Kenneth Grubb, 19 July 1966; Clark, *Letters*, 111–112.

241. Cicely Saunders letter to The Right Reverend the Lord Bishop of Stepney, 27 July 1966; Clark, *Letters*, 112–113.

242. Cicely Saunders letter to The Rev Dr Almon Pepper, 25 October 1966; Clark, *Letters*, 116.

243. Saunders C. M. *Report of Tour in the United States of America (Spring)*, unpublished, 1963.

244. Cicely Saunders interview with David Clark, 2 May 2003.

245. Saunders, *Report of Tour in the United States of America*.

246. Feifel H. *The Meaning of Death*. New York: McGraw Hill; 1959.

247. Florence Wald interview with Neil Small, Hospice History Project, 29 February 1996.

248. Buck J. 'I am willing to take the risk': Politics, policy, and translation of the hospice ideal. *Journal of Clinical Nursing*. 2009; 18(19): 2700–2709.

249. Cicely Saunders letter to Esther Lucille Brown, 16 February 1965; Clark, *Letters*, 78–80.

250. Frankl V. *Man's Search for Meaning*. London: Hodder and Stoughton; 1964.

251. Esther Lucille Brown letter to Cicely Saunders, 30 November 1965. King's College London Archives, SAUNDERS, Dame Cicely (1918 – 2005), Correspondence and related papers, 1948 – 2005, K/PP149/3/1-5.

252. Esther Lucille Brown letter to Cicely Saunders, 17 November 1966. King's College London Archives, SAUNDERS, Dame Cicely (1918 – 2005), Correspondence and related papers, 1948 – 2005, K/PP149/3/1-5.

253. Saunders C. Unpublished text of lecture at Yale School of Nursing, 28 April 1966.

254. Cicely Saunders interview with Neil Small, Hospice History Project, 14 November 1995.

255. Saunders C. St Christopher's Hospice. *The British Hospital Journal and Social Service Review*. 1967; LXXVII: 2127–2130.

5 | The Expansive Years of Hospice in the World (1967 – 1985)

I suppose with my background I wasn't necessarily going to be the easiest person . . . but I was totally concentrated on getting the patients right and I was doing a lot of talking and I was doing a lot of writing and I was doing a lot of travelling[1].

The Hospice Movement

From the summer of 1967 to the autumn of 1985, a period of eighteen years, Cicely was the medical director of the hospice she had founded. Even before it was up and running, St Christopher's was attracting interest from many countries and, especially, as we have seen, from the United States. Although formulated in the specific context of London's hospitals and homes for the dying as well as Cicely's cultural world of Anglican belief and practice, her ideas met with support from American liberals, civil rights supporters, and those of different faiths. Many others from various corners of the globe were drawn to her as a source of inspiration. During these years, Cicely connected to and helped form a global community of activists who promoted hospice ideas. They campaigned against the twin undesirables: terminal neglect of the dying on the one hand and the medicalisation of death on the other. They spoke up for disenfranchised patients locked inside bureaucratic systems where personal narratives and experiences were so easily lost as death approached and the medical industrial complex took over. In time, they gained recognition from the health professions and established a body of specialist knowledge that was documented in the literature and supported, if only to a modest extent, by the evidence of research.

It is now clear that during the years leading up to 1967, the Hospice Movement was already in formation[2]. The opening of St Christopher's in July of that year should not be seen as the start of the modern hospice initiative, but rather as the culmination of a project that made that initiative possible. Although the term 'Hospice Movement' had not yet appeared in the lexicon of terminal care in 1967, its foundations were firmly established. From 1958 to 1967, between the ages of forty and fifty, Cicely had undertaken a remarkable personal project. Harnessing her own faith, her private sorrows, her professional skills, and her indomitable energy, she had gathered around her the support of friends and colleagues who, with her, made St Christopher's Hospice a reality. This marked the high point of one aspect of her vocation, but also the mere beginning of its true purpose. For now the work of the hospice had to be developed in earnest, and its ideas and principles would require testing in practice. The job would involve a huge volume of daily clinical work and numerous organisational duties, as well as ongoing responsibilities and concerns about finance, staffing, and sustainability, that were never far away. There was also the unfolding process of change taking place in the wider environment itself which had an impact on local services — the creation of the Department of Health and Social Security in 1968 by the Labour government, the restructuring of health authorities introduced by the Conservatives in 1973 and 1982, and the gradual drift towards an internal market for health care. During these years as medical director, Cicely experienced six changes of government and observed the efforts of four different prime ministers, culminating with the start of Margaret Thatcher's extended period in 10 Downing Street, that began in 1983.

St Christopher's Gets Going

We have seen how the formation of St Christopher's took place over nearly a decade. Its opening was also a process rather than an event. During the later period, the hospice had to be commissioned. It needed fixtures and fittings, equipment, furniture, and all the accoutrements required in a modern, metropolitan, purpose-built facility. It also required formal statements about governance, management, clinical practices and procedures, admission and discharge policies, principles for staff support, training and ongoing education, as well as a vision for the research that would be conducted there. Cicely thrived on this. She was a detail terrier for whom no issue was too small. In the autumn of 1966, she was involved in a lengthy discussion and correspondence with Council member the Reverend A.E. Barton — about the altar rail in the hospice chapel. He took the view that there should not be one. She wondered how, with her stiff knees, she would be able to get up again after taking communion. She thought that residents of the hospice Draper's Wing, planned for the long-term care of elderly residents, might have the same problem. Eventually they compromised on a moveable bench which could be placed in front of the communicants[3]. With the Bishop of Stepney she had exchanges about the form of the daily prayers. Both she and Helen Willans, of the Church

Army, who was to be in charge of Draper's, thought the book of the Church of South India might be an interesting innovation. She was also keen to introduce daily communion in the chapel and ward prayers, following the tradition of St Thomas's, which are taken by the Sister or nurse in charge, both morning and evening[4]. In this context it might seem surprising that she seemed to pay so little attention to the physical aspects of David Tasma's 'window', although she referred to it constantly within her creation of the founding narrative of the hospice. It had no special decorative features, being just one panel in the modern glazing at the entrance to the hospice. The plaque which marked it was mundane in the extreme and in a style favoured by high-street engravers of nameplates and sports trophies. As a memorial to the 'founding patient', it seemed under-whelming in the extreme. Nevertheless, as Cicely became fond of saying, she had 'built the hospice round the window' and would often be photographed there in years to come, even if visitors found the iconic spot somewhat mundane.

Staffing

Appointing staff to work in the hospice was the single most important aspect of the commissioning process. Here, Cicely's methods were individual and un-orthodox, even by the standards of the time, though it seemed no one called 'foul!' or cried 'nepotism!' Eschewing advertisements, selection processes, and appointment panels, her favoured approach was to select personally people she thought would fit the bill. These could be long-standing friends as well as those whom she had got to know in the context of her own clinical work. They included a friend of a god-daughter, or people who identified themselves to her through her lectures, teaching, and public speaking. Cicely had done lots of talks in local churches and these led to a stream of volunteers offering their services. The organiser of volunteers, who was the first ever to work in a hospice, was a friend of Colin Murray Parkes and came onboard before opening. The first Night Sister was asked to come after hearing a talk at the Royal College of Nursing. More notably, the first matron, Verena Weist, had been Ward Sister to Mrs G. and, as early as the spring of 1964, Cicely was writing to Sir George Godber, Chief Medical Officer, at the Ministry of Health, about her suitability, based on twelve years of experience at the Waterloo Hospital and then time as assistant matron at the Lambeth Hospital[5]. Thinking she might have a research role as well, Cicely unlocked funds from the World Health Organization (W.H.O.) to enable Miss Weist to travel with her to the United States in the summer of 1965, visiting a number of hospitals and research centres. She 'was the sort of matron who would go round and make a bed and get a patient comfortable and speak with the nurse, and knew if she needed a bit of help or something'[6]. Not only did she land the top nursing job at the hospice, she actually went on to marry Mrs G.'s widowed husband, Jack Galton, whom Cicely had in fact appointed as chief steward. The whole hospice attended the wedding, but the match created problems, as the matron protected her husband and he became sensitive about his status: '[Q]uite a tricky situation even for those egalitarian days'[7]. Then there was Helen Willans, whom Cicely had met when she made a donation to St Christopher's in memory of a friend. She was shown round the unfinished building by Cicely, promptly opted to work in the Draper's Wing, and then personally visited and selected all the residents, 'quietly working all the hours'[8]. She went on to be matron from 1971 to 1983, after the sudden death of Helen Galton from cancer. Mrs Cherubim, Cicely's cleaner at Connaught Square, was also taken onto the staff. Likewise, there was the G.P. Mary Baines, who had lost touch with Cicely after medical school, but then heard her giving a radio appeal for St Christopher's in 1964. When she and her husband moved to Sydenham the next year, she was quickly offered a job at the hospice and soon took on a key clinical role beginning in April 1968. That same year, Cicely's old friend from Connaught Square, Gillian Ford, began what became a twenty-year stint of providing medical cover one weekend in four. A few years later, Tom West, one of Cicely's closest friends and with whom she already had a complex personal relationship, was taken on as her medical deputy. In 1966, as she made some of these plans, she wrote to Colin Murray Parkes, expressing her ideas for a 'non-hierarchical staff structure' (it wasn't to be) and her enthusiasm for appointing friends, patient's relatives, and others, all of whom she considered to 'fit entirely naturally into the St Christopher's group'[9]. Looking back, Cicely felt her methods worked well enough: '[O]n the whole, with no appointments committee or anything like that, I don't think we made any more mistakes than are made now, with all the hassle that goes on about appointments'[10]. Her overall approach was captured in the maxim 'Employ the unlikely but not the unstable'[11].

The First Patients to Arrive

The first patient to be admitted to St Christopher's was to be for 'long stay'. It had been agreed that ten per cent of patients (excluding the residents of the Draper's Wing) would be in this category. This was the kind of person particularly dear to Cicely's heart and familiar to her from St Joseph's. Mrs Medway had syringa myelia, a chronic condition that compresses or destroys the surrounding nerve tissue of the spinal cord. She had lived all her life in Bermondsey, but after the death of her husband had moved to be with a cousin in Southend. Things were not going well there and when Cicely bumped into Mrs Medhurst's former district nurse from London after one of her lectures, they discussed the possibility of admission to St Christopher's. The Hospital Board agreed to the arrangement on the grounds that Mrs Medhurst had been a London resident: '. . . so she arrived in a car with two nieces and her lovely mattress with a hole in it so she could spend a penny through it at night, her favourite chair, and her favourite picture of *Christ I Am the Light of the World*, and there she was'[12]. In Cicely's view, 'God sent us Mrs Medhurst. She was the first to be admitted and she was with us for eighteen months and she would have made anywhere in the world home, and she did as much as anybody to make the place a community'[13]. Cicely never again saw a patient with this condition at St Christopher's.

Three terminally ill cancer patients were admitted on the same day as Mrs Medhurst. Alexandra Ward was opened first to accommodate them and they were pictured with Princess Alexandra at the official opening on 24 July 1967. On that day, the other two wards and the reception area were packed full of well-wishers, supporters, and secretaries from relevant grant-giving trusts. The princess unveiled a sculpture of St Christopher, crossing the stream with the Christ-child across his back (Figure 5.1). The work had been commissioned from Witold Kawalec, whose alabaster figure of the kneeling woman had been acquired in 1964 by Cicely to go in the entrance to the hospice and to be in memory of her Aunt Daisy, who died in that year[14]. A Polish exile who had served in the Royal Air Force in the Second World War before studying sculpture at Nottingham College of Art, Kawalec had met Cicely through the Drian

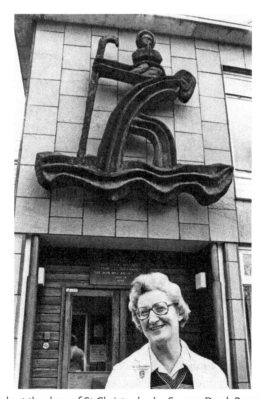

FIGURE 5.1 Cicely at the door of St Christopher's. *Source: Derek Bayes.*

Gallery connection. His sculpture of St Christopher came to be his best-known work. The saint was a paradoxical symbol — yes, the patron saint of travellers, who might be journeying through illness and beyond, but also associated in other beliefs as the saint whose name must be heard each day if death is to be avoided, thus accounting for his popularity[15].

With the opening complete, everything lay before them.

> And we then just got down to the work, and of course I was really the only person in the house who'd ever done whole-time hospice care, and so it was a continual learning curve for everybody. And we had a lot of big staff meetings talking about how do we do breakfast and basic things like that. Chapel had been dedicated in June and so we started out with having services there. We gathered in a lovely Irish cook who really made us really welcome in the dining room and gave us really very good food. And we started out with volunteers, and they were a very interesting group, and worked very hard . . . chief steward gathered in one or two stewards; a very nice local woman came as the most perfect receptionist, like a lovely blonde barmaid, she was a wonderful receptionist; Peggy and her husband, who was a police inspector, used to come in and out. You know, we just gathered it up. It sounded terribly haphazard and indeed it was[16].

By October, Alexandra Ward was full and they were feeling stretched as they opened up City Ward as well. Each ward had eighteen beds and they were aiming to have at least one nurse per bed. Draper's Wing had sixteen people living there. By March 1968, Nuffield Ward was also open. It was a gigantic effort from a standing start.

St Joseph's — Ongoing Links

If all this was not enough, the links with St Joseph's were also re-kindled. After Mother Dolores moved on from Hackney, she was followed by Sister Claude de la Colombiere, described by Cicely as 'a nun large enough to fit that name'[17]. Cicely was invited back and began a Saturday afternoon session in her former stamping ground. True to form, she managed to bring someone else in to help. Richard Carter was a pathologist at the Royal Marsden Hospital and had offered his services as a volunteer at St Christopher's, but Cicely persuaded him to come to St Joseph's with her. So each Saturday afternoon, he admitted patients, she did a ward round, and afterwards they met up for tea. Together with Sister Mary Antonia, whom he came to adore, they had 'a hilarious time' together, full of laughter[18]. It was a re-engagement and also a symbol of moving forward. Cicely could go back with a new assurance to the place where she had learned so much. She had also moved on in some ways since the death of Antoni and now had Marian in her life, if only on elastic.

By the end of 1970, a new houseman, Richard Lamerton, was installed at St Joseph's. He had first visited the hospice as a Bart's medical student and attended one of Cicely's ward rounds. On qualification he asked Cicely if he could come to train at St Christopher's. She considered it no place for a trainee at that time, but soon she was worrying about medical cover and praying for more help. He called again and she took him on, in answer to her prayer. The chirpy Yorkshireman did a year of training at St Christopher's before moving to Hackney on Cicely's recommendation. She came to regard him as something of a maverick. On one occasion she told him: 'I don't know who we were praying for, but it wasn't you!'[19] Nevertheless, she had confidence in Lamerton, and when she was too busy to accept an invitation to write a book on the care of the dying, she handed it to him and kept a close interest in his efforts thereafter, writing the foreword to the first edition[20]. She ensured he was properly supervised at St Joseph's, and she organised for the more experienced Dr Ron Welldon at St Christopher's to do a ward round with Lamerton twice a week. Subsequently, Dr Robert Twycross took on a similar role at St Joseph's. After a period from 1965 to 1967, when medical work at St Joseph's had 'fallen back', now with help from its much younger sibling it was again on a positive trajectory. It was typical of Cicely that, in the midst of her many new responsibilities at Sydenham, she was not prepared to see Hackney lose out.

Growing Demands

It was all 'frightfully hard work'[21]. She was on duty in the hospice every second weekend and would often have some kind of speaking engagement on her weekend 'off'. She was the only full-time doctor, along with Albertine Winner in a very part-time role and Colin Murray Parkes doing one day a week and Ron Welldon mainly deployed on research work. In March 1968, more part-time help came when Mary Baines joined the medical team. There were three wards to look after, four beginning in 1975. Despite the workload, Cicely had to learn to give up some responsibilities and to let go. During the planning years she had been everything to St Christopher's; now she had to devolve duties to the matron and the bursar. It was soon obvious they were short of staff in those early days. On one occasion a nurse came out of Alexandra Ward and told her: 'Dr Saunders if you don't have more nurses, you won't have any nurses'[22].

Despite this, there was a sense of commitment amongst the staff that was palpable. It seemed to be made more so by the fact that those coming to work at St Christopher's from the National Health Service were somehow burning their boats. Investing their careers in a small charitable endeavour, would they ever get back into the mainstream system? It didn't seem to matter. There were patients to be looked after and a constant ebb and flow of new arrivals, deaths, losses, and separations. Cicely began to feel that St Christopher's, at this point, could not do without her. She became less eager to accept some invitations which involved extended periods of absence. It was partly about a reluctance to be away, but it was also the avoidance of returning to find some problem or difficulty which had arisen in the interim and needed her attention. So in June 1969, on getting back from Yale, she had to write to her friend Esther Lucille Brown in San Francisco, explaining she would have to put off the trip planned for that autumn:

> I have come back to the Hospice to find that, although it has managed well enough in my time away, it is not yet really established sufficiently to be happy with my absence for more than two or three weeks at a time. This probably sounds as if I have not managed to establish a viable institution, but you must remember that we are not quite two years old. I know that other people can do pretty well everything, but a child of two years old does rather need its mother to feel sufficiently secure[23].

The reception desk staff called her 'mum'. Draper's Wing had continuity and the familial atmosphere she had found at St Joseph's. Just as in Hackney, Cicely became devoted to special patients there who buoyed her up in times of difficulty. Some of the staff encouraged other members of their own families to work at the hospice. It became common to talk about the whole of St Christopher's as a family. The long-stay residents volunteered in the hospice and had meals in the dining room. By the early summer of 1968, St Christopher's was making nursery provision available for children of the staff. The childless woman now had offspring.

But unlike a family, St Christopher's was also a community of interest and of purpose. Cicely knew this needed to be nurtured and curated. She brought in stimulating speakers to explore challenging questions. She used the ungainly term 'community of the unalike' to capture the diverse tissue of belief and orientation which was held together by something in common. They were also supported by the hospice 'visitor'; first and before opening, this was Evered Lunt, who had been Bishop of Stepney since 1957. As we have seen, Cicely had first met him at St Joseph's in 1960 and visited him at home to discuss her ideas. Recovering from an appendix operation at the time, he greeted her in cassock over pyjamas, something which endeared him to her. When the St Christopher's group first gathered together two years later, he was the one she wanted everyone to meet. He was generous with his time at their regular planning days spent together. If Cicely majored on practical matters, he would follow on with more spiritual concerns. He gave wise counsel on the type of community the hospice should become. He was hugely appreciated for his role at the various dedications and ceremonies that took place as the site was acquired and building progressed. Cicely quizzed him on the forms of prayers, worship, and ritual that should be adopted by the hospice, and he took a keen interest in individual patients as they began to arrive. He, along with others like the Orthodox priest Metropolitan Anthony and Sidney Evans from King's College London, contributed to a series of talks for the hospice staff in the early days — on the nature of persons. He continued to be involved with the hospice after his retirement in 1968. Although the hospice had no official chaplain at first, through Lunt's manner of influence, it was nevertheless a place of religious and spiritual reflection from the start. Nor was this bounded by Cicely's own denominational parameters. There were agnostics, even atheists amongst them, as well as those of other faiths such as Albertine Winner, who was Jewish. For Cicely, 'the idea that there's only one way . . . sort of fell off gradually I suppose'[24].

Specific Influences

Several key people stand out for their role at St Christopher's in the early years. Some had long-standing positions at the hospice; others made temporary visits but produced a big impact. One such was Sister Zita Marie Cotter, a Sister of Charity working as a nurse and administrator at St Vincent's Hospital, New York, where Cicely had first met her in 1963. They subsequently stayed in touch through the formative years of St Christopher's, maintaining a regular correspondence and meeting up in the United States, even when Sister Zita Marie moved to Kansas and New Mexico. By late 1966, they were planning for Sister Zita Marie to make an extended visit from about the time the hospice opened. Cicely was delighted with the six months they had together. She found in Zita Marie someone who made a contribution to the 'foundation stones' of daily life and prayer in the hospice. Zita Marie worked directly with patients, encouraged the staff, and was a skilled facilitator. When she left, Cicely wrote: '[W]e feel at the moment rather as if a light has gone out'[25]. She was the first of many to come from the United States and elsewhere, brought in by Cicely's open-handed invitations, given practical tasks to do, and encouraged to help shape the life and work of the hospice through their individual ideas and skills. No sooner had she left, than Florence Wald herself was arriving for a stint and being warned by Cicely: 'How I am looking forward to it, but I hope you have a good holiday first because we are quite hard work!'[26] In fact it was a very significant time for Wald. She was in the process of making the decision to give up the role of nursing dean at Yale and devote her energies full time to hospice work. She arrived at Sydenham with her husband Henry and their children and stayed for four weeks, working on the three wards and conducting surveys of the various departments. When she returned to the United States in October, she joined with her colleagues Morris Wessel, Ray Duff, and Ed Dobihall to formulate a plan for the New Haven Hospice. Clearly, the influence of St Christopher's was spreading[27].

Barbara McNulty had trained as a nurse at St Thomas's and then became a district nurse in the rural Cotswolds, working for a religious community. She had been part of the original St Christopher's group and, when matron and Cicely asked her to join them at St Christopher's, she took the decision to drop everything in Gloucestershire and move to Sydenham. She was the first Sister in charge of Alexandra Ward. It was a role she had never taken on before, but Cicely was confident in her. Certainly a person who had the measure of Cicely and her approach — she recognised the modus operandi — and the attention to detail which could be over-bearing, but she also saw how it was coupled with a bigger vision in Cicely, that was often rationalised as the workings of the Holy Spirit[28]. One such example came out of a conversation between them about a female patient with severe pain from bone metastases who had made the choice to go home. Due to fear that the patient might become addicted to her medication (a moderate dose of diamorphine, or heroin), the G.P. had reduced and then stopped the dose on which she had been established. The pain returned, the situation worsened, and within ten days the patient was re-admitted, never to leave the hospice again[29]. Reflecting on the case, Cicely was galvanised into doing something.

Home-Based Care

Although a district nurse, McNulty had never considered that St Christopher's could reach beyond its inpatient wards. Cicely, by contrast, already had such an idea in formation, though she in turn had never worked in the community. Their discussion led to the genesis of the domiciliary care service, that began in October 1969. McNulty and Mary Baines (as an experienced G.P.) were the obvious people to take it forward. Now the hospice, already discharging patients home in some numbers, could reach out to the wider community of need, to patients and families at home, to the local G.P.s, and to the district nurses. McNulty took on the challenge with skill and energy. She began by making personal contact with literally hundreds of local family doctors, explaining what the hospice was about and what it could offer. The district nurses also had to be won over and convinced they were not 'losing' their patients. This was made clear by emphasising the 'advisory' nature of the service; it did not provide direct nursing or medical care and was not a sub-stitute for existing services. At first, McNulty was largely a one-woman show. She had to make herself available twenty-four hours per day. Baines added more capacity, as well as the necessary medical knowledge. Another nurse from the wards was then drafted in. Baines ran an outpatient clinic in the hos-pice and members of the team made home visits when they were requested. They took on patients from within the locality, but also from farther afield — Brighton, Gravesend, and Guildford.

As the team expanded, its members spent more and more time outside the hospice. They saw how quickly things could change for patients at home as their symptoms suddenly worsened or as the strength of a family carer ebbed away. They had expertise to bring into the home, but they also had the back-up of admission to the hospice, should it be needed. They could likewise conjure up all manner of other resources. One day, Cicely was having lunch in the dining room with the Rev David Sheppard, the Bishop of Woolwich since 1968, a Left-leaning clergyman and well known as a former England cricket captain. Barbara McNulty rushed in, enquiring if Cicely knew a faith healer, as a patient on the domiciliary service had asked to see one. Sheppard immediately proffered a number to call, that she followed up soon afterwards. To her astonishment, it took her straight through to Buckingham Palace, where a chaplain there, with faith-healing interests, was able to help and subsequently went out to see the patient at home[30]. During the early 1970s, McNulty was travelling to the United States with Cicely and, in close discussion with Florence Wald and her associates, helping to shape the strategy of the New Haven Hospice. By 1973, New Haven was up and running and Sylvia Lack, one of Cicely's early registrars, was working there, in an approach that favoured domiciliary services over the inpatient care model. As we shall see, however, it was not until 1980 that Colin Murray Parkes published the results of an evaluation of the St Christopher's domiciliary service, supported by monies from the King Edward's Fund.

In a paper presented in 1970, Cicely gave a wide-ranging overview of the work of St Christopher's and, with it, a sense of the responsibility the hospice organisation had quickly become[31]. Despite a continuing reliance on charitable grants and gifts, the National Health Service now contributed two thirds of the running costs; indeed, the research programme together with the experimental outpatient and domiciliary service were, at that time, wholly supported by National Health Service funding. A teaching unit was also under construction. By this time, some four hundred patients died at the hospice each year, and between forty and sixty patients were discharged home, at least for a short time.

Soon a majority of patients had their first encounter with the hospice's services in their own homes. A couple of years later, Cicely and Albertine Winner provided more data on the levels of service being provided[32]. The outpatient arrangements at St Christopher's allowed G.P.s to refer patients for pain control, along with an opportunity for them to become familiar with the hospice prior to admission. There were 504 outpatients in 1969 to 1970 and 673 in 1970 to 1971. In addition, home-care service visits were up from sixteen in 1969 to seventy-nine in 1971. St Christopher's had doubled the number of people in its care at any one time simply by the establishment of its outpatient service.

Education

Another component of the vision which Cicely had long anticipated was the provision of a formal programme of education at St Christopher's. This would be one of the things which marked it out from the other hospices which had preceded it. She saw how skills and knowledge could be advanced through practise. Her ambitions for research would steadily bear fruit in the first decade after opening. In addition, education and teaching were also essential to consolidate new approaches and, most important of all, disseminate and build capacity beyond the staff group of St Christopher's itself. By 1969, there were twelve medical students, twenty nursing students, and eleven others spending time at the hospice. They were each allocated to a ward and mainly given practical duties. It was clear they needed a more structured educational experience.

Given the stresses of raising funds to build the hospice, it had been an inspired move to purchase the plot at 57 Lawrie Park Road in 1964. From the outset it was earmarked for a Study Centre, that would be pushed forward when funds could be obtained. These eventually came from two foundations — Wates and Wolfson. The leadership of the centre was patchy during the early days. Cicely acknowledged this new line of development did not always rub along easily with the growing clinical commitments of the hospice. Initially, there was a nurse tutor, Miss Neville, who got the Centre up and running and organised the first conference before moving away in slightly unhappy circumstances to another post at St Thomas's. At that point there were fears the Centre might become a white elephant, an extravagance which would not pull its weight. Cicely moved quickly to address the situation. Two nurses, Dorothy Summers and 'Squirrel' Young, had been coming to the hospice from the outset as weekend volunteers and brought a vast amount of practical knowledge as well as a huge reputation for hard work. One Saturday morning, to Summers's enormous surprise, she was summoned to Cicely's office and asked if she would leave her existing job as a nurse tutor at London's Mayday Hospital and take over the Study Centre. A more formal interview soon followed. Shocked and delighted in turn, Summers accepted immediately[33].

The Centre got going in 1973 and Princess Alexandra was again there for its official opening the following year. For ten years Dorothy Summers was its coordinator (she eschewed the title of director). Quite quickly, Miss Young was also added to the staff complement as another nurse tutor, and Peggy Miller took up duties as a clinical teacher. Summers realized early that if people were to come in from outside for education and training, then it was important the St Christopher's staff members themselves should not be neglected in the process. She introduced a more formal induction for new colleagues, followed up with quarterly study days. Initially a nervous teacher, Mary Baines soon became a very popular contributor to these sessions. Weekly sessions led by Miller were introduced for nursing auxiliaries. A course for volunteers followed next and was widely appreciated, with Cicely herself a key speaker. A regular slot was set up for international visitors. More formal nurse programmes were introduced, such as the Joint Board of Clinical Nursing Studies course on 'Care of the Dying Patient and Family'. Both external students and existing hospice staff benefitted from this. A therapeutics course became an annual event. Tom West introduced an intensive five-day course for G.P.s. Contributions were made to the post-ordination training of Anglican ordinands. Gradually, they moved towards multi-disciplinary education. The hospice became a key centre for education and training at a time when there were few places where it could be found. There was growth and activity, but perhaps an absence of strategy. 'Co-ordination' needed to give way to leadership, and Cicely became increasingly convinced it should come from medicine.

The change got underway in 1980, when American psychiatrist and gay rights activist Dr John E. Fryer spent a year at St Christopher's. He was well known in the United States as the person who, in 1972, had challenged the American Psychiatric Association over its classification of homosexuality as a mental illness. A large, outspoken figure, Cicely had first met him through the International Work Group on Death, Dying and Bereavement, that he had helped to found. Initially, she did not warm to him, but he was persistent in his requests to come and spend time at the hospice and review its educational programmes. At first she told Fryer that St Christopher's wasn't ready for him. He was an 'enfant terrible' who would only be allowed to come when she expressly invited him to do so[34]. He first visited in 1978, carefully watched over by the hospice founder, who the following year asked him to make a more extended stay. Her eventual confidence in him says much about Cicely's openness to new influences and approaches during the 1970s, particularly those inspired through her American networks. Later (and despite her deliberations at the time), she may have considered the invitation to Fryer a 'rash act', but she also acknowledged he did a lot of imaginative things and 'got us thinking a bit more'[35].

He was there from August 1980 to June 1981, took part in senior staff meetings, and also had patients referred to him by Colin Murray Parkes. When he returned to London from his Christmas vacation in Philadelphia, he sensed the turmoil which was erupting around him. He was making Dorothy Summers unhappy; senior colleagues were worried about his influence. There was discontent and rumblings. He quickly defended himself, declared that Cicely had mandated him to make changes and to strengthen the role of medical education. He stayed on as planned and some accommodation was found between the conflicting viewpoints. Cicely's colleagues may well have been ruffled by the preferential treatment he was given — paid salary, an apartment with colour television, and extended conversations in her office over glasses of malt whisky. In turn, they had to endure his outbursts, his use of strong language, and his encouragement to staff to let out their emotions when the stresses of hospice work became too much for them. Yet his restructuring went ahead and even led to some more mundane developments, such as the first conference for hospice administrators. Crucially, he also identified Dr Kerry Bluglass to take over from him as director of the Study Centre when he returned to the United

States, with Dorothy Summers staying on as co-ordinator until her retirement in 1984. Also a psychiatrist and with links at Birmingham University, Bluglass was director of studies until 1985. She was then succeeded by Gillian Ford, who came on secondment from her post as Deputy Chief Medical Officer at the Department of Health, just as Cicely stood down as medical director. By then, the medical leadership of the Study Centre had reached its zenith.

Relationships in the Hospice

As the 1970s advanced, there was a continuing need to attract appropriate staff, and in this, Cicely's methods remained direct and pragmatic. We have seen that her long-standing friendship with Tom West, begun at medical school, had survived physical separation and the experience with Antoni. When Cicely heard he was resigning from the mission field and from his work in Nigeria, she quickly wrote, offering him a job as her deputy at the hospice[36]. He was delighted and flattered. Why she felt she wanted to do this is not clear. Cicely and West had corresponded intensely during his time in Nigeria. In the interim, he had been back periodically. He had attended the laying of the foundation stone, and both Cicely and his mother kept him informed of developments at Sydenham. But, he couldn't come back permanently for two years. It seemed a long time. Cicely told him she would wait. Then, in 1972, on an impulse she sold a rug she had inherited from her father and bought an airline ticket to Nigeria. He returned to Britain six months later and started at St Christopher's in 1973. He wasn't in with the bricks, but nor was he part of the 'second wave' of appointments. His new role concerned his mother. She worried her son was too caught up with Cicely, who might in turn scupper Tom's prospects of marriage. By Cicely's account, he remained very fond of her in what was always a platonic relationship: 'I *knew* that we couldn't ever really say what we felt because that would break what we had, and what we had was safe as long as we didn't get on to a really deep level'[37]. It was a precarious and risky platform on which to build a day-to-day (and hierarchical) professional re-lationship, not least in the charged emotional atmosphere the hospice could sometimes generate. Inevitably, there would be repercussions. Whilst West found the practice of hospice medicine to be relatively straightforward, he was expected to do a degree of organisation and management of the hospice which came less easily[38], and Cicely was constantly looking over his shoulder.

It was an awareness of the tensions that could arise between people in the hospice environment that saw Cicely leaning on Evered Lunt for guidance and succour in the early years. Then a new line of support suddenly opened up. Belgian-born, American psychiatrist and former Jewish seminarian Dr Sam Klagsbrun had first heard Cicely speak on her visit to Yale in 1963. It would be several years until they met again. On this occasion, she was attending a talk he was giving to a conference of Protestant Chaplains in the United States. He was speaking about Job, under the title 'The Man I Hate Most in the Bible'. His purpose was to explore how people of faith respond to anger, often rather ineffectually. He received a tepid response to his talk, except from Cicely. At the end of his address, stooping low and apparently 'ready to pounce', she walked to the podium. Klagsbrun knew who she was. In what he recalled as an impressive and aristocratic tone, she said to him: 'That was the most outrageous presentation I've ever heard'. He apologised if he had offended anyone and explained that his intention had simply been to stir up the audience. Her reply surprised him: 'No, no, no. You mis-understand me. It wasn't offensive; it was really provocative and challenging, which I understand is what you deliberately tried to do'. She went on: '[Y]ou know, we British are very stuffy, and at St Christopher's we're terribly filled with ourselves and I'm beginning to worry about that. We need someone like you to come over there and stir us up the way you've upset this whole audience'. He accepted immediately and set in train a series of annual visits that went on thereafter for thirty-five years, at first engaging in some clinical rounds, running sessions with staff, and talking with senior management, but increasingly working in the role of what he saw as 'management consultant', or in the St Christopher's terminology 'visitor', which was his official title beginning in 1985, when he took over the role from Philip Edwards, who had previously been the hospice chaplain. The appointment of Klagsbrun broke several moulds — Jewish, American, a clinician — yet he quickly became a part of the culture of St Christopher's, to the extent that staff would hold on to tricky issues, tensions, and conflicts to discuss with him on what became increasingly enervating and exhausting visits for him each year[39]. Klagsbrun's involvement from this stage onwards was very important. Only seen for a matter of days each year, he was nevertheless well known to the staff. He also gained special access to the thoughts, feelings, relationships, and tensions that existed within the senior team. If he self-confessedly adored Cicely, he could nevertheless see her strengths and weaknesses, and was candid in reflecting them back. He also maintained a rich correspondence with her between visits, covering not only updates and practical matters at St Christopher's, but also literary, religious, and philosophical ideas which they shared and which served to enrich Cicely's thinking and her work in the hospice and beyond over many years.

Friends, Family, and Marriage

Cicely had good friends from her evangelical days who stayed with her in the years that followed. Notable among them were Rosetta Burch and Madge Drake. Rosetta and her husband Martin moved to Norwich in 1976, where, following a career in business, he was appointed lay chaplain to the bishop. He died in 1978, but Rosetta continued to live in East Anglia, where Cicely would visit her with Marian. Rosetta was an underlying source of good advice about St Christopher's at some crucial moments. Madge too was an 'awfully good listener'[40]; Cicely and she spent long hours in conversation in Madge's caravan in the New Forest, where they had bird-watching holidays. Gillian Ford remained close to her as a friend from their flat-sharing days during the late 1950s, as a holiday companion, and as a colleague who would first volunteer and then be on the staff at St Christopher's. From her early visits to America in 1963, Cicely also forged several deep friendships with people who remained close to her until death intervened. Among these, and in addition to Florence Wald, there was Grace Goldin, Carleton Sweetser, Sister Zita Marie, and Marty Herrman. With each of these she maintained not only regular contact through visits whilst on work-related trips, but also shared holidays and, in particular, regular and sustained correspondence. Cicely's correspondence with Grace Goldin is voluminous and worthy of study in its own right. They first met on Cicely's visit to Yale in 1966, when Goldin was working with a public health colleague on a book about the history of hospitals[41]. Goldin, who lived in Swarthmore, Pennsylvania, was interested in the wider history of medicine and also wrote an entry on 'British hospices' for *Encyclopaedia Britannica* in 1980, and the following year published a substantial piece on St Luke's, Bayswater, and the growth of early homes for the dying during the nineteenth century, that she termed 'proto-hospices'[42]. She was also an accomplished poet and photographer and took many pictures of Cicely, Marian, and life at St Christopher's as well as produced a picture history of hospitals which included some striking images of hospices, patients, and staff[43]. Despite the distance that separated them across the Atlantic Ocean, Goldin was, as we shall see, a person in whom Cicely confided, shared important news, and detailed the day-to-day challenges of life with Marian. In turn, Cicely encouraged Goldin in her own work, commenting on drafts and read her poems with a keen and supportive interest.

Another Bereavement

The spring of 1968 saw Cicely's mother suddenly fall ill. Still living in Highgate at age seventy-seven, she had a mild sub-arachnoid haemorrhage and Cicely arranged for her to be admitted to St Thomas's for treatment. She then went to St Christopher's to convalesce. Meanwhile, Cicely postponed a planned holiday to Edinburgh with Marian to visit some of his Polish friends. Chrissie settled well. Safely ensconced in a single room, and in the words of the Ward Sister 'throwing her weight about in the nicest possible way,' she seemed on the road to recovery and, as Cicely put it, 'she was behaving beautifully and I was getting on beautifully with her'[44]. Thus reassured, Cicely and Marian left for Scotland. As they were driving north in the afternoon, Miss Packer from the Draper's Wing, who knew Chrissie well, went in to visit and found Chrissie writing a letter to Lilian. Suddenly, as the two of them chatted

Chrissie cried, 'Oh my head!' — and collapsed unconscious. It was a major haemorrhage. The consultant from St Thomas's was called; Albertine Winner slept in the hospice overnight to keep an eye on things, but the outlook was poor. On reaching Edinburgh after the long drive, Cicely was allowed time to settle with a glass of her favourite Scotch before she was given the news that had been telephoned through from the hospice.

When Cicely called St Christopher's at eight o' clock the next morning, 16 May 1968, she was told her mother had died at around 2 am. Cicely was three hundred miles away, so her brother Christopher set about making the necessary arrangements. She stayed another twenty-four hours in Edinburgh to recover from the journey, then returned to Sydenham. Up to a month before, Chrissie had been well and driving her car. In Cicely's view, her mother had never been happier in her life than in those last years. How ironic then that, thus reconciled, Chrissie should die in the hospice Cicely had created, whilst her daughter, the medical director, was far away in Scotland, about to begin a spring holiday.

Chrissie's funeral and cremation took place on 21 May 1968 at Beckenham Crematorium, and a service was held for her on the same day at St. Christopher's. In the subsequent weeks, Cicely received many letters of condolence, that rather softened the picture of Chrissie as a shallow, friendless, and difficult person. Some were from friends who had found in her significant wisdom when reflecting on the challenges of life. Others were from clubs and charities grateful for her involvement, deep interest, and support. Three masses for her soul were said at Buckfast Abbey, arranged by the Reverend Mother at Holy Trinity Convent in Bromley, Kent. After some prodding of her brother John by Cicely, a headstone was installed for her at Eton Parish Churchyard, adjacent to Gordon's memorial. In Rubislaw granite, it was inscribed: In Him is our Peace. Chrissie's estate had a value of £38,220 net of charges. It included four properties. In this context, Cicely, John, and Christopher did not overlook Lilian. She was provided by them with an annuity and also a house at 147 Cranley Gardens, in north London. Another curious administrative duty that Cicely undertook after her mother's death was to return three cheques to the Burgersdorp Branch of the Standard Bank in South Africa; they had been made out in favour of Fred Knight in 1919 and somehow had remained in Chrissie's possession. It was the end of an era. As Cicely put it, after that 'I never worried about my parents again'[45].

Over the subsequent years, the three Saunders siblings maintained good contact and Cicely took a keen interest in her brothers' six children, being happy to use her position to lobby for them when she could. In January 1978, she asked her friend and colleague Balfour Mount in Montreal if he knew of anyone looking for an au pair who might take on the middle child of her brother, describing her as a 'bright girl who has done extremely well with riding in Pony Club trials and is gaining confidence all the time', but who 'needs something extra to give her a boost as her older brother and younger sister are bouncing, cheerful extroverts who find life considerably easier than she does'. There were family gatherings of the Saunders and anniversaries spent together. Cicely also maintained diligent contact with her various godchildren like Rosetta Burch's daughter, Rosemary, who much later was to care for her at St Thomas's when she developed breast cancer.

Marian

Since 1963, Cicely's relationship with the artist Marian Bohusz-Szyszko had been developing, slowly and intermittently. She had fallen in love with his paintings and then with him. She became his patron, and his work was prominently displayed in the hospice from the outset. He had professed his love for her, but declared himself not free to marry. His long-estranged wife in Poland was still alive, he continued to support her financially, and his Catholic faith precluded any divorce. It seemed an arrangement that suited him. He also had a son, Andrei, living in Warsaw. There was indeed a lot to piece together about his circumstances.

In the early days, 'he was fairly forthcoming. More forthcoming than I was particularly prepared to be to begin with'. Cicely is referring here to the level of intimacy in their relationship. She was clearly fascinated by this wild, romantic, sexually assured artist, but held back by concerns over his commitment to her and the strong possibility that they might not be able to marry. She readily admitted that 'he was playing fast and loose with me when he was being very much the free artist'[46]. He also seemed light on material resources, with little by way of regular income and insufficient prospects for that to change. As part of a loosely formed Polish University in Exile, that had been established in London in 1952, he gave lectures on Sunday afternoons in various galleries around the city and he saw his pupils on Saturday afternoon and Sunday morning. He adopted the title of professor, that stayed with him for the rest of his life and was used by others, if slightly improbably in the British context. He was clearly highly intelligent. If his English was idiosyncratic, he was fluent in German and Russian. He was also an accomplished mathematician and had taught the subject at a high level during his years of wartime internment. On one occasion, one of his captors, himself an accomplished professor of mathematics, heard Marian explaining an aspect of his own work to Marian's fellow prisoners. Afterwards the officer told Marian it was the clearest exposition of that particular theorem he had ever heard. Cicely attended Marian's London classes whenever she could, even when they were in Polish, and found him to be 'a brilliant, brilliant teacher'[47].

It was through these encounters that she eventually learned he had an Italian daughter. At the end of the war, ahead of the advancing Russians, Marian was in a long march along the Baltic, from East Prussia to the port city of Lübeck.

There, by Cicely's account, he had a 'terrific affair' with a poetess. His lover's cousin was second-in-command to General Anders, whose Polish forces had played an important part in the Italian campaign. Apparently to get out of a heated situation, it was arranged for Marian to go to Italy by army lorry. Staying in a hostel in Rome with other Poles, he soon met Maria Flagiole, who had lost her fiancé during the war. The story goes that she picked out Marian from the rest to be the father of her child. He seems not to have had a problem in assisting her. When a baby girl was born, Marian hastily arranged for his daughter to be baptised near St Peter's. She was given the Christian name of Daniela, but took her mother's surname. Marian then borrowed as much money as he could (he was still paying it off years later when he and Cicely first met) and gave it all to Maria for their daughter's safe keeping. He told Maria he had been offered a professorship in Poland but would not accept it because of his anti-Communist sentiments. He then high-tailed it out of Rome and went to London: '[H]e just walked out and left them'. Daniela never saw her father for years and was told by her mother that he was in prison in Poland. But as a teenager, she learned that Marian was in London and, at the age of eighteen, she went there to find him. Although Cicely and Marian were acquainted by this time, it seems Cicely wasn't told much (if anything) about these past events. As she rather under-stated years later about his daughter: 'I wasn't much in the picture about her'[48].

Two years later, Daniela was back in London and was at one of the weekend lectures. When she suddenly felt unwell, Cicely offered to drive her to where she was staying with friends of Marian. There, sitting on the floor, Daniela poured out the whole account to Cicely, who was by now beginning to have inklings of what was going on. Daniela had brown eyes, fair hair, and was strikingly beautiful. Cicely could see she was Marian's daughter. Daniela was also very angry. Unaware of the story about the money, all she knew was that Marian had abandoned his child and her mother, and for years had not been seen again. At the same time, Marian was drawn to his estranged daughter and wanted to see her more. Over the years, Cicely helped Daniela and her father to understand each other. When Daniela moved to Florence, away from her mother, Cicely and Marian visited her, but the encounter was tricky. Daniela then became successful in the conference-organising business. Eventually, she moved to San Francisco, where in 1980 she had a child of her own, named Maximiliana. Cicely and Marian travelled to see them the following June, when Cicely was in the United States for other visits. In time, Cicely came to think of Daniela as her step-daughter and they maintained contact in the future.

During the stumbling years of Cicely and Marian's relationship, his means of support were tenuous. He was living in the dilapidated environment of the Polish White Eagle Club in Balham, south London. When it was hit by fire, his name card on the door was scorched, but he and his paintings were safe. He then moved to the Polish Y.M.C.A., north of the Thames, near Ealing, where he had a big room from which he could run his classes and also entertain female friends. Things were improving from his early days in England, when he had supplemented his meagre earnings by painting naked girls on ties to sell to sailors. As his income picked up, he sent his wife over-the-counter drugs to sell for money in Poland. He seems to have been the most unlikely suitor for Cicely, the Roedean– and Oxford–educated Christian. Yet, she bought his paintings, quickly drew him into her circle (he features prominently in Cicely's photographs of the St Christopher's foundation stone ceremony of July 1965), and no doubt subsidised his day-to-day expenditures. For Cicely, it seems to have been worth it: '[H]e was fun, he was maddening, he was affectionate'.

Marian had good Polish friends who lived in Edinburgh and to whom he introduced Cicely. Wladek and Hanka Jedrosz had known each other in Poland before the Second World War. He was sixteen years older than her, had left his home country as soon as hostilities broke out, and later saw action in France before moving to Liverpool. Hanka was the daughter of a bridge builder and had joined the secret army in the Warsaw Ghetto. She was among the first group of women ever to be taken prisoner of war. When hostilities ended, she moved to Brussels, where she was the subject of extensive publicity. Wladek read the story in the Polish press and went to Belgium to find her. From there they made their way to London, before an opportunity arose in forestry work for Wladek in Scotland, at Carrbridge in the Cairngorms. As peacetime began to consolidate, he moved to Edinburgh and established his own business beginning in late 1947. A trained forester, with a degree, he set about making pit props. Hanka then began training as a psychiatric nurse, but lost a baby when she was struck by a patient. She decided to re-train as a teacher and went to Moray House teacher training college. They had a son, Aleksander, born in 1952, and Marian was his godfather. It was to this household that Marian made regular visits, especially at Easter and Christmas. Although Wladek's business was not always going well, he faithfully sought to help Marian, keeping him well supplied with canvases of old works that he purchased in Edinburgh's Grassmarket, as well as paints to use on them. On this basis, Marian was able to paint extensively when in Edinburgh — and seems always to have left the paintings behind when he returned to London. This environment, at once unfamiliar to Cicely, also gathered her in. The Polish language, the food, the powerful spirit of people in exile with no hope of ever going home — these were all rich cultural experiences for her. It was a very far cry from Hadley Hurst, but it was compelling, visceral, and a way to understand Marian better — who he was, how his friends saw him, and why they were attracted to him.

The 'Kibbutz'

Cicely began to ponder a way forward for her Polish artist, one that would bring him closer to her on a day-to-day basis, but would fall short of the marriage she really wanted and which he seemed so reluctant to consider. Over time, a suitable solution evolved in Cicely's mind. She was fond of Wladek and Hanka. Like Marian, Wladek too was a colourful character, but his business was not going well and enforced retirement was looming. So, true to form, she offered Wladek a job as head of maintenance at St Christopher's, whilst Hanka got a teaching job in the local Sydenham area. They moved to London in 1969, with Aleksander staying on in Edinburgh to complete his schooling.

In late 1968, Cicely decided to move from Restmorel House in Lambeth to Sydenham, where she could live closer to the hospice. She wrote to her landlord at the Duchy of Cornwall and gave notice of her intention to quit. The move took a whole year to realise, and it was just before Christmas 1969 that she left her rented flat behind, paying dilapidations of £84 16s in the process[49]. It was a practical relocation, but there were also other motives behind the move. For £11,000 she bought a comfortable house at 50 Lawrie Park Gardens, on a pleasant street just round the corner from St Christopher's. There, with Marian and the Jedrosz's, the two couples began a new life together under the same roof. As Cicely explained, the arrangement would bring 'a degree of respectability for Marian and me, but also made it possible for them, because Wladek only had about £1,000 to put into the house'[50]. Characteristically, her brother John supervised the legalities, to ensure everything was in order, though Marian appeared to have nothing to contribute to the financial arrangements.

On moving in, Cicely had the ground floor mostly to herself, whilst Wladek, Hanka, and Marian lived upstairs (Figure 5.2). In time, Aleksander joined the household when he commenced college in England. Hanka took care of the meals and various domestic matters. They thought of it as their 'Polish kibbutz', and after some initial changes it was to prove a lasting domestic arrangement. The difficulties surfaced early but were quickly resolved. Tensions began to rise between the two women of the household. Cicely found Hanka interfering and possessive. Hanka found Cicely ungrateful and overbearing — points she later conceded were true[51]. Pragmatism prevailed. The house was split in two and henceforth they lived more separately. Marian moved downstairs to be with Cicely. He had his own room cluttered with the inter alia of his painting. Her friends and colleagues were tactful enough not to say much about the arrangement[52]. Though she and Marian never shared a bedroom until they were eventually married, she had indeed travelled quite a long way from the evangelical Christian and Billy Graham counsellor of the 1940s and '50s. The estate agent's daughter had at last bought her first property, albeit on a shared basis. She would live there for the rest of her life. Cicely and Marian were perhaps unusual even by the standards of the late 1960s; he was sixty-eight and she was fifty-one. Moreover, he seemed to come and go as he pleased and even kept on his room at the Y.M.C.A. for another dozen years until 1982, when he had his first stroke.

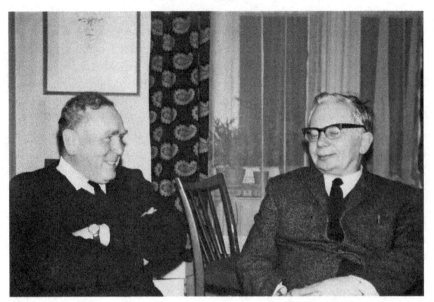

FIGURE 5.2 Wladek Jedrosz and Marian Bohusz-Szyszko at Lawrie Park Gardens. *Source: Aleksander Jedrosz.*

In the years that followed the new arrangement, Marian continued to paint and to be productive. He had space to work on the fourth floor of the hospice, as well as at home and in the Y.M.C.A. Cicely bought him a car, though he was a dreadful driver and burned out the clutch several times in the first few months. He enjoyed holidays with her and foreign travel together, as well as getting to know her friends in many parts of the world. In 1971 they took a three-week holiday in Africa. But doubts would flare up in her mind. In 1972 she was feeling mixed up — still unsure of her ongoing feelings for Tom West but also uncertain of her future with Marian. To disturb her emotional landscape further, on the night of 13/14 February she had a vivid dream about Antoni[53]. She had gone to bed feeling 'all of me is wrong' and dreamed that Antoni had come back. Cicely was going to China to give a lecture and he was in some kind of retreat in Japan. They met and walked through lovely dark trees. 'I didn't tell you I'd come back', he said. 'You've got your other life to do'. Cicely thought to herself, 'Oh, I'll have to tell him about Marian but I won't do that yet'. Then they got to an unfinished town, with red gravel everywhere, and walked across a plank. Cicely turned to Antoni and said, 'Well I'm going to have to go back and you won't come with me, but it will be all right'. Yet they kept on walking and walking, something they had never done together in his lifetime. She woke up feeling 'completely washed over' and would not dream of Antoni again for another five years.

Marian's wife, Zofia Lubienska, was still alive in Poland, a nervous and troubled person who constantly feared for her own safety, rarely leaving home.

Their son Andrei was also there, having taken up the academic career that his father had never realised, teaching in the University of Krakow. Then in 1975, Marian's wife died suddenly in a house fire. If Cicely expected a proposal of marriage to be soon forthcoming, she was wrong. It was not until the beginning of 1980 that Marian padded into her room in the early hours and asked for her hand in matrimony, as long as it was kept secret. In a contradiction typical of her relationship with Marian, she wasted no time in accepting and quickly arranged a special licence for the ceremony to go ahead within two weeks. It was not the kind of compromise she would have accepted in her professional life. Seventeen years after they first met, Marian Bohusz-Szyszko and Cicely Saunders became husband and wife on 31 January 1980. She was sixty-one and he was seventy-nine. At the parish church of St Phillip in Sydenham, she was 'given away' by Gillian Ford, who also provided the celebratory lunch, and Tom West was the best man[54]. The only other guests were Wladek and Hanka Jedrosz. Cicely joked with Marian that the patrician Pole had waited for the English bourgeois, to become a Dame of the British Empire — announced just days earlier — before he would propose marriage to her. Another explanation might be that he was sensing his failing health and wanted to be sure that, in Cicely, he had someone to look after him when the time came, and indeed that would not be long. At first their news was kept from all but a tiny group of close friends. Marian, it seems, was still sensitive about how his Polish friends in London would react. Cicely told the whole story to her friend Grace Goldin in a letter of 15 February 1980. It had been a 'most delightful mixed wedding for a mixed marriage, with two young priests, one Anglican and one Roman Catholic, and four friends only. It was very special (Figure 5.3). It makes more difference than you might think and is altogether splendid'[55]. Marriage was soon consequential for Cicely's schedule and it placed increasing constraints on her travel. She quickly cancelled a planned trip to Israel, using the pretext that her new husband had a commitment at the same time that would be impossible to break[56]. It seems an odd inversion, given her role and status compared with his. Even more remarkable was news of the engagement of Tom West — and not to Cicely, as she repeatedly told people. In late middle age, and almost simultaneously, they had both found married life, but not with one another.

Marriage

She later described her marriage as 'fifteen years which were very happy — deeply, deeply happy'[57]. For most of those years, Marian's health was a concern. At the end of 1980, in early December, he had a prostate operation but was soon recovered and busy organising an exhibition with one of his students and getting ready for his eightieth birthday in February. Just two years after they married, he had a stroke, in January 1982[58]. It hit his speech centre and for a few days he found all talking difficult. Cicely took him to

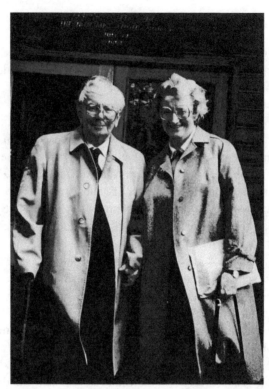

FIGURE 5.3 Cicely and Marian leaving for their wedding. *Source: kept by Cicely Saunders.*

a senior neurologist. His Polish gradually came back, but his English was 'like talking though treacle'. Cicely was 'thanking God' that Wladek and Hanka were upstairs and able to see to him during the day when she was at St Christopher's. She also gave notice that foreign travel would now be severely curtailed. Alarmed at his vulnerability, Marian quickly called on his friends to empty his things from the Y.M.C.A. From now on he would make the hospice his main space for teaching, and Cicely would rarely be far away if she could possibly avoid it. In July she wrote to Balfour Mount, pulling out of her talk at a planned autumn conference in Montreal. Marian was now breathless on walking but still managing to paint. 'I just wish to keep him this way and he feels so insecure when I am away that I hate to rock the boat for him'[59]. By early September, Cicely was even refusing dinner engagements in London, on the grounds that Marian did not like going out in the evening[60]. Following a 'mild transient ischaemic episode' later that month, he was shaky on both legs, wouldn't eat when at the Jedrosz's alone, and declared himself 'very weak' when Cicely was out in the evening. Her marriage was closing in and she declared to Grace

Goldin: 'I have now made the decision never to spend a night away'[61]. Soon, all long-haul travel for Marian was also ruled out of the question. In the coming years, many invitations were declined or sometimes cancelled at the last minute. Cicely would write regularly and in detail to her American friends on the ups and downs of the situation. Marian's speech came and went with his vigour, his painting likewise. On one occasion when they were in Norwich to see Rosetta Burch, he visited the Catholic Cathedral and made a confession which did him 'the power of good'[62]. He was reported to be 'extremely happy and as long as I keep him feeling secure he looks well and paints well and enjoys himself'. Cicely had painted *herself* into a corner of her own volition, and now could adopt the caring role — not as nurse, almoner, or doctor — but as wife and companion. Despite its constraints on her movements, she was deeply fulfilled in her situation. Cicely had always known that one day Marian would need help, and had long determined that it would be she who would provide it:

> Marian is fine, but only so long as he has the constant attention of his wife. It really is intensive tender loving care and he looks fit, has just completed a magnificent Resurrection for the Vatican, and is in the midst of a series of portraits. However, he really hates it when I am away, even for a day. Although he does not come in and out of my office very much while he is painting upstairs, he likes to know I am about in a splendidly demanding way[63].

Soon she made changes to their home, installing a shower off his room when he could no longer use the bath. She dealt with the 'Polish gloom' that could accompany even a minor tummy upset[64], yet felt fully affirmed in their marriage and found in him 'a most enchanting husband'.

Despite his problems, Mariam continued to paint 'with as great strength, conviction, and creativity as ever'[65]. They holidayed with Cicely's friend Carleton Sweetser and his partner Dieter, in 1981, just as she came into a handsome legacy from her father's estate, that paid for all the drinks[66]. In summer 1983, after a holiday of two weeks together with them on the Isle of Wight, Marian painted a portrait of Sweetser in just four sittings[67]. There were also enquiries about Marian's work from farther afield, and a collection of postcards and reproductions was made to capture his achievements. He was interviewed by Shirley du Boulay for Cicely's biography; but, according to Cicely, he did not come across 'in his full glory'[68]. By the spring of 1985, however, Marian had developed 'heart block'[69]. In May he was fitted with a pacemaker, that brought about significant improvement, allowing him to walk into the hospice to paint in his studio there. Despite this, in August a trip to Lake Maggiore was cancelled when Marian had a series of nose bleeds. If he was relieved not to go, Cicely was not, and 'could have done with a break myself'[70]. Indeed, it turned serious and Marian had to be admitted to St Thomas's Hospital for three weeks. She even feared she might lose him, but he rallied and, in due course, by late December, he was home. The following month he was back to painting, gathering together a large collection of pastel works made during his illness and convalescence, and planning an exhibition. It was a pattern of rise and fall that would continue for much of the next ten years.

Clinical Themes and Issues

During these years as medical director of St Christopher's, Cicely maintained the flow of her clinical writings. An article that appeared in 1968 in a Catholic quarterly 'for the sick and those who care for them' elegantly captured the hospice orientation to care in the last stages of life[71]. It called for a positive approach at a time, not of defeat, but of life's fulfilment. Such an approach could recognise the many possible paths to life's ending, in which comfort and care become the prominent aims through a 'middle way' between too much and too little treatment, and where understanding and empathy are vital. We can also see in this article a theme that Cicely had first picked up a few years earlier — the growing attention to notions of personhood, particularly in the family context. Influenced by ideas from Colin Murray Parkes, along with colleagues in the United States, this notion had also been explored in the group discussions at the hospice. The greater focus on families was regarded as an important distinction between care at St Christopher's and the approach Cicely had seen at St Joseph's. The emphasis on person speaks in turn of a growing influence from psychology and theology. It was developed more extensively a few years later.

Psychological Dimensions

Cicely had become pre-occupied with the person as someone in *inter-relationship* with others and how the person, thus seen, is 'being' in the face of physical deterioration. At such moments, 'full-time concern for the patient' becomes essential. This is neatly captured in the statement that professional work in this area has two key dimensions: 'We are concerned *with* persons and we are concerned *as* persons'[72]. This notion of 'being' also found its way into Cicely's everyday language and she became fond of using phrases such as 'she was being very bereaved' or 'I was being rather lost about things'. It is an odd syntax but cropped up so frequently (for example, during interviews) that it tells us something important about Cicely's orientation to the world and, indeed, her own manner of 'being' within it.

'Being' in this approach to caring could be costly to those who gave it. At St Christopher's, the emphasis was upon the development of a multi-disciplinary team which could work together to explore the needs of individual patients at the deepest level, but which could also support and enrich itself not only through the inclusion of a range of professional perspectives, but also by the involvement of volunteers, as well as the children of staff and the elderly residents who were accommodated in the Drapers' Wing. In this way, a sense of community was fostered and enriched which might also serve to ameliorate the consequences of work involving constant exposure to loss, sorrow, and bereavement. In addition, specific attention was also needed to support the staff, and this was fostered through small-group discussion and the regular involvement and psychiatric perspective of Colin Murray Parkes.

We have seen that Parkes had been part of Cicely's development since the earlier years of the 1960s, when they met in London and Boston. Initially, he was suspicious of this evangelical Christian and her motivations with regard to dying people. Would she exploit their vulnerability for religious ends? At the same time, he was drawn to her enthusiasms and drive. He thought of her ambition for St Christopher's as a kind of therapeutic community, and he encouraged her in thinking about it that way, drawing on the ideas of Maxwell Jones and others[73]. She also became interested in the work of Jean Vanier and his L'Arche communities for people with learning disabilities, something that was reinforced when Vanier's sister, Therese, came to work as a doctor at the hospice. Somebody once drew a cartoon of Cicely with a castle in the clouds, it was called 'St Christopher's Hospice' and she was underneath pulling the castle down to earth. The image resonated with Parkes, who felt this was exactly what she was trying to do, to create something almost heavenly on earth. There was a mutual sense of apprehension between them when she invited him to do sessions at the hospice, but he nevertheless agreed. She was glad that he accepted. He was well known and conferred a sense of respectability on St Christopher's at a time when it badly needed to establish a good reputation. At the same time, she was showing him the way, what could be done, and that there was no such thing as 'the hopeless case'[74], a phrase used by C.J. Gavey in the early 1950s, and for whom Parkes had actually worked. Parkes sensed there was so much more which could be done for the dying and bereaved, but he approached Cicely and the new hospice with a degree of caution nevertheless.

The week before he began at St Christopher's, Parkes had a nightmare[75]. He was going from bed to bed in a hospital where people were being tortured and there was nothing he could do about it. His feeling of utter helplessness in the dream made him question what he was going into. Though Cicely could bring about quick results with her knowledge of pain relief, the psychological suffering of the patient was less amenable to rapid transformation. Parkes was drawn to the idea that a community could be created which would be helpful to patients and families. He was interested in families and family psychiatry, and had a lot of knowledge about grief and loss which had obvious relevance in the hospice. On one occasion Cicely told him:

> The worst minute for me is when I have to say goodbye to the families because, during the patient's illness, I've often got to know those family members very well, and then the patient dies and they all come and say goodbye and I realise, just when they need me most, I'm losing them, or they're losing me. I want to change all that. I want somehow to retain a link with the families, particularly those who need it, so that we can continue to help them[76].

This was what Parkes wanted to hear. He was interested in reaching out to relatives before they were bereaved, when he thought he could anticipate their problems. He wanted to get across the idea that the unit of care in the hospice is not the patient, with the family as an optional extra, but should be the family, of which the patient is a part. But Parkes soon realised that he was set to be inundated by the referrals he was receiving at St Christopher's. He could not see them all individually, nor was it appropriate that he was asked to deal with psychological matters whilst physical problems were attended to by others. It was a false dichotomy and ran counter to the inter-related conceptualisation of 'total pain'. Moreover, he was only there one day a week, and yet every other patient was being referred to him. A different approach was needed. Parkes was a realist. He took the view that holism was a 'pious dream'. There needed to be a more effective way to deal with all the problems that were being presented. So, he set about supporting the nurses, doctors, and other staff to deal more directly with psychological problems. If he saw a patient, it was to advise on what others could do to help and to use the opportunity to teach about his ideas and methods. In the same way, he set up an association for bereaved families who wished to come back to the hospice. It was quite informal and was known as the Pilgrim Club. They were trying new things, experimenting, taking risks.

Science and Art

Cicely was coming at the issues from all sides. From the outset, there was an emphasis on the science and the art of caring at the hospice. She knew that there would have to be some kind of recognisable research to validate the work they were doing. But, she was also aware that the process of the work was as important as its outcomes. She was determined that this 'community' would be a place to do things differently, to think differently, and where volunteers, staff, patients, and families could find some sort of meaning at a time of great demands on the human spirit. But in a pamphlet published in 1967, Cicely had also mapped out the need for evaluation of the St Christopher's approach[77]. She saw that research was needed to under-pin the work in a structured way. For the first five or six years, very little was published. However, by 1978, some important evidence was emerging from research studies. She was fortunate to have Parkes's skills as a researcher as well as a clinician. Over time, he built up a cohort of cases consisting of 276 patients who died of cancer in two London boroughs, forty-nine of whom were still under active treatment at the time of death. He found among them much unrelieved pain, whether the patient died in a hospital or at home, and, as patients came into the study, he was able to show that people with serious pain problems were referred from the start to the hospice, and their pain was largely relieved[78]. Unrelieved pain, as reported later by families, was found among only eight per cent of patients at St Christopher's, compared with twenty per cent of those in local hospitals and twenty-nine per cent of those being cared for at home[79]. The work was repeated ten years later as part of the ongoing evaluation of the hospice. Although pain and symptom control improved in the hospital setting over time, psychosocial needs and continuity of care continued to be better approached in the hospice[80]. Parkes also conducted an important evaluation of the domiciliary service. It was based on evidence taken from surviving spouses of those who had been supported at home, as well as a comparison group of those who had not. Published in 1980, it drew upon interviews carried out in 1974 through to 1976, usually about thirteen months after the patient's death. Even though those receiving the service appeared to have more problems and a greater burden of symptoms than those in the comparison group, the results were compelling. Those on the service were able to stay at home longer before they died and spent less than half the amount of time in hospital. The costs of the home-care service were about one quarter those of the inpatient care which it avoided. Family members also reported very positive feelings about the help they had received and the reassurance it had provided[81].

Such work was badly needed. In 1973, in a volume on health services research, Cicely and Albertine Winner presented the problem quite starkly: 'The position of terminal care in this country is at present unsatisfactory'[82]. Although interest in research into this work was growing, much of it remained descriptive and anecdotal, and high-quality studies were desperately needed to promote a rational approach to the care of the dying. Small achievements could be significant, such as when Cicely was asked to write a chapter on terminal care for a volume on the scientific foundations of oncology[83], and the editors thought it necessary to explain their reasons for including a contribution from such an underdeveloped medical field with scientific foundations which were only just being laid.

October 1970 saw Cicely in the United States for a high-powered symposium on 'catastrophic illness'. Elisabeth Kübler-Ross was a fellow contributor, speaking on coping patterns of patients who knew their diagnosis. In the published proceedings, Cicely's article on 'the patient's response to treatment' contains thirty-five clear black-and-white photographs taken at St Christopher's and in patients' own homes. They show patients and staff singly, in groups, and with relatives. Three of the photographs are of artwork produced by patients. One shows a drawing of her pain made before admission to the hospice and is contrasted with another made three months later, when the patient was about to return home. A third, made four days before a patient died, shows a child standing fearlessly before a dragon (of death) which is being fed flowers. Taking up the theme of the conference, Cicely advanced the notion that, whilst catastrophe is defined in the dictionary as 'a disastrous end', it can bring good from people and serve to bind them together — something seen repeatedly at the hospice. Seven photographs, with associated commentary, reveal a range of dispositions in response to illness: feelings of threat, doubt, longing, anxiety, depression; denial; resolute cheerfulness; weariness; and fighting back. In one example, Cicely says: ' "Mrs E., . . . couldn't you just let go?" Her reply: "Well, you know I might if you went away" was astringent as ever but came from real friendship. Next morning she died quietly'.

In this tour de force, Cicely emphasised the inter-connections of science, art, and religion in the care of those with life-threatening illness. The science at St Christopher's, she explained, was in a programme of research which included psychosocial studies of grief and bereavement as well as pharmacological work on the relative merits of different narcotics and their management, plus planned studies on the control of symptoms other than pain. The photographs show how the relief of pain and these other symptoms can sub-serve important work which patients and families may need to undertake in the final weeks and months of life. But whereas 'science tries to look at things in their generality in order to use them, art tries to observe things — and people — in their individuality, in order to know them'. It was a powerful distinction.

The photographs illustrate the importance of welcoming patients to the hospice and the involvement of the staff's own children in the life of the community. One shows a patient busily writing her life story. Here, Cicely is making it clear that 'the art of medicine is concerned with values and therefore judgements. It is the way we look at the essence of a situation, at people with their particular needs and at what is relevant treatment for them'. This is further amplified in the distinction between 'the path of vigorous treatment' and 'the way of doing nothing', both of which are judged to be wrong. Instead, Cicely states in a memorable phrase: 'we are called on to find the middle way of responsibility and judgement'.

Finally, the dimension of religion is explored, surprisingly defined as 'the field of personal relationships between people prepared to give themselves to each other in the context of a common life'. In this context, the relationships between staff and patients and between patients and their relatives are of particular importance. 'We are a community, and this kind of caring and involvement is a religious commitment for many of us.' Cicely suggests here that there is too great a division between the well and the ill, which masks the unity that exists between them. Illness and suffering should not simply be accepted without trying to help, 'but it does mean that we are not the only givers'. Just three years into the operational life of St Christopher's, the founder had succeeded in framing its purpose and values with remarkable richness and clarity.

'Palliative Care'

In 1976, *Nursing Times* published a revised and updated set of Cicely's articles which had originally appeared in 1959 and caused so much interest at that time. There was a sense that the field of terminal care was beginning to consolidate. There were opportunities to review changes that had occurred during the previous seventeen years and to address new debates, issues, and contexts. By now, the increasing use of the term 'palliative care', was coming to denote the transferability of ideas developed in the hospice into other settings, including hospital and home, as well as a broadening reach beyond those imminently dying.

The new terminology had originated with Balfour Mount, a Montreal-based surgeon working at the Royal Victoria Hospital. His first contact with Cicely started inauspiciously. In 1973 he was developing an interest in the care of the dying at his own hospital. He had read Elisabeth Kübler-Ross's book *On Death and Dying* and noted the references there to Cicely Saunders and her publications. On impulse he decided to telephone her at the hospice. Connected immediately, Cicely told him she was on her way to lunch and he should call back in an hour. He dutifully did so. 'Now exactly what is it you want to do?' she asked. He explained he would like to come over for a visit for a few days to take a look at the hospice and how she worked. 'I know you', she replied, to his bewilderment. 'You want to come over with your wife, see a few plays, drop in and take a look around, and then go back. Well I won't have it. Leave your wife at home, come over prepared to roll your sleeves up, stay for a whole week, and I'll have you'[84]. Astonished, Mount was instantly in her thrall. He arranged a visit immediately and was at St Christopher's within days. Completely impressed by the care being delivered at the hospice, he was concerned nevertheless that the approach could never meet the great level of need that existed in the wider healthcare system. He suggested to Cicely that a pilot project should be conducted to see if the hospice approach could be transplanted to the hospital context. 'That would never work' was her initial reaction. Undeterred, he returned to St Christopher's the following year for an extended visit. His medical colleague Ina Cummings also undertook a period of training there. Indeed, it was her calming, clear perspective and presence which were so important in drawing together the team in Montreal and helping to decide how the St Christopher's model could be integrated into a teaching hospital setting[85]. By 1975, they were operational with a service in the Royal Victoria Hospital.

It was in this context that, musing as he shaved one morning, Mount came up with a new name for this whole approach. At one level he liked the term 'hospice' — as an adjective as well as a noun — mainly because he thought no one would know what it meant. But then he became aware that 'hospice' had less-attractive associations in the French language, being more associated with institutional, even custodial, care. He also knew that medicine often made use of 'palliative' treatments when disease could not be reversed. He hit on the idea of 'palliative *care*' that could be delivered in a specially designated unit. Cicely was uncertain about the new term at first, as was Dr Robert Twycross, her research fellow. She told Twycross that some Canadians, like John Scott, didn't like it either, preferring the more positive and community orientation of 'hospice'[86]. But sensing its possibilities, she quite quickly embraced it in the coming years and readily cited Mount and Montreal as it source. In truth, the neologism was to prove hugely consequential as it entered into use across the world and sounded out the message that hospice principles could be practised in many contexts. It was not the setting that was important, but rather the approach to care that was being adopted.

Beyond Cancer

One aspect of this changing approach was to think about how it could be applied to people with conditions other than cancer. This is something often overlooked by commentators on the history of hospice who fail to acknowledge that, whilst the main appeal of places like St Christopher's in the early days was particularly in relation to those with advanced malignancy, there was a concern too for those with other conditions. Until the arrival of Tom West, Cicely had a very part-time deputy in Albertine Winner. It was another of Cicely's informal appointments and served as a measure of support and practical help to the medical director in busy times. Upon her retirement, Winner moved from her government post back into clinical work, via a refresher course at the London Hospital. The two then shared an office together at the hospice. A trained neurologist, Winner began exploring how the work with long-stay patients could develop. They were mainly cared for in Nuffield Ward. At first, Mrs Medhurst was there, along with 'Chuckles', who was meant to have cancer but perhaps didn't. Then, quite quickly, there were two then three people with motor neurone disease (M.N.D.), and one with Parkinson's disease. Winner saw that these patients had their own particular needs and the hospice should be doing something for them in a more concerted way. They came to be an important aspect of the life and culture of the place, creating a cadre of influence not unlike those influential and inspiring patients Louie, Alice, and Terry at St Joseph's. They also brought with them new kinds of clinical challenges.

Winner and Cicely could see there were special issues with this group of patients. Communication was uppermost. For those with M.N.D., speech was almost inevitably impaired. Then came the heavy nursing load as they became more physically dependent and problems of breathlessness became more intransigent. An early patient was Valerie, who had been in the Girl Guides. One Christmas, two former Guides were volunteering and spending time with Valerie. The two worked out that they could communicate with her by blinking in Morse code. Cards were created with each of the letters in code. Cicely would ask on a regular basis if Valerie had any special needs and then Miss Packer would come in to transcribe painstakingly the 'coded' messages of reply. In Cicely's view, this combination of volunteers, an inspired solution, and the involvement of someone from the Draper's Wing could 'all knit together' in a way that made the hospice approach effective and special. Looking back years later, she could remember the M.N.D. patients by name. Ted Hole and Sydney Fellows spent five years each at the hospice. They became 'absolutely enshrined' in her memory. She wrote about some of them extensively — Barry, who was only twenty-eight, and William, the police sergeant. 'They were patients but they were very profound friends'[87]. They were also becoming a second specialist area of interest within the hospice, in addition to the care of those with advanced cancer, and by 1981 it was possible to write up a publishable account of the first one hundred patients cared for at St Christopher's with M.N.D[88].

There were forty men and sixty women in the group. Twenty of the patients had been in the care of the domiciliary service before admission. Mostly the clinical picture was one of progressive wasting of the muscles, especially those of the upper limbs, combined with corticospinal tract degeneration. The patients were admitted to four or six bed bays and were encouraged to become part of the hospice community. The majority had a considerable insight into their condition and welcomed discussion of it. But at the same time, 'truth may be implied but not discussed, may be deliberately avoided or spoken of apparently realistically but with no real comprehension'[89]. These ambiguities and subtleties had become so typical of Cicely's thinking about the situation of those with advanced cancer. Now in the protracted course of a neurological disease, they seemed even more relevant. Sharing fears could help sort out those which were realistic from some of the unrealistic horrors which could surface. Many worries had a constructive response, especially when explored with the patient, doctor, and nurse together. It was found that '[t]he capacity of most people to adjust gradually to an unwelcome situation and finally face it has given the staff courage to trust them with truth when it has been demanded'[90]. This was rarely a cause for regret. In short, Cicely learned that patients with neurological disorders, and their families too, seemed able to benefit from the hospice setting. Most integrated well into the hubbub of St Christopher's, and accepted the deaths of cancer patients that occurred frequently around them, but some found this wearing and were, in time, given single rooms. Children and grandchildren were regularly present in the hospice wards, and there were frequent days out and visits. Most of the families appreciated that St Christopher's did not have visiting on Mondays, and they could regard this as a day of rest. That said, if anyone arrived from a long distance, then the Monday rule was relaxed and visitors were made welcome. As one relative put it, 'there were rules and no rules'[91].

Two of these patients produced articles for publication in healthcare journals[92], one making use of a Possum apparatus which he controlled from the only movement he had, his head, and which lit up the letters he selected. Cicely spent many hours with him as he painstakingly set out his ideas. But despite the strong presence of these patients in the hospice and the contribution they made through their time there and, in some cases, the writing they did about their experience, such an approach became less favoured over the years. Whilst Cicely had made a central notion of the hospice as a community which would include longer term patients and residents, in due course changing clinical norms and cost pressures conspired to reduce the time such patients spent there. Modern palliative care would make the inpatient hospice a place for specialist pain and symptom management, after which many patients would return home or move on to other forms of residential care. But, during the first dozen years of St Christopher's, there was scope to experiment. Cicely and her multi-disciplinary team, that included the physio- and occupational therapy so important to these patients, found for them new ways of living with life-threatening disease. There was painting, chess, typing, writing or dictating poetry, a listening library, collage, even a wine-making set. If the long-term presence of the M.N.D. patients at St Christopher's was to diminish, Cicely was nevertheless doing two important things. First, she demonstrated such patients did belong within the hospice philosophy and, second, she provided practical examples of supporting them which could be used and adapted in other settings. It could be captured in the words of one of the patients to Cicely, towards the end of his two years in St Christopher's: 'not a catastrophic illness, a coming together illness'[93].

A Landmark Volume

In 1978, Cicely's first book — for which many had waited so long — finally appeared. So busy had she been that she had let in Richard Lamerton with a first volume on the hospice approach to care of the dying. He wrote to stimulate both professional and public interest, and a revised and expanded version of his book was later published by the popular Pelican imprint[94]. Hers was a more technical document of record, an edited volume with contributors who had been involved directly with the work of St Christopher's. This is the book which, over a long period, so many had been encouraging Cicely to produce. It was to go into multiple editions, with additional editors, in the years that followed. In the first edition, Cicely wrote the preface, an opening and a closing chapter, and she also inserted detailed editorial notes at the beginning of some chapters and addenda at the end of others. These were all characteristics of her passion for detail, or even an over-weaning predisposition to intervene. Her beginning chapter was important in opening up a debate about the relationship of terminal care to the 'cure' and 'care' systems, arguing that no patient should be inappropriately locked into one or other system[95]. From there, a broad definition of terminal care was outlined — an absence of suffering, preservation of important relationships, an interval for anticipatory grief, relief of remaining conflicts, belief in timeliness, the exercise of feasible options and activities, and consistency with physical limitations, all within the scope of the dying person's ego ideal. As in earlier written works, a subtle and non-dogmatic approach was proposed by Cicely on the issue of truth-telling, that she saw as a matter, based on a relationship, of finding 'the particular truth which is fitted to our patient's need'.

Thereafter came chapters from others on pathological, physical, and psychological aspects of care; on pain and other symptoms; on radiotherapy, chemotherapy, and hormone therapy; and on surgery; as well as on inpatient, outpatient, and home care; plus the National Health Service, the law, and ethics. The contributors included many who had been involved with the work of St Christopher's and others with a substantial interest in the field. The frontispiece reproduced a painting by a St Christopher's patient, used subsequently in teaching, to illustrate the concept of 'total pain'. The book, *The Management of Terminal Malignant Disease*, was the first in a series, and the editors noted that: 'Some of the material is controversial, and no effort has been made to iron out what are sometimes quite marked differences in opinion'.

The concluding chapter, 'The Philosophy of Terminal Care', began with Cicely's re-statement of the concept of 'total pain', including a reply to one of its detractors. It also explained how, following a conversation with a patient, she ceased to use the expression 'terminal patients' in favour of 'patients with terminal illnesses'. The chapter emphasised the need to focus on patients wherever they happen to be. It was not a manifesto for hospice as panacea; indeed, Cicely clearly states its role in relation to other elements within the care system:

> A few hospices will be needed for patients with intractable problems and for research and teaching in terminal care, but most patients will continue to die in general hospitals, cancer or geriatric centres or in their own homes; the staff they will find there should be learning how to meet their needs.

In this first book, she had already seen the wider context and what would become the 'mainstreaming' of palliative care in the future. Thus contextualised, she detailed the essential elements in the management of terminal malignant disease: concern for the patient and family as the unit of care; management by an experienced clinical team; expert control of the common symptoms of terminal cancer, especially pain in all its aspects; skilled and experienced nursing; an inter-professional team; a home-care programme; bereavement follow-up; methodical recording and analysis; teaching in all aspects of terminal care; imaginative use of the architecture available; a mixed group of patients; an approachable central administration; and the search for meaning. The chapter was the distillation of twenty years of detailed clinical practice, self-reflection, and research. The book may have been slow in coming, but it was a hugely solid landmark in the evolution of her approach and a demonstration of how others were developing it. Within a few more years, in a chapter Cicely wrote for a book edited by Manchester–based pain expert Mark Swerdlow, she went to even greater lengths to suggest that the 'terminal' condition of a patient may not be an irreversible state, and 'active', 'palliative', and 'terminal' care could each be seen as overlapping categories[96]. The idea of hospice as a place to tuck up terminally ill people quietly, out of harm's way, was steadily pulled apart — and reconstructed as something far more consequential.

The Maturing of Ideas

There could be no straightforward and simplistic blueprint for the hospice which had been established around the 'window'. The rise of hospice and palliative care in a distinctly contemporary guise was now taking place against a backdrop of modest but growing clinical, educational, and research interest[97]. For Cicely, this effort was about establishing the modern science and art of caring for patients with advanced malignant disease, as well as drawing attention to those with many other conditions who might benefit from the approach. In particular she was eager to see studies on the science of pain control and the underlying pharmaco-kinetic mechanisms at work in the administration of strong opiates. This began with close scrutiny of the methods of pain relief favoured within the early hospices and terminal-care homes, in particular the use of the so-called Brompton Cocktail[98], that had been gaining popularity throughout the twentieth century — a mixture of morphine hydrochloride, cocaine hydrochloride, alcohol, syrup, and chloroform water, but with many local variants and names.

The Demise of the Brompton Cocktail — Robert Twycross

Such mixtures had become widely adopted and were made available for the patient to drink on demand or at regular intervals. In 1952, the Brompton Hospital had produced its own supplement to the National Formulary and the mixture appeared in print for the first time under the name 'Haustus E.' ('Haustus' meaning a draught or potion, and 'E.' perhaps 'elixir'). This version was then listed in Martindale's Extra Pharmacopoeia in 1958. In 1976, buoyed by its use in the newly opening hospices, it had appeared in the British National Formulary and gradually had come to be known by several different names: Brompton Cocktail, Brompton Mixture, Mistura euphoriens, Mistura pro moribunda, Mistura pro euthanasia, even 'Saunders' Mixture'. Some practitioners in the United Kingdom favoured diamorphine over morphine; some even dropped the cocaine and used morphine and diamorphine together in the mixture[99]. It was not universally favoured or understood. Much of the fear came from a lack of knowledge about how to use morphine properly. Professor Duncan Vere, reflecting back in later life on his experience in London in the mid 1960s, refers to the formula as 'Mist Obliterans' —'a matter of patients being rendered so that they did not know what they were doing by doctors who certainly did not know what they were doing'[100].

In her early writings, Cicely had been eager to promote this rather exotic formulation, but it was St Christopher's research fellow Robert Twycross who set out to scrutinise the potion in detail in what became a series of classic studies, the first of their kind undertaken in the hospice setting. Twycross had first met Cicely in the freezing winter of early 1963 at an international Christian student conference where she was one of the senior members in a workshop on 'health and healing'. Her contributions and reflections resonated with him. The following year, whilst still an undergraduate at Oxford University, he created the Radcliffe Christian Medical Society simply to give a pretext for inviting her to speak there on the management of pain in terminal cancer. Cicely stored away these things — as we have seen, from quite early days she was on a personal recruitment campaign to attract the right people to St Christopher's. So it was that five years later, in 1968, an invitation was duly made to Twycross to join her team at the newly opened hospice. Perhaps surprisingly, he declined the offer, in favour of completing his Membership of the Royal College of Physicians, and it was not until 1971, and following the death of Ron Welldon, the first clinical research fellow, that with further encouragement from Cicely, he finally began work at Sydenham. It was typical of her tenacity — a talent like Twycross first identified in 1963, eventually brought into the coop eight years later[101].

Now, Twycross subjected the Brompton Cocktail to unparalleled clinical and scientific scrutiny. Over the next few years his work focussed on a number of areas: standardisation of the mixture, the relationship between the active constituents and the vehicle, the keeping properties of the mixture, the role of cocaine within it, and also the relative efficacy of the morphine and diamorphine. Indeed, between 1972 and 1979, Twycross produced thirty-nine publications on these and related themes. Towards the end of the period, he reported on an important breakthrough in a controlled trial of diamorphine and morphine in which the two drugs were administered regularly in a version of the Brompton mixture containing cocaine hydrochloride in a ten-milligramme dose[102]. A total of 699 patients entered the trial and, of these, 146 crossed over after about two weeks from diamorphine to morphine, or vice-versa. In the female crossover patients, no difference was noted in relation to pain or other symptoms evaluated, but male crossover patients experienced more pain and were more depressed while receiving diamorphine, suggesting the potency ratio was lower than expected. Twycross concluded that if this difference in potency is allowed for, then morphine is a satisfactory substitute for orally administered diamorphine, but the more soluble diamorphine retained certain advantages when injections were required and doses were high. In a second trial[103], that was described in a letter to the *British Medical Journal*, the morphine and diamorphine elixirs were compared with cocaine added and without it. There were forty-five satisfactory crossovers, and because the trends within the morphine and diamorphine groups were similar, they were combined for purposes of analysis. The study showed that introducing a ten-milligramme dose of cocaine after two weeks resulted in a small but statistically significant difference in alertness; but, stopping cocaine after this period had no detectable effect. Twycross adjudged that, at this dose, cocaine is of borderline efficacy and tolerance to it develops within a few days.

As a result of this work, in May 1977 — almost exactly a decade after opening — the routine use of cocaine with patients at St Christopher's was abandoned and, in particular, morphine was prescribed alone in chloroform water, together with an antiemetic when indicated. Cicely, through the work of Twycross, had tested her intuitions and found them wanting. She had then acted on the consequences. In 1979, as one of three chapters he wrote for the important trilogy *Advances in Pain Research and Therapy*, edited by John Bonica and Vittorio Ventafridda, Twycross drew together his summative statement on the matter[104]. There had been, he suggested, a tendency 'to endow the Brompton Cocktail with almost mystical properties and to regard it as the panacea for terminal cancer pain'. Generously, he allowed that if the physician is aware of the potential side effects of the main ingredients, then its use might be maintained. But set against this was the disadvantage to the pharmacist, the potential unpalatability to the patient, the higher financial costs incurred, and the restricted potential for the physician to manipulate the doses given. The Brompton Cocktail was about to depart from the received wisdom of the new palliative-care community. Cicely and Twycross, with support from Duncan Vere at the London Hospital, began to see the wider implications of all this. It became clear that simpler, more predictable means of pain control could be adopted; that narcotics could be used safely; and, in particular, that morphine was just as effective as diamorphine.

At St Christopher's, Twycross and Welldon before him, had been early in a sequence of talented doctors who began to forge both the clinical and the evidence base for the new field of hospice medicine. In 1976, Twycross moved to Oxford to lead his own National Health Service hospice. There he continued the pain work with new fellows working under his direction, first Dr Geoffrey Hanks and then Dr Claud Regnard — two doctors who later had a significant impact on the field in their own right. Initially, the junior doctors at St Christopher's were graded as senior house officers. Then the hospice began to take registrars for training, and for a period it was the only place that did so. In the years leading up to 1987, before the specialty was formally recognised, it became a magnet for young doctors seeking to be trained in this new branch of medicine. In total, thirty-three doctors availed themselves of this opportunity until a formal training programme in palliative medicine became available through the medical Royal Colleges[105]. Many of these early registrars moved on to become medical directors in other places as the great expansion of independent hospices got underway during the 1980s, when ten new hospices opened every year. The teaching of these people fell mainly to Tom West and Mary Baines, and, to a lesser extent, Cicely, who for much of the time was now pre-occupied with things beyond the immediate clinical realm.

Total Pain Further Explored

During the early years at St Christopher's, Cicely's concept of 'total pain', first laid out in the important papers of the mid 1960s, was further elaborated by researchers, clinicians, and indeed patients themselves. It was important to Cicely. She drew on it heavily in her teaching and writing, and she was keen to develop it further, sensing that it resonated with many people. The concept entered into the fabric of daily life at the hospice and became a defining feature of its philosophy and approach. By 1985, and her retirement as medical director, palliative medicine was just two years away from specialty recognition in the United Kingdom. It is not unreasonable to view the concept of total pain as a major element within the armamentarium of the new discipline. Its influence was powerful and wide-ranging.

When considering Cicely's writings on total pain and related subjects, several publications in the period 1968 to 1985 merit attention. The notion that chronic pain presents particular challenges to the clinician is regularly stated in her work at this time. In particular, it is seen as a problem on the level of meaning, for such pain can be timeless, endless, meaningless, bringing a sense of isolation and despair[106]. This is in stark contrast to the acute pain, familiar in teaching hospitals, which so often is seen as purposive — for example, in the diagnostic process as an indicator of problems or post-operatively as a staging post on the road to recovery. An important chapter published in 1970 describes chronic pain as 'not just an event, or a series of events . . . but rather a situation in which the patient is, as it were, held captive'[107]. Cicely saw that in terminally ill patients, a major challenge is to avoid the onset of such pain by active strategies of prevention — in particular, the regular giving of strong analgesia in anticipation of, rather than in response to, the onset of pain. She had first seen this in action at St Luke's, and in her days at St Joseph's she had adopted the oft-repeated maxim: 'constant pain needs constant control'. At the same time, she always emphasized the value of listening, as in the patient who said 'the pain seemed to go by just talking'. If terminal pain could be regarded as an illness in itself, then the use of drugs would not simply be a matter of technique, but also the expression of a commitment between one person and another. She was also being encouraged by Mary Baines to ask more about the causes of pain[108]. In short, Cicely's thinking and practice were moving to new levels of sophistication and subtlety.

Crucially, she saw the relief of pain as the most vital component in confronting the issue of euthanasia, for pain in the final stages of cancer is something that had attracted the imagination of the public and was a regular theme in public debate[109]. It was therefore important to demonstrate to the public that pain could be avoided. The use of moderate doses of strong opiates was a core feature of this. For example, during the 1970s, only ten per cent of patients cared for at St Christopher's Hospice needed a dose of more than thirty milligrammes of diamorphine. Moreover, it was found that by providing physical relief, opportunities then arose for communicating with the patient on a much deeper level, not least on the complex issue of what to disclose about the prognosis.

But Cicely also had to beware of mis-interpretations of her approach. There was unwelcome publicity following the screening on German television of a film about the hospice in 1971, in which St Christopher's was portrayed as some kind of 'death clinic'. That same year, she cautioned one American correspondent that she was not intending to induce a 'high' in her dying patients and was certainly not in favour of the use of L.S.D., that she regarded as a dangerous drug she would never use[110]. Despite this, and to Cicely's dismay, St Christopher's was linked to the use of L.S.D. in articles which appeared in *The New York Times* and *Newsweek* in December 1971[111]. The following year she wrote a slightly hectoring letter to Elisabeth Kübler-Ross requesting that she did not use the phrase 'hospice for the dying' when referring to St Christopher's[112]. By the late 1970s, enquiries from journalists about visits and interviews were mounting. She was particularly anxious that foreign-language pieces gave an accurate representation of the work of the hospice. When a Swedish journalist made a request to visit, she pointed out rather sharply that a more economical use of time would be for him to talk to nurses in his own country who had already been to Sydenham and were well acquainted with the St Christopher's approach[113].

Despite such concerns and irritations, over time there was a growing confidence within the world of hospice that the complex and multi-layered symptoms associated with terminal pain could be attended to effectively by a combination of the well-informed use of narcotics and a sophisticated understanding of the emotional, spiritual, and social problems which might also occur for those with terminal illness. 'Total pain' had become firmly established as a central concept within the emerging palliative care specialty and was proving useful in clinical work, in teaching, and (to a lesser extent) in research.

The New Science of Pain Relief

By 1973, it had become possible for Cicely to refer more fully to some of the research on pain being carried out at St Christopher's[114]. Pain was acknowledged to be a problem still inadequately tackled, whether in the patient's own home or in the busy general hospital ward. One part of the difficulty was that the constant pain of terminal cancer was not alleviated by earlier teachings to the effect that doses of narcotics should be spaced as widely as possible to avoid the onset of dependence. Fears about dependence also limited the availability of morphine and diamorphine in some countries, and double-blind trials at St Christopher's were designed to shed light on the relative merits of the two drugs. Another problem was that of titration, the careful grading of the dose to achieve the desired effect, that was largely seen as a subjective process, although by 1976 it was possible to refer to the use of radio-immunoassay as a method for measuring the level of drugs in the body, thus allowing Twycross's research to show that the use of opiates with terminally ill patients does not escalate continually, and might even decline[115].

The liberal use of pain medication could alarm doctors who had been socialised into using morphine with extreme caution. Since the early twentieth century, greater regulation of the use of opiates in several countries meant that patients could find it difficult to get adequate pain relief. Both doctors and patients were concerned about the possibility of addiction to strong drugs. Reinforcing this perspective, the endurance of pain without resort to powerful narcotics was portrayed as a test of moral fortitude and, in the case of cancer, an inevitable aspect of advanced malignancy. Prior to the 1970s, cancer pain had generally received little international attention as either a clinical or a public health problem, and it was often regarded as an intractable, not fully controllable, consequence of the disease. Since then, John Bonica had been driving the development of the International Association for the Study of Pain (I.A.S.P.). He had gathered together an international group in 1973, in Issaquah, Washington, near his base in Seattle. Buoyed with enthusiasm, it held its first World Congress in Florence in 1975 and the first issue of the journal *Pain* was published that same year. Pain specialists Dr Kathleen Foley from the United States and Dr Vittorio Ventafridda from Italy organised a follow-up meeting specifically on cancer pain immediately after the Congress in Florence, and this was attended by 150 people. Research presented at this and subsequent meetings suggested physicians had the means to relieve even severe cancer pain and that the principal factors contributing to poor pain management were legal barriers against opioid use and a lack of knowledge in pain management on the part of clinicians. Soon the National Cancer Institute in the United States was supporting work on the epidemiology of cancer pain in a collaborative study involving five centres. Following the close links that Twycross and Cicely had developed with these groups, St Christopher's also became involved in the programme. Some of the participants went on to contribute to the first International Symposium on Cancer Pain.

Held between 24 and 27 May 1978 on one of the Venetian islands, the meeting became a landmark event in the history of the field and resulted in a hefty volume, edited by Ventafridda and Bonica. Famously, it was the site of a stand-off between Twycross and Ray Houde of Memorial Sloan Kettering in New York. They clashed on three key issues: the question of 'tolerance' to opiates, the rule of giving analgesia 'by the clock', and the benefits of parenteral versus oral administration of morphine. Perhaps urged on by Cicely's presence at the meeting, and eager to get across the British hospice perspective, Twycross argued there was little evidence of tolerance, advocated for careful titration of the drug, and pressed forcibly for a rigid approach to regular giving. Despite the controversies, both Cicely and Twycross were asked to write chapters for one of the volumes reporting the proceedings[116]. Cicely took the unusual step of using patients' paintings and drawings, case histories, and research in combination to develop her argument. One individual series of pictures was particularly telling. It showed the feeling of being impaled by a red hot iron, of total isolation from the world, of the implacable heaviness of pain or, in one case, the feeling that 'I am a scrap heap'. Another woman who had experienced a year of relentless pain from carcinoma of the pancreas drew it as a small rodent eating into the side of a tree trunk. The few traces of green at the top were described as 'my life trying to get through'. By attention to all aspects of such pain, the possibility of its relief came in sight. So, rather unusually, Cicely was able to state, 'Vital signs in a ward specializing in the control of terminal pain include the hand steady enough to draw, the mind alert enough to write poems and to play cards, and, above all, the spirit to enjoy family visits and spend the last weekends at home'. This was revolutionary and almost an ironic take on the 'vital signs' normally observed in hospital wards at that time — temperature, heart rate, respiratory rate, and blood pressure. She went on to argue that good care using this approach could also be delivered in a variety of settings and was not dependent upon the availability of an inpatient hospice facility.

At the beginning of the 1980s, another substantial chapter on pain management at the end of life appeared from Cicely's pen (she seems hardly ever to have used a typewriter and never a computer), this time in Mark Swerdlow's collection *The Therapy of Pain*[117]. There she cited examples from published studies conducted between 1954 and 1978 which gave evidence of unrelieved terminal pain. By contrast, data on a series of 3,362 patients cared for by St

Christopher's between 1972 and 1977 — significantly exceeding the numbers she had so impressively generated at St Joseph's — showed that only one per cent had continuing pain, though more than three quarters presented to the hospice with such problems. The achievement of these results, however, could occasion the phenomenon of 'staff pain', resulting from prolonged exposure to the suffering of patients and families facing death. Although the need for formal staff support was acknowledged and described, it was argued that 'the resilience of those who continue to work in this field is won by a full understanding of what is happening and not by a retreat behind a technique'. The same chapter made the important point for those countries in which diamorphine was unavailable, that morphine was now the preferred analgesic of the two. The issue of morphine versus diamorphine had been significant. If the Americans in particular were anxious about morphine, most of the world, it seemed, was more concerned about diamorphine — heroin.

So important was the issue in Cicely's mind that she had a grant lined up to compare the two even before St Christopher's opened. There had been close discussions about it with Sir George Godber, the government's chief medical officer, beginning in 1964, and Gillian Ford had also intervened to help. The work was initiated in 1969 by Ron Welldon, St Christopher's Sir Halley Stewart Clinical Research Fellow, who in due course identified the equivalent dose of the two drugs. Then, one year later, in November 1970, he died suddenly and the work came to a halt. As we shall see later, in a place where death was all around, his passing was particularly hard to endure. But in due course, Twycross came in and completed the study[118]. It was terribly important work. Cicely had become enthusiastic about the properties of diamorphine whilst working at St Joseph's, but she knew it was essential to test this out, not least with a drug that was not available in most parts of the world and was also heavily demonized as the preference of addicts and misfits. Much later she expressed some pride in what had been done:

> If you're going to be proved to be wrong, which I was, because there was no clinical observably difference between the two drugs, it's very nice if you set the study up in the first place, which I must say I've said an awful lot of times, I'm afraid, in a rather boastful way. We could say to the rest of the world, 'we haven't got a magic drug that you haven't got' and 'it's not the drug that you use it's the way that you use it'. And that was a completely new look in the pain research field as far as I know[119].

Social Work at the Hospice

Given Cicely's history as an almoner, it is surprising that social work did not figure prominently in the St Christopher's team from the outset. It is perhaps a marker of how far she had become absorbed in the medical and nursing dimensions and their linkage to aspects of spiritual care and personhood that she could appear to overlook the important skills and family casework knowledge which she had learned as an almoner. Eventually, more than a decade after opening, a social work position was advertised, albeit at a rather junior level. Characteristically, it was filled in an unconventional manner. Elizabeth Earnshaw Smith had read Social Science as a mature student at Edinburgh University and then gone on to a career in social work. She worked in hospitals in Edinburgh and London, rising to a senior position at St Charles's, Notting Hill, where she saw how abject poverty and social disadvantage were intertwined with health, illness, and the role of social and medical services. Ten years away from retirement, she felt she was getting too far from the coalface of clinical practice. In late 1979, she saw that St Christopher's was looking to make its first social work appointment. She had followed the progress of the hospice with interest, having first heard Cicely speak in Edinburgh. She had also been in the habit of sending social work trainees to Sydenham for a day of orientation, but was disappointed that they were always looked after by nurses. She sensed a possibility and so contacted Cicely and Helen Willans, and made an arrangement to see them one Sunday. She explained she was interested in hospice social work, but the position as advertised was too junior and didn't make sense when there was so much leadership, teaching, and policy to develop in relation to the role of social workers with the care of the dying. St Christopher's, she felt, should be taking a key role in this for the whole of London. Cicely listened with interest. She was used to this approach to hiring staff and, soon afterwards, took the case to the St Christopher's Council, which agreed to the appointment of Earnshaw Smith at the same level as her existing post. She took up her new role at the hospice in January 1980[120]. Within a few months, this extremely experienced social worker was asking challenging questions — about the triumvirate of Cicely, Willans, and West which ran the hospice but seemed remote from the rest of the staff, and about why social work and physiotherapy seemed to be appendages to the core professions. Most significantly, she began to bring a reverse logic to the care of the hospice patients, asking the staff to focus on the strengths of their patients and those of their family members, encouraging them to use these and to build a sense of capacity rather than of deficit in their orientation. They used family trees to help visualise this, and learned more about the importance of previous illness, losses, deaths, and bereavements, and how these affected the current situation. Encouraged by Cicely's emphasis on the importance of 'endings', they also looked more closely at the immediate circumstances of death, its continuing importance for those left behind, and the need to consider this in any bereavement care that followed. St Christopher's was now strengthening its approach to this type of work and moving well beyond the model Cicely had first seen demonstrated at St Joseph's.

An International Showcase

In June 1980, St Christopher's held a special conference involving participants from seventeen countries. The idea had come from Dorothy Summers, Co-ordinator of Studies at St Christopher's. She wanted to demonstrate that the hospice, that had 'taught Bal Mount all he knew', could also, like him, put on a successful international meeting. They took the theme of a Bar Mitzvah as an explicit salute to David Tasma, the Jewish 'first patient' and also an acknowledgement of how the hospice had now 'come of age'. Cicely hand-picked the speakers from her extensive international address book. There were three days of sessions and then another day spent visiting some of the hospices in southern England that had opened in the time since St Christopher's got going, as well as St Joseph's. The last day was a huge celebration of the collective hospice endeavour.

The contents of the event were captured in a subsequent edited collection[121]. Its eight chapters were written by no less than twenty-eight contributors, from the United Kingdom, Canada, the United States, South Africa, Australia, Holland, and India. The contributions included extensive discussion of hospice philosophy and practice, but also some critical self-reflection on the state of the Hospice Movement worldwide. Cicely noted in the preface:

> It was obvious that the conference believed that their work should be inte-
> grated with general medical practice, forming a complementary local resource
> and service. They recognised that much excellent 'hospice care' was carried
> out without use of the title and that the greatest impact of the movement was
> already being seen in the way that people were being cared for in conventional
> settings.

The section on hospice philosophy made explicit reference to David Tasma as 'St Christopher's founding patient' and contained one of the first detailed accounts of his legacy — in particular, his 'window in your home'. This was followed by Cicely's later much mis-quoted comment: 'We moved out of the National Health Service with a great deal of its interest and support, in order to build round that window. We moved out so that attitudes and knowledge could move back in . . . .' The Hospice Movement therefore continued to be concerned both with the sophisticated science of treatments and with the art of caring, bringing competence alongside compassion. This, in turn, raised other dichotomies, such as balancing the needs of the individual with those of society as a whole, and the creative tension between the assurance of faith and the flexibility of tolerance.

Cicely and St Christopher's were also stimulating other developments, some of them close to home. Thelma Bates was a consultant radiotherapist who had re-trained at St Thomas's after years of clinical experience in Britain and New Zealand[122]. She visited and took an interest in St Christopher's soon after its opening. Then, in 1974, Cicely suggested that Mary Baines should spend a week at St Thomas's to see how a radiotherapy department worked. Baines came away much impressed by the value of radiotherapy and the benefits, in some cases, of just a single dose for pain and symptom relief. Bates was duly invited back to Sydenham on an occasional basis to see patients, and she began referring some for radiotherapy or chemotherapy. The two parties were learning from each other in ways which might have seemed surprising. This was a big step forward from patients 'growing fat' in their beds, that Cicely had seen at St Joseph's and that she was clearly so keen to move beyond. It was another example of the way the 'palliative-care' approach was building on the hospice model and taking it in new directions. When Bates learned from Cicely that a team had been established to bring hospice principles into St Luke's Hospital, New York, her interest was further stimulated. The work had been spearheaded by the hospital chaplain, Carleton Sweetser, who had spent time at St Christopher's and had been able to mobilize his colleagues to look at ways to foster hospice skills across the hospital, rather than to designate specialist beds for terminal care. The idea was refreshing and new. Bates went to New York to see how it worked, then came back to London and began devising a plan. When the first hospital support team in palliative care got going at St Thomas's in 1976, Bates had been able to secure the involvement of nurse Barbara Saunders and doctor Andrew Hoy — both trained and highly experienced from their years at St Christopher's. The concept was also spreading in New York, and a working group to plan a similar team was now underway at the prestigious Memorial Sloan-Kettering Cancer Center[123].

By 1980, in her early sixties and recently married, Cicely was entering, albeit unknowingly, into her final five years as medical director. She was enjoying a period of significant personal and professional fulfilment. It was a moment to feel more expansive, to think freely, and to try out new ventures. In this spirit she started to bring together a small collection of writings in a volume called *Beyond All Pain*, that was published by S.P.C.K. in 1983[124]. It was the product of her diligent daily reading over several years. The compact book of eighty-eight pages comprised a personal selection of poems, prayers, and other writings which Cicely had found helpful both in her work and in her own personal encounters with illness, loss, and sorrow. It was offered to those who face death and suffering, and also those who care for them. The writings were grouped under five headings: the search for meaning, anger, suffering, dying, and resurrection. There were contributions from the work of writers of diverse orientation and character, including the founder of logo-therapy and concentration camp survivor Viktor Frankl, theologian Teilhard de Chardin, and novelist D.H. Lawrence. Also present were some poems by patients cared for at St Christopher's. Although the publisher reduced the emphasis on bereavement which she had wanted for the book, taking out three sections in the process, Cicely was pleased with her 'little volume' and sent it enthusiastically to many friends and colleagues. It was, at one level, a personal indulgence, but at another it was a symbol of her breadth of spirit, depth of vision, and awareness that these ideas needed a wider public. In due course, she would revise and further extend the collection.

A Global Influence

Between 1967 and 1985, Cicely produced, individually and with others, around eighty-five publications, appearing in several languages and in numerous countries[125]. She wrote for clinical journals and prestigious textbooks, for religious publications, and for the wider public. Three clinical and organisationally oriented books on hospice and palliative care appeared, one of them was soon produced in a second edition and another was translated into French. Her work appeared in the proceedings of symposia and conferences, it was described in magazines and newspapers, and it became the subject of documentary films. Links with overseas colleagues produced a growing cross-fertilisation of ideas.

Early Origins and Contemporary Scene

During this period there began to be a degree of reflection on the state of the phenomenon which was developing around hospices and related activity. Perhaps the first published work to use the term 'Hospice Movement' is the revised 1980 second edition of Richard Lamerton's book on the care of the dying, that devoted an entire chapter to the subject[126]. Cicely also became interested in the early origins of homes and hospices for the dying. In preparing the hospice's annual report for 1972, she wrote to Grace Goldin[127], asking her for more insight into this. Goldin's entry on 'British hospices' in *Encyclopaedia Britannica* defined 'hospice' as '[t]he name frequently given to the guest houses established for the reception of pilgrims and travellers within the precincts or upon the property of religious houses'[128]. Cicely was intrigued by this welcome to weary travellers who might thus have found a way to paradise by dying whilst en route to their pilgrimage destination. By 1983 she had learned of the work of the *Dames du Calvaire*, established by Jeanne Garnier in Lyon in 1842 to create homes for the dying in France, and had to acknowledge to a French Sister: 'You were the first of all of us I think. I am sorry it has taken me so long to find out'[129]. She saw the value of the historical associations of hospice, but was also challenged to link this to the modern context in which the new hospices were beginning to make a mark. It was a theme she would enjoy returning to in later life.

Building on her experience of people with M.N.D., Cicely had increasing evidence that hospice could be developed in many modes and settings — extending beyond initial successes with cancer patients — to include those with non-malignant conditions. In due course, the challenge of caring for people with A.I.D.S. would arise and, by the spring of 1985, this was being discussed at the hospice and with the Royal College of Nursing and the Department of Health and Social Security — if only in language which stressed the importance of infection control and the safety of members of staff[130]. Above all, a major purpose came to be seen as the improvement of care for the terminally ill within the mainstream setting, not through the continuing proliferation of hospice units, but rather through education and training and the broader diffusion of appropriate knowledge, skills, and attitudes.

Of course, St Christopher's had a vital role to play in this. Initially it was the only centre for specialised education and training in the new field of terminal care. As early as 1969, Cicely had written to Sue Ryder, her fellow charitable founder and innovator, commenting on a successful training visit from a Polish doctor of their mutual acquaintance and noting: '[H]e has made us realise how blessed we are in the amount of space, equipment and so on we have here; one should not be ashamed of one's blessings but only continue to give thanks and try to use them with proper responsibility'[131]. But building on such successes, there was soon a tidal wave of requests from around the world to visit, to work, and to spend time at the hospice. Initially these were encouraged, even fostered (she was keen for American colleagues like Avery Weisman and Elisabeth Kübler-Ross to visit, even when they did not find time in their schedules to do so). But she could be extremely snippy with others who sought to impose themselves when it did not suit. One American would-be visitor got a particular lashing: 'I think only a psychologist without clinical responsibility could ask a medical director to take him round a hospital over Christmas. I am sorry to sound so unwelcoming but have you any idea how many things one has to do at this time and how many staff have to sort out their own Christmas with their families and the work with patients?'[132] By 1975, there were two thousand visitors per annum; special hours were set aside for them each week, and in due course, some tours were conducted in French. This was one way of dealing with the flood of interest, but Cicely was not well disposed to those who made extravagant journeys to St Christopher's at the expense of over-looking growing expertise nearer to home[133], and she also complained to Elisabeth Kübler-Ross about the constant requests for information from the United States that were not matched by any willingness to meet the postage or printing costs[134]. She seemed inconsistent in these areas — very willing to solicit visitors when they suited her purpose, but at times churlish (though in letters she at times protested the contrary) to some who wrote seeking advice or entrée to the special environment she had created at Sydenham.

In Demand Around the World

There were also many who asked Cicely to come to them. In these years as medical director, she visited North America around a dozen times, developing and extending her close professional links as well as her enduring friendships. Often the two combined, as with Balfour Mount and the palliative-care service at the Royal Victoria Hospital, Montreal, and at the international conference he hosted every two years starting in 1976. Theirs was an extended and close relationship. Enthused by what he had seen at St Christopher's, Mount now had his own palliative-care unit in Montreal. He also fostered a controversial study in which a medical anthropologist starved himself to gain entry to the hospital wards and the palliative-care unit to contrast and compare covertly the care he received in the two settings[135]. Despite these, at times, maverick approaches, Cicely gave much encouragement to Mount's work, speaking at the first meeting and staying with the Mounts at their home. She found him to be an excellent clinician, rather fanciful in his ideas, and sometimes prone to temper tantrums with hospital administrators when he didn't get his way. She admired Bal Mount hugely (Figure 5.4), knew him through a divorce and remarriage, and considered his work to have an excellent philosophical base[136]. Over the years, they maintained an enormous correspondence, full of newsy items, family updates, abstract and spiritual reflections, as well as gossip and chitchat. Undoubtedly, he was one of her favourite visitors to her office, though most were graciously welcomed (Figure 5.5).

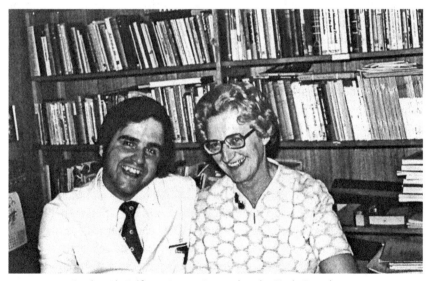

FIGURE 5.4 Cicely with Balfour Mount. *Source: kept by Cicely Saunders.*

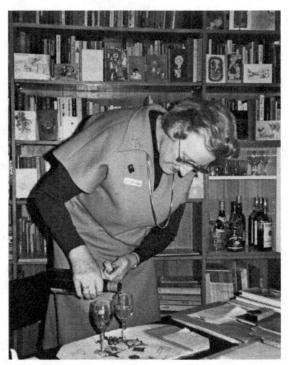

FIGURE 5.5 Pouring drinks. *Source: kept by Cicely Saunders.*

Cicely also made visits to many other countries, including Yugoslavia, Belgium, Australia, Israel, and South Africa. Her network of collaborators expanded, and her influence and reputation grew as she was acknowledged increasingly as the 'founder' of the modern Hospice Movement. She took an extremely close interest in the many services and settings to which she was introduced on these trips and would often comment on them in great detail in later correspondence. By 1977, and after several visits to the United States, she had discovered the pleasures of first-class air travel and asked that this be provided when she made a visit to Western Australia: 'I am six feet tall and getting arthritis in my knees and last winter had a crush fracture of my spine. I think I am not fussing when I say that a trip of these dimensions has got to be done in this way'[137]. Her time there, in September, included a rigorous schedule of visits to clinical centres, public meetings, and showcase lectures, as well as a few 'wildflowers, birds, etc.'[138]. Australia was immediately followed by a holiday in Israel (the first of three visits there) with Tom West and Marian, but of course there were also meetings with hospice enthusiasts, contacts to be made, and advice to be given[139]. In the summer of 1978, she returned to Poland and, through meetings in Warsaw, Gdansk, and Cracow, was astonished at the progress which had been made since her previous visit in 1962. If she still found it hard to see how a hospice like St Christopher's could be created there, given the demands of the acute medical system, nevertheless, improvement in pain control was a goal worth pursuing[140]. She noted to Halina Iwanowska, the hospice activist in Gdansk:

> The more I talk with people in Poland, the more I realize the situation is just the same as we found in Italy — that people have no idea at all about the effectiveness of that kind of pain control. Consequently one hears a lot of demanding techniques which will only be done by a few and only reach a few whereas I am quite sure those patients we saw together with unrelieved pain could be helped without any extra use of people or time[141].

She visited South Africa in 1979 and continued to encourage clinicians there like Dr Henrik Venter and Dr Richard Scheffer. In 1982, she was invited to lay the foundation stone for the first hospice in India, but was unable to attend, though she stayed in regular contact with its founder, Dr L.J. de Souza.

It is apparent that Cicely did not see her vision as something which could only be bounded by the discipline of medicine. The concept of 'total pain' took into account physical, emotional, psychological, social, and spiritual elements, and required to be addressed through the combined skills of a multi-disciplinary team of carers, including volunteers, with active attention to family involvement. It also became clear that the resulting possibility of 'staff pain' must likewise be attended to. In establishing a foundation outside the parameters of the British National Health Service in the form of an independent, charitable hospice, Cicely also displayed a degree of scepticism about the ability of the mainstream healthcare system to foster her ambitions. For Cicely, moving out of the National Health Service to let new influences flow back, had meant establishing an inpatient hospice and then a home-care service that had become a centre for the development of three activities: clinical care, teaching, and research. In Britain, others began to follow along similar lines, though few combined these three elements at the same level. Hospices modelled substantially upon St Christopher's — as independent charitable institutions — opened in Sheffield, Manchester (she was there for the opening of St Anne's Hospice in June 1971), Worthing, and elsewhere. There was a constant flow of communication between the staff of St Christopher's and others across the United Kingdom who shared similar aspirations, and a great deal of emphasis on the active relationship between hospices and their local communities. As the work developed, it took on the character of a reformist social movement, challenging prevailing attitudes, practices, and modes of organisation. Nevertheless, quite early Cicely could be stern in cautioning those who sought to embark on such a path. For example, in May 1970, she wrote to a would-be hospice founder in Woking, Surrey, stating rather bluntly:

> I think in the first place you must realise that it is going to involve much more work and much more expense than one can possibly envisage at the moment.

I feel strongly myself that a project like this should not be embarked upon unless one literally cannot help it because the compulsion that it is the right thing is so strong[142].

She also commented with concern on the failure to adopt more modern approaches to terminal care at the long-established Hostel of God, in Clapham. One of the first of the nineteenth-century hospices, with encouragement from Cicely it was eventually able to make the transition into the new era of hospice and palliative care, but not before she had laid down some strong concerns in 1975 to the Bishop of Southwark about its mode of organisation and working: 'The Sisters have not had the support of either imaginative doctors or trustees and, although they have done a marvellous job in many ways, it is terribly sad to see the present standards of care'[143].

Recognition at Home

The enthusiasm for hospice nevertheless continued to grow and, in time, caught the interests of policymakers who began to take a closer interest in the subject, leading to the first national symposium on the care of the dying, held in London in November 1972, with the proceedings published in the *British Medical Journal*. It was a level of recognition that could scarcely have been imagined almost exactly a decade earlier, when Cicely had hesitantly presented her paper on the treatment of intractable pain in terminal cancer at the Royal Society of Medicine. In 1972, actor Sheila Hancock gave a lay view on 'death in the family' as a counterpoint to Cicely and Professor W. Ferguson Anderson, a Glasgow geriatrician, who gave professional perspectives. One of the many detailed pieces was from Eric Wilkes, characteristically self-effacing and urbane, paying a well-rounded tribute to Cicely: 'Our small, eccentric unit in Sheffield, with which I am associated, is only a faint shadow of St Christopher's Hospice, but it does demonstrate the possibility of what can be done without leadership of the quality of Dr Cicely Saunders'[144]. Cicely's own contribution began with an account of how patient and family 'are often separated by unshared knowledge' and went on to describe how the experience of pain can cut off patients from those around them[145]. She outlined the known methods for the control of pain using a combination of analgesics, adjuvants, and other methods, including listening to 'the various facets of distress'. She argued that the inpatient unit can provide a place where families may be reunited, such as in the case of the sons of a dying man who, after admission, 'met their father again, when at home they had been refusing to speak to him, resentful and uncomfortable with the illness of which they were so frightened'. Cicely explained how it can then become a matter of helping to produce 'a climate in which the patients can find their own meanings'. This may be a matter of listening without necessarily knowing the answers, whilst at the same time persevering with the development of practical skills. Simplicity and simply being there may be all important. Her piece concluded with the phrase so significant to this overall approach and so often quoted afterwards: '[Y]ou matter because you are you'. In these ways, she stated, patients can live until they die, and the relatives may go on living afterwards.

Inspired in part by such language, this was the start of an era of *emotional planning* in hospice and palliative-care services in Britain. Ideas and proposals for new services often came forward at the local level, sometimes despite (rather than because of) the support of local health bureaucrats. Only gradually did formal guidance begin to appear, sometimes hastily cobbled together in the face of a rising tide of local hospice developments led by specially formed charities and local zealots. Hospices were mushrooming, and this brought more and more demands upon St Christopher's. Some services were also being formed within the National Health Service — for example, in Oxford and Southampton. In 1977, Cicely was called to help in Aberdeen 'where they have a Continuing Care Unit opening with little public relations done with the doctors beforehand and a great need of an open meeting'[146]. The year before, she had set up a 'think tank' of hospice doctors and some clinicians from elsewhere, such as Kenneth Calman, who was undertaking a Medical Research Council clinical fellowship at the Royal Marsden Hospital. They met at St Christopher's every few months to share questions and clinical problems, stimulating development in the emerging field of hospice medicine and preparing the ground for later recognition as a specialty. In 1979, Cicely was responding to suggestions from Oxford that a special service for children should be established there: 'On the whole I do not believe in Hospices for children, but I may be wrong'[147]. She was a landmark of policy recognition came in 1980 with the report of the Working Group on Terminal Care produced by the Standing Sub-Committee on Cancer of the Standing Medical Advisory Committee, chaired by hospice founder and later professor of community medicine Eric Wilkes[148].

The 'Wilkes Report', as it came to be known, was a response to the significant developments that had taken place since the work two decades earlier of H.L. Glyn Hughes. Notwithstanding his role as a hospice founder within his own locale, Wilkes gave a cold shower to expansionist tendencies among hospices. The report argued that these were neither affordable (in cash) nor sustainable (in personnel). Rather, the focus should be on encouraging the principles of terminal care throughout the health service and with good coordination between the sectors. If prescient in orientation, it did little to stem the immediate tide of enthusiasm for the creation of new hospice organisations. The decade that followed was unprecedented for hospice growth in Britain, with one hundred new hospices coming into existence, each seeking to negotiate some kind of grant or subvention from its local health authority.

Within this wider culture of recognition, important developments were taking place internationally. There was increasing acknowledgement that the benefits of hospice and palliative care should not be confined to those in the affluent nations of the world, but that the epidemic of cancer in developing countries also required attention. Gradually, interest in these issues was spreading throughout many societies and cultures.

An International Forum

November 1974 saw the first full meeting of the International Work Group on Death, Dying, and Bereavement, in Columbia, Maryland. It emerged from the activities of *Ars Moriendi*, a multi-disciplinary association focussed on the professional response to death and loss, and that had been established by John Fryer. Cicely was among the founding group of 'I.W.G.', as it became known, and subsequently it was organised into a pattern of bi-annual meetings around the world, seeking to be catalytic, sharing knowledge and experience, and working in a collegial manner, albeit in a group whose membership was by invitation only. Colin Murray Parkes, Tom West, and Thelma Bates were other people from within the St Christopher's sphere who became involved. It had a glittering membership of academic thanatologists and death-oriented clinicians who fostered a particular style of engagement, that, Cicely remembered, could involve frank discussion and often robust language. On one occasion, she returned from a meeting to take part immediately in a prize-giving event for nurses in London. As each recipient came up to the podium, Cicely could not shake out of her head, the repeated exclamation of the I.W.G. discussion: 'bullshit, bullshit, bullshit'[149]. It is a mark of her approach that she stayed with I.W.G., only missing meetings as Marian became more dependent, and after his death resuming her interest and travelling long distances to attend. She held an iconic place in the group, and her high-toned contributions, laconic observations, and generally patrician aura were much loved by its members.

If I.W.G. existed in the rarefied atmosphere of closed discussions in luxurious settings, other international organisations were engaging with issues of pain and terminal care in ways which might yield more obvious policy and practice benefit. In 1982, under the leadership of a new chief of cancer, Dr Jan Stjernsward, W.H.O., enlisted the aid of hospice-care leaders and cancer pain specialists, plus pharmaceutical manufacturers to develop a global Programme for Cancer Pain Relief. It would be based on a three-step analgesic 'ladder', with the use of adjuvant therapies, and incorporating the use of strong opioids as the third step. The key meeting of the group, in which Robert Twycross played a prominent role, was at the Villa d'Este on Lake Como outside Milan in October 1982. The members were becoming very focussed on the global scale of the problem associated with cancer pain, the lack of medical education on the subject, the wariness of clinicians in engaging with the use of strong opiates, and the major barriers that existed in laws and established procedures which combined to restrict access to appropriate medication in many parts of the world. On the back of these efforts, W.H.O. representatives launched an international initiative to remove legal sanctions against opioid importation and use, relying on national co-ordinating centres to organize professional education and to disseminate the core principles of the newly formulated 'pain ladder' — simple guidelines for pain relief which could be operationalised in many settings. The interest of W.H.O. raised further debate about the relationship between palliative care and oncology. It was increasingly recognised that curative care and palliative care were not mutually exclusive, and that as long as few options for curative oncological treatment existed for many patients in the developing world, the allocation of resources should shift towards a greater emphasis on palliative care. Cancer pain was coming to be defined as a public health issue and, as that occurred, the scope for wider involvement — beyond the immediate world of hospice — was in turn opening up. By the spring of 1986, Cicely was writing to Stjernsward, eagerly awaiting a copy of the W.H.O. technical report[150] which would outline this entire programme and eventually lead to — and this was a huge landmark — its own definition of the emerging field of palliative care, published in 1990[151]. The momentum was growing and formal recognition from the medical establishment now came within the grasp of its founders. Britain would be the first to achieve this, and as we shall see in due course, Gillian Ford, Cicely's long-established and dear friend, would be in the vanguard of developments.

Honours and Plaudits

During her years as medical director at St Christopher's, and with increasing frequency, Cicely was showered with an array of honours and prizes. Things got underway with an honorary doctor of science from Yale in 1969. The build-up to and aftermath of the visit were painstaking. Cicely fussed endlessly over protocol on the day; the cap; the gown; the hood; the 'sub-fusc'; the colour of shoes, stockings, and dress; and the possibility of having the whole academic outfit made in London for subsequent use[152]. It was a momentous occasion for Cicely, in which she took the view that every single patient she had ever looked after was present with her[153].

Media Engagements

During the mid 1970s, Cicely had got into dialogue with television presenter and transatlantic celebrity David Frost. It resulted in a thirty-minute 'Frost Interview' with Cicely, broadcast by the B.B.C. on 19 September 1974. He took a keen interest, visited the hospice, and on the programme spoke to some of the patients from St Christopher's. Cicely was pleased with the result and saw it as a buffer against other programmes, and the wider debate on euthanasia that was building up at the time. In the months that followed, as assiduous as ever, she provided him with updates on some of the patients and families he had met and tried to tempt him (without result) into other collaborations[154].

Following the success of the Frost Interview, the B.B.C. took further interest and the idea that Cicely might feature on the television programme *In the Light of Experience* was first discussed in 1976. She explored it with producer Angela Tilby of the B.B.C.'s Religious Department and, despite initial worries, became more relaxed about the possibility. The programme was broadly in the 'religious affairs' category and focussed on the life and work of a particular individual. Lasting a full half hour, it was again a serious opportunity for Cicely to explain herself and to draw wider attention to her hospice ideals. She decided to use it as the moment to become more public about Antoni Michniewicz, their relationship, and the importance of it all for the development of St Christopher's. Quite why she chose this time was never explained. It was a busy period of consolidation and development. The work of St Christopher's was becoming more widely known and its status as a hub of expertise was now established. She could feel more confident in her achievements. It was a year in which she published almost a dozen items. Perhaps most significant was that these included her re-workings of the *Nursing Times* articles. In doing that, she had been taken back to 1959, the year of their first publication, but also the period just before she had known Antoni, who had been admitted to St Joseph's in January 1960 and died there in August. Sixteen years later to the very month, her 'sub-conscious quietly got to work' and she wrote a draft script for the programme over a weekend. Sending it to Tilby, even if it were not to be used for some time, she explained: 'I think I have needed to get it off my chest for quite a long time . . . . This is the first time I feel I have told the story of how St Christopher's began truthfully'[155]. The idea stayed with her for the next few years. On the night of 16 – 17 August 1979, again coinciding with the anniversary of his death, she dreamed again about Antoni. He was in Rugby Ward at the hospice, but alive and well following the intervention of 'a healer'[156]. There would be no further dreams of him until after Marian had died, but before that the programme was broadcast — on 20 August 1980, marking the twentieth anniversary of Antoni's death. Her most compelling story was now in the public domain and would become synonymous with the maturing narrative of her life, loves, and work. But it was not laid to rest. She would revisit the story in earnest almost twenty years later.

Awards

Beginning in the late 1970s, some major award was conferred upon Cicely every year; sometimes there were several close together. In 1977 she received the Lambeth Doctorate of Medicine from the Archbishop of Canterbury; in 1979 she became the first woman to receive a Gold Medal in Therapeutics from the Worshipful Society of Apothecaries. There were also honorary degrees from the Open University in Britain as well as from Columbia University and Iona College in the United States. In 1981 she was made a Fellow of the Royal College of Nursing, to add to her fellowship from the Royal College of Physicians of 1974.

Then, in 1980, the Queen's New Year Honours list again contained Cicely's name. She had been made a Dame and was clearly delighted in all that it conferred. She regarded the honour as a salute to the whole of the Hospice Movement and constantly reaffirmed that belief in all of the wider recognition she received. By the end of January she had replied in acknowledgement to more than five hundred well-wishers who had written, sending their felicitations. She explained to her American friends that this was something like being knighted and that, although she had not yet been to Buckingham Palace to be invested, the title should be used from now on. Friends could go on calling her Cicely, but 'acquaintances and enemies' should use 'Dame Cicely' and most certainly not 'Dame Saunders'[157]. Despite this, Americans continued to use the latter for the rest of her life when referring to or meeting her, perhaps to her amusement if not slight irritation.

The following year saw her awarded the Templeton Prize for Progress in Religion. It was enormously prestigious and marked her out not only as a great clinician and service innovator, but also as one who had made a contribution to understanding the importance of religion to individual life and to society. Its founder had established the prize in 1972 to honour living persons who could be described as 'entrepreneurs of the spirit'. For Cicely, it was recognition not only of her faith, but also of her works and the practical ethic that linked the two together. It also brought a handsome financial contribution, and this was put towards a new day centre at St Christopher's. As she noted to a colleague in Poland: 'We find ourselves increasingly involved with the elderly and lonely bereaved in our community and there are people with chronic diseases other than cancer near to the hospice who would, I think, benefit from attending any such centre with our patients'[158]. At the public ceremony in London's Guildhall on 12 May 1981, and in the presence of H.R.H., Princess Alexandra, Patron of St Christopher's, Cicely was described as 'the woman who has changed the face of death'. In her own address, she took time to review her personal history of involvement in the field as well as the evolution of places called 'hospices' over the centuries. She also provided a striking definition of the modern hospice:

> [It is] a skilled community working to improve the quality of life remaining for patients and their families struggling with mortal and long-term illness. Some also include the frail elderly. Hospice is about a special kind of living

and in a sense is still concerned with travelling; patients, families, elderly residents and the staff and volunteers who meet them, all find they are drawn into a journey of the spirit[159].

From 1981 to 1984 there were no less than nine more honorary degrees from prestigious universities in Britain and America. Academia was saluting her achievements, and Cicely, who had never held a substantive post in a university and who had not completed her M.D. thesis, relished the recognition.

Meeting Her Biographer

The initial conversations at the B.B.C. had drawn Cicely to the attention of Shirley du Boulay, who had worked on the highly successful 'Woman's Hour' radio programme and then moved into television before leaving Broadcasting House to work as a freelance writer, and in time became an accomplished biographer. The two worked together on *In the Light of Experience* and also a televised panel discussion. When the time came, du Boulay saw in Cicely a complex and challenging subject for her first book and began discussions with her about it in the summer of 1981. By August it was agreed, and Cicely gave her biographer leave to look at all the available material. She was relieved that the book she had been thinking of writing about her own story, and which had sat in the back of her mind for so long, would not have to be attempted. du Boulay was encouraged to speak with Cicely's closest colleagues and friends, and the follow-up international conference to the Bar Mitzvah in 1982 was a good opportunity for this. By March 1983, Cicely was reading drafts of the early chapters. She liked the material and could see that du Boulay would help strike a blow for 'all the right things about hospice'[160]. Once again the opportunist, she also persuaded du Boulay to include a whole chapter of extracts from the diary of a St Christopher's patient, Ramsey, who was at the hospice between 20 June and 8 September 1978, when he died at age forty-eight. Arguably, it badly interrupted the flow, as the book moved back and forth in the later chapters from a narrative of Cicely's life to an account of the day-to-day workings of the hospice as an organisation. But it was typical of Cicely's keen-ness, always to seize an opportunity to advance some argument or point of view. When the pre-publication copy arrived in January 1984[161], Cicely wrote to the publisher, praising du Boulay 'with the feeling that she knows me better than I know myself, but glad that this part of the story of St Christopher's has been so sympathetically told'[162]. At age sixty-four, she could feel content to be one of perhaps just a few female doctors to see a biography published in their own lifetime. Widely reviewed, it celebrated her contribution; but, more important to Cicely, it was a lucid, insightful, and robust account of her work and that of the hospice she had founded. An early review in *The Lancet* from Derek Doyle of St Columba's Hospice in Edinburgh, was upbeat. He began by questioning the motives of someone who would allow a biography to be written whilst 'very much still alive'. He was reassured that this was born of a 'quiet assurance allied to courage'. For him the book did not contribute to 'canonisation in her lifetime', that he nonetheless felt was taking place in some settings. Rather, he found in it both a candid account of her life and character along with the best description yet of the philosophy and practice of hospice: 'She is revealed as intensely human, often uncomfortable to work with, at times intolerant and unable to suffer fools, sometimes insecure and sharp of tongue, but always fascinating and inspiring, to the point of being electrifying'[163].

All in all, by the 1980s, Cicely was enjoying a period of significant professional and personal fulfilment. As the plaudits accumulated, she could be modest about her achievements, as she opined in a letter to Grace Goldin:

[T]here are not many original ideas in the world. One only brings together things culled from here and there, shakes the kaleidoscope and finds a new pattern. That I have said often enough and it is really my feeling about the originality or lack of it of St Christopher's[164].

It was a reasonable, if under-stated, description. Likewise, on another occasion, she reflected: 'Periodically as I look at this building I am astonished at the effrontery of thinking we could build such a place around the window'[165]. But others thought differently and wished to see Cicely honoured and recognised for her achievements. There was no doubt she took pride in this, and it perhaps fuelled her vanity, but always she deflected the praise and turned it, in the end, onto the achievements of the whole world of hospice and everyone who contributed to it.

Challenges — Personal and Professional

The professional and clinical achievements of Cicely's years as medical director cannot be allowed to mask the organisational issues and difficulties which also had to be overcome, as well as the personal obstacles and dilemmas which had to be faced throughout these many and varied years.

In the summer of 1968, with the hospice open for just a year, Cicely reached her fiftieth birthday. She would do some reflection on what had been achieved, and was able to go over things with Florence Wald, who came for a working visit. But soon her health was giving her problems. She took medication for fibroids and tried to battle on. Then, in August 1969, the hospice staff 'put down their collective feet' and she accepted that she would have to go into hospital for an hysterectomy[166]. An early casualty was a planned visit to the United States in October. She explained to her chairman, Lord Thurlow, that it was nothing serious, but she would be off for two months, a locum would be brought in, and she would convalesce at St Christopher's rather than 'in a flat on my own'[167]. As we have seen, it was in late 1969 that the 'kibbutz' was established in Lawrie Park Gardens. So this combination of new living arrangements and recovery from surgery must have been demanding for Cicely, both emotionally and physically. In any event, the period of absence was much longer than expected and she did not get back to work at the hospice until 23 March 1970. To compound the problem, her back then started to give her trouble and in June she told Marty Herrman: 'I am not exactly blooming as I am, at the moment, supported by a most uncomfortable surgical corset!'[168] Cicely's health continued to trouble her at various times. She injured her spine in 1977 and had a bad fall on some wet steps in early 1985. But mostly, in the 1980s, it was Marian's well-being, rather than her own, which took priority.

The Death of Ron Welldon

There were also losses and stresses from time to time that affected the whole of St Christopher's. A major one was on 9 November 1970, when Dr Ron Welldon, the hospice's first research fellow, died suddenly, the news reaching Cicely by cable in Lexington, Kentucky, just as she was about to take a ward round and give a lecture. Welldon left a widow, psychiatrist Estela D'Accurzio, and a child of nine months. For a whole year he had been in severe pain from a slipped disc, and four months earlier had undergone a laminectomy. The circumstances of his death seem unclear. Cicely wrote that he had mistakenly taken an overdose of sleeping pills: 'No doubt at all that it was a mistake'[169]. But Richard Lamerton, many years afterwards, offered a different account. Welldon was taking large quantities of the newly marketed drug paracetamol to treat his pain, whilst seeking to avoid drowsiness and maintain his work output. In Lamerton's view, Welldon died of an overdose of a drug which was not known at the time to have hepatoxic properties[170]. Whichever was the case, it was tragic that a mix-up over drugs should occur in a doctor experiencing chronic pain, and who had extensive knowledge about the use of powerful opiates.

Cicely spoke about Ron Welldon in Lexington on the night of his death. She had two thoughts: 'death is an outrage' and 'death is alright'. She explored his 'fascinating way of turning things upside down', how she had found solace herself in being with him, and also of his extraordinary personal qualities as a physician. In the days following, now on holiday, she visited with her friend Sister Zita Marie Cotter, first near Gethsemane, a Trappist Monastery, and then a centre run by the Sisters of Charity of Nazareth. In these places, and without fore-planning, she found herself going into retreat 'and somehow it all got gathered up'. She had avoided this kind of situation for almost a decade, knowing that her father had died whilst she was at Grandchamp. But now, having been given retreat without volition, 'all was well'[171].

On returning to London, however, she found the hospice in shock. The Rev Ed Dobihall, an associate from Yale who was spending time as a chaplain at St Christopher's, took a memorial service in the chapel with family and colleagues all packed in together and with Welldon's little son gurgling away throughout[172]. In the days that followed, Ron was missed dreadfully. On Christmas Eve, Cicely wrote to Elisabeth Kübler-Ross with the news. Cicely also stayed in touch with Welldon's wife and ensured that his obituary was published in *The Lancet*[173].

No sooner had the obituary appeared, and before 1970 had even come to an end, Cicely was in touch again with Robert Twycross and making active plans for him to come as Ron Welldon's replacement. Twycross visited the hospice on 22 December and met with Albertine Winner, the chair of trustees, as well as Colin Murray Parkes and Duncan Vere, at the London Hospital. By 29 December, everyone involved was agreed that he should be offered the post. He had no research training, but his reference was excellent and Cicely was convinced of his 'real concern about terminal care and of his very courteous and considerate personality'[174]. She, as always, and even in the wake of tragic loss, was the pragmatist and the planner.

Further Losses, Worries, and Criticisms

The following year, the death of Lord Thurlow after a period of illness took away a chairman in whom she had great confidence and who had been such a support to her in the pre-operational years of St Christopher's. He had joined Cicely at a time when they were struggling for money and he had been willing to sign the contract to proceed with building even though only half the needed sum had been raised. When the hospice opened, he visited whenever he could, chairing meetings, but also getting to know the long-stay residents of the Draper's Wing as well as the staff and patients. His old dog Tammy was looked after at the hospice when he was away, and as his condition deteriorated, Albertine Winner and Cicely both made sure to visit him[175]. When his obituary appeared in *The Times* on 1 June 1971 but contained no mention of St Christopher's, Cicely was quick to write to the newspaper editor asking for an addition to be made[176].

There were more mundane challenges occasioned by relations between the staff and the particular circumstances of those involved. Miss Neville was deputy matron at the beginning, but left in 1973 when the Study Centre opened. The leaving was only partly mutual and left Cicely, who had intervened directly, feeling uneasy. As she later put it, '[h]iring is alright; firing's terrible'[177]. The arrangements in the hospice could be awkward. If a member of staff didn't get on well with matron, there were other ramifications. Matron was married to the chief steward. If a colleague had a family member who received care from the hospice, and the medical director was involved, further complications could ensue. In addition, sometimes staff could become over-involved with patients. Cicely was aware of this on the small number of occasions when it happened, and knew she was vulnerable, especially as in these years she became much more open about what happened with Antoni, but she took the view that such involvement would only be inappropriate if it stepped out of the boundaries created by St Christopher's as an organisation and a community. That was the strength of the hospice approach: Teamwork could protect against over-involvement and serve to mitigate potential risks. Looking back in the mid 1990s, Cicely reflected:

> [W]e've had some casualties along the way. I wouldn't say we were always terribly good at handling them, but somehow we have kept going, although I think there were one or two hurt people, and [Miss Neville] certainly was, that I've felt guilty about and responsible for, and think that, you know, I didn't really handle that as well as I should have done[178].

There were also periodic financial crises, including a major one in 1974. This had been building up steadily in the prior period. The annual accounts of the first three years each showed an operating deficit. The hospice was spending more than it generated and the gap was not being filled by the relatively modest fund-raising efforts that existed at the time. An organisational review undertaken by students at Cranfield School of Management urged more prudence on financial matters and greater devolution of budgetary powers and responsibility[179]. Other visitors to the hospice, on writing about their experiences, said critical things about staff morale and the management culture, describing it as authoritarian and inflexible, and concerned only for the patients and not for the staff. One such account produced by a visitor in 1974 resulted in a caring but firm reply to its American author:

> I made no comments about your report at the time as I did not know what to say. You were here at a particularly difficult time when Marian Newell, Sister Spears, and Nurse Cosser were all going to leave for various reasons, and I know you had problems of homesickness .... I am very unhappy about the idealistic image of St Christopher's which some people produce and perhaps what you say will be a good corrective[180].

In particular, though, Cicely objected to the phrase 'much hostility' in the report and asked for it to be changed, though she did acknowledge that 'anger' was a component of the St Christopher's culture. Such observations stimulated the creation in 1979 of a Foundation Group to look again at the early statement of *Aim and Basis* that had been drafted by Olive Wyon, but the members could find little reason for any significant re-orientation. Always there were links back to the origins and initial vision. Sometimes these were personally painful, such as the next year when Cicely lost her great stalwart from the early days, Jack Wallace, who died after a minor operation. His confidence in her vision and willingness to play a supplementary role to it had been crucial to the success of the enterprise.

Continued Opposition to Euthanasia

In her years as medical director, Cicely continued to oppose the legalisation of euthanasia whenever the opportunity arose, affirming a position she had first set out in 1959[181]. In 1972, she challenged a Dutch colleague on the wisdom of promoting what was then being termed 'active euthanasia'. She described a recent example of a patient in the hospice who had been asking for her life to be ended. Cicely had gone to see her, explained it couldn't be done, but were such a course of action legal, would the patient like it to be done now?

> [T]he instant response was 'no, not now'.
> 'When would you want me to?' I asked.
> 'If the pain got too much or if I got desperately fed up with it all'.
> I replied to the effect that we would certainly be able to control pain . . . I said we would certainly help feelings of anxiety and desperation . . . and I told her she could certainly send for me if she wanted to do so. She went on to say that was really what she wanted but added how hard she found it for her husband to see her like this . . . and asked me not to tell her husband.
> I said, "[W]ell we have only been talking about pain haven't we?"
> I think that was the truth of the matter . . . . Never when I have asked 'Do you want it now' have I been given the answer 'Yes'[182].

She opposed euthanasia on several grounds. As in this example, she thought it was mostly something that could be avoided by good palliative care. She thought it imposed too much pressure on the surviving family, arguing that it was more significant even than the trauma of suicide. She was also at pains to clarify some of the terminology in use at the time — for example, to make it clear that desisting from inappropriate treatment or ceasing to strive for the prolongation of life in the irreversibly dying constituted 'proper medical care' and should not be described as 'euthanasia'. Rarely did she invoke arguments about the sanctity of life, relying instead on the power of her clinical experience to argue against assisted dying. But here she was in a clinical grey area, where evidence was difficult to marshal, and anecdote tended to be the main line of her reasoning: 'I do not believe in taking a deliberate step to end a patient's life — but then, I do not get asked'[183]. As she noted in her preface to a volume prepared by Sylvia Lack and Richard Lamerton, from papers presented in 1973 at a St Christopher's conference — 'If a patient asks to be killed, someone has failed him'[184].

Between 1970 and 1974, a working party of the Church of England Board for Social Responsibility sought to develop an Anglican contribution to the debate on euthanasia[185]. The group had seven members, though the first chairman, the Right Reverend Ian Ramsay, then Bishop of Durham, died suddenly in October 1972. Two chapters in the report were drafted by Cicely, who 'for her sins' as she put it to A.N. Exton Smith, had been invited to serve

as a member of the group[186]. The report recommended that the law on euthanasia should not be changed. All members endorsed the recommendations,
including (1) the undesirability of extending the term 'euthanasia' to incorpo-
rate the withdrawal of artificial means of preserving life or to include the use
of pain-relieving drugs that may marginally shorten life; (2) the assertion that
if all care of the dying was at the standard of the best, then there would be no
prima facie case for euthanasia; and (3) the belief that such standards are more
hindered by ignorance than by money and staff shortages.

In 1976, when Cicely came to revise her articles from 1959 which had
appeared in *Nursing Times*, the changes she needed to make to the paper on euthanasia — in light of growing public debate and possible legislative change —
were so extensive as to require publication in two tranches over consecutive
weeks. The first article[187] began with a discussion of euthanasia debates in the
House of Lords, from 1936 to the most recent concerning Baroness Wootton's
Incurable Patients Bill (1976). In Cicely's view, many of the 1976 proposals
should already have been available to patients, though she acknowledged that
not all patients receive the help they need. The danger of Wooton's proposal,
albeit produced by those with 'a manifest concern for the relief of suffering'
was that patients deemed 'incurable' may feel they not only had the right, but
also the duty to choose a quick end. Rather than concentrate on assertion and
counter-assertion, the article focused on the argument that people are suffering
when they need not. She noted the many therapeutic advances in the seventeen
years since the original article was written, and accepted that some added to
the problems — particularly when no clear rationale for continuing treatment
exists. She took strength from Pope Pius XII's Allocution of 1957, that states
'in a case in which death is deemed certain and life can be prolonged only by
artificial methods, the physician is not absolutely obliged to prolong life by
extraordinary means'. In this context, the emerging notion of 'Living Wills'
seemed to have some merit and Cicely offered a brief discussion of the debates
around 'furore therapeutics' and 'meddlesome medicine'. More positively,
she also noted that the intervening years had seen valuable additions to the
pharmacopoeia and a sounder knowledge of the use of appropriate drugs — as,
for example, in the work pioneered at St Christopher's. Much more thought and
consultation were required on the question of euthanasia. In particular, two additional questions need to be answered: 'Do patients ask for euthanasia?' and
'What would they do and feel if mercy killing became a legal option?' Cicely
found strength in the case of Captain Oates, as described in Scott's journal of
his last expedition to the Antarctic in 1912. Like Oates's companions, who
cared for him throughout and until he left voluntarily to die on the ice, those
caring for the dying must convey the sentiment: 'You matter because you are
you. You matter to the last moment of your life, and we will do all we can to
help you not only to die peacefully, but also to live until you die'[188]. The article
of the following week[189] argued that frank requests for euthanasia, even among

those who apparently 'believe in' the idea, are still very rare. Sometimes it is a question of disentangling 'the real question' from a 'somewhat confused story'. At times, relatives may question the purpose of continuing to care when the situation is deemed by them to be 'hopeless'. Cicely took the view that legalising 'the right to die', with attendant procedures and safeguards, would likely hinder proper terminal care, that was now developing at scale in many places, and could impose traumatic decisions on both patient and family.

Cicely feared increasingly that the *right* to die might be interpreted by some as a *duty* to do so. In 1977 and 1978, she took part in debates at the Royal Society of Health and the Union Society, Cambridge, where in each case motions in support of the legalisation of euthanasia were defeated. She did acknowledge, however, that both sides in the euthanasia debate have a vendetta against pointless pain and impersonal indignity, though their solutions were radically different in character. She was supportive but concerned when the still neophyte I.W.G. organised a meeting in 1977 with the Euthanasia Education Council, writing to John Fryer that, in pressing for the withdrawal of unnecessary treatment at the end of life, the Council might shade into endorsing 'mercy killing'. 'If we keep talking together with our definitions clear, there would, I think, be less need to polarise and have the Euthanasia Education Council on a totally different side of the fence from the ordinary Hospice workers'[190]. Those who opposed new legislation had a responsibility to work towards a situation where no one should be so desperate as to feel the need to request euthanasia[191]. As she had showed in a 1982 discussion of definitions from active, to palliative, to terminal care, these could be overlapping and even reversible categories, making the appropriate moment for the consideration of euthanasia far less clear. Her clinical reasoning was becoming stronger and more in tune with the competing claims of modern medicine and the conflicting attitudes this could bring in patients who might continue to hope for improvement, even when their disease was advancing. Therefore, '[t]o accept a situation when treatment is directed to the relief of symptoms and the alleviation of general distress will no longer mean an implicit "there is nothing more we can do" but an explicit "everything possible is being done"'[192]. This, for Cicely lay at the heart of the opposition to euthanasia and would be a position she maintained for the rest of her life, even as the medical landscape continued to change and become more complex.

Changing Roles

The year 1985 saw key changes at St Christopher's. Albertine Winner stood down as chairman and became president of the hospice, succeeding Lord Amulree, who had died the previous year. This enabled Cicely to take over as chairman and Tom West to replace her as medical director. Cicely's change of role proved to be an unfolding process and was accompanied by much painful and personal deliberation. As she explained to John Fryer: 'There came a time when it was right to go to Albertine and talk to her on the basis of a long discussion which Tom and I had with Sam while he was over, and indeed on the basis of what we have been thinking about over the past months'[193]. There was much rational talk with Klagsbrun about 'the changing of the guard', about her worries concerning Tom West, and about the need to develop a stronger senior management team. There were also less rational, more emotional exchanges about a terrible sense of conflict, of being pushed away, edged out, dismissed, and of losing control[194].

Three factors can be discerned in the process of Cicely giving up her role as medical director of the hospice she had founded.

First there was Marian and marriage. Cicely quickly realized and submitted to the fact that Marian's health was in decline. She could not, however, predict the trajectory which it would take. In the event, it was intermittent and extended. She rightly judged that if she wished to care for him in his last years — however many of these there may be — then she would need seriously to draw back from the many responsibilities which came with her role. She had to start disappointing her admirers around the world and to decline their invitations. Equally, she appeared at times increasingly impatient with the many acolytes who wanted to come to St Christopher's, to have their photograph taken with its founder, and to take up the time of the staff. Wifely devotion to Marian was an escape from the undesirable elements of her situation, as well as a barrier to continuing with the aspects which gave her pleasure.

Second, in stepping back from the role of senior doctor, she averted the growing possibility that her clinical acumen might be diminishing. Even in the not very rapidly developing field of hospice and palliative medicine, Cicely was in danger of getting out of touch. The syringe driver for continuous infusions of analgesia, the development of slow-release formulations of morphine, and the newer generation of anti-depressants were all areas with which she was less familiar. It would be embarrassing to get something wrong or to have to rely too heavily on others to cover for her. Likewise, when teaching and lecturing farther afield, if her material was less informed by contemporary clinical practice, then embarrassment could result.

Third, there were the growing pressures inside the hospice. Her colleagues could see Cicely was not only slowing down herself, but was also becoming more absorbed with her responsibilities towards Marian. His well-being was a constant preoccupation to her and was affecting day-to-day matters. In particular, Tom West was concerned the place should be run differently.

Tellingly, when West became medical director, Cicely remained in her office, right over the entrance to St Christopher's, and from which — with an eagle eye — she watched over its comings and goings. Tom moved in next door. She was in the chapel most mornings and continued with her long-standing practice of taking the prayers herself on Mondays. She was regularly in the dining room and, after a pre-prandial sherry, took a rather dignified promenade through the building to go to lunch and then return to her office. She did weekend on-call work in the hospice, often subtly backed up by the second doctor who checked carefully on her activities. She took a hand in fund-raising and did a measure of administrative work. There was an unambiguous message that Cicely was still at the helm and must be closely consulted on any matter of significance. She remained a continuing presence on a daily basis and would do so for some years to come. It was clear that she was not retiring.

Notes

1. Cicely Saunders interview with David Clark, 16 May 2000.
2. Clark D. Originating a movement: Cicely Saunders and the development of St Christopher's Hospice, 1957–67. *Mortality*. 1998; 3(1): 43–63.
3. Cicely Saunders letter to The Rev A.E. Barton, 10 November 1966. Clark D. *Cicely Saunders: Founder of the Hospice Movement: Selected Letters 1959–1999.* Oxford: Oxford University Press; 2002: 117 (hereafter *Letters*).
4. Cicely Saunders letter to The Right Reverend the Lord Bishop of Stepney, 23 January 1967; Clark, *Letters*, 119.
5. Cicely Saunders letter to Sir George Godber, 16 April 1964; Clark, *Letters*, 68–69.
6. Cicely Saunders interview with David Clark, 16 May 2000.
7. Cicely Saunders interview with David Clark, 16 May 2000.
8. Cicely Saunders interview with David Clark, 16 May 2000.
9. Cicely Saunders letter to Colin Murray Parkes, 14 June 1966; Clark, *Letters*, 107–108.
10. Cicely Saunders interview with David Clark, 16 May 2000.
11. Cicely Saunders interview with Neil Small, Hospice History Project, 7 November 1995.
12. Cicely Saunders interview with Neil Small, Hospice History Project, 7 November 1995.
13. Cicely Saunders interview with Neil Small, Hospice History Project, 7 November 1995.
14. Cicely Saunders letter to Sister Zita Marie, 13 August 1964; Clark, *Letters*, 74–75.
15. When the author discussed this version with Cicely on 12 December 2001, she seemed never to have heard of it and was indeed somewhat taken aback by the notion.
16. Cicely Saunders interview with Neil Small, Hospice History Project, 7 November 1995.
17. Cicely Saunders interview with David Clark, 11 May 2004.
18. Cicely Saunders interview with David Clark, 11 May 2004.
19. Richard Lamerton interview with Michelle Winslow, Hospice History Project, 14 October 2004.
20. Lamerton R. *Care of the Dying.* Hove: Priory Press; 1973.
21. Cicely Saunders interview with David Clark, 11 May 2004.
22. Cicely Saunders interview with David Clark, 11 May 2004.
23. Cicely Saunders letter to Ester Lucille Brown, 27 June 1969; Clark, *Letters*, 138.

24. Cicely Saunders interview with David Clark, 15 December 1999.

25. Cicely Saunders letter to Mother Leo Frances, 13 May 1968; Clark, *Letters*, 134–135.

26. Cicely Saunders letter to Florence Wald, 18 June 1968; Clark, *Letters*, 135.

27. Neil Small interview with Florence Wald, Hospice History Project, 29 February 1996.

28. See du Boulay S. *Cicely Saunders: The Founder of the Modern Hospice Movement*, 2nd ed. London: Hodder and Stoughton; 1994: 151–152.

29. Baines M. From pioneer days to implementation: Lessons to be learnt. *European Journal of Palliative Care*. 2011; 18(5): 223–227.

30. Barbara McNulty interview with Neil Small, Hospice History Project, 23 January 1996.

31. Saunders C. The patient's response to treatment: A photographic presentation showing patients and their families. In *Catastrophic Illness in the Seventies: Critical Issues and Complex Decisions*. Proceedings of the Fourth National Symposium, 15–16 October 1970. New York: Cancer Care; 1971: 33–46.

32. Saunders C., Winner A. Research into terminal care of cancer patients. In McLachlan G., ed. *Portfolio for Health 2: The Developing Programme of the DHSS in Health Services Research*. Nuffield Provincial Hospitals Trust. London: Oxford University Press; 1973: 19–25.

33. Dorothy Summers interview with Neil Small, Hospice History Project, 13 December1995.

34. John Fryer interview with Neil Small, Hospice History Project, 26 February 1996.

35. Cicely Saunders interview with Neil Small, Hospice History Project, 7 November 1995.

36. Tom West interview with Neil Small, Hospice History Project, 28 January 1997.

37. Cicely Saunders interview with David Clark, 20 September 2000.

38. Tom West interview with Neil Small, Hospice History Project, 28 January 1997.

39. Sam Klagsbrun interview with Neil Small, Hospice History Project, 27 February 1996.

40. Cicely Saunders interview with David Clark, 20 September 2000.

41. Thompson J.D., Goldin G. *The Hospital: A Social and Architectural History*. New Haven, CT: Yale University Press; 1975.

42. Goldin G. A proto hospice at the turn of the century: St Luke's House, London, from 1893 to 1923. *Journal of the History of Medicine and Allied Sciences*. 1981; 36(4): 383–415.

43. Goldin G. *Work of Mercy: A Picture History of Hospitals*. Erin, Ontario: The Boston Mills Press; 1994.

44. Cicely Saunders interview with David Clark, 25 September 2003.

45. Cicely Saunders interview with David Clark, 25 September 2003.

46. Cicely Saunders interview with David Clark, 23 August 1999.

47. Cicely Saunders interview with David Clark, 16 May 2000.

48. Cicely Saunders interview with David Clark, 16 May 2000.

49. King's College London Archives, SAUNDERS, Dame Cicely (1918 – 2005), K/PP149/1/24.

50. Cicely Saunders interview with David Clark, 16 May 2000.

51. du Boulay, *Cicely Saunders*, 216.

52. Cicely Saunders interview with David Clark, 2 May 2003.

53. Described in Cicely Saunders interview with David Clark, 23 August 1999, and also in a handwritten photocopied text, in possession of the author.

54. Gillian Ford, pers. comm., 4 September 2017.

55. Cicely Saunders letter to Grace Goldin, 15 February 1980; Clark, *Letters*, 198.

56. Cicely Saunders letter to Dr Arnold Rosin, 21 February 1980; Clark, *Letters*, 199.

57. Cicely Saunders interview with David Clark, 2 May 2003.

58. Cicely Saunders letter to Grace Goldin, 25 January 1982; Clark, *Letters*, 220–221.

59. Cicely Saunders letter to Balfour Mount, 22 July 1982; Clark, *Letters*, 225–226.

60. Cicely Saunders letter to Elsa Perkins, 2 September 1982; Clark, *Letters*, 228.

61. Cicely Saunders letter to Grace Goldin, 30 September 1982; Clark, *Letters*, 229

62. Cicely Saunders letter to Grace Goldin, 28 October 1982; Clark, *Letters*, 230.

63. Cicely Saunders letter to Marty Herrman, 10 March 1983; Clark, *Letters*, 235.

64. Cicely Saunders letter to Grace Goldin, 22 December 1983; Clark, *Letters*, 243–244.

65. Cicely Saunders letter to Hilde Berenbrok, 8 June 1983; Clark, *Letters*, 238.

66. Cicely Saunders letter to Carleton Sweetser, 23 June 1981; Clark, *Letters*, 209.

67. Cicely Saunders letter to Grace Goldin, 20 June 1983; Clark, *Letters*, 238–239.

68. Cicely Saunders letter to Grace Goldin, 4 May 1983; Clark, *Letters*, 248–249.

69. Cicely Saunders letter to Professor Eric Wilkes, 25 March 1985; Clark, *Letters*, 258–259.

70. Cicely Saunders letter to Carleton Sweetser, 28 August 1985; Clark, *Letters*, 262.

71. Saunders C. The last stages of life. *Recover.* 1968; Summer: 26–29.

72. Saunders C. A therapeutic community: St Christopher's Hospice. In Schoenberg B., Carr A.C., Peretz D., Kutscher A.H., eds. *Psychosocial Aspects of Terminal Care.* New York: Columbia University Press; 1972: 275–289. Italics added by author for emphasis.

73. Manning N. *The Therapeutic Community Movement: Charisma and Routinization.* London: Routledge; 1989.

74. Gavey C.J. *The Management of the "Hopeless" Case.* London: H. K. Lewis; 1952.

75. Colin Murray Parkes interview with David Clark, Hospice History Project, 10 January 1996.

76. Quoted by Colin Murray Parkes in an interview with David Clark, Hospice History Project, 10 January 1996.

77. Saunders C. *The Management of Terminal Illness.* London: Hospital Medicine Publications Limited; 1967.

78. Murray Parkes C.M. Home or hospital? Terminal care as seen by surviving spouses. *Journal of the Royal College of General Practitioners.* 1978; 28: 29–30.

79. Murray Parkes C.M. Terminal care: Evaluation of in-patient service at St Christopher's Hospice part 1: Views of surviving spouse in effects of the service on the patient. *Postgraduate Medical Journal.* 1979; 55: 517–522.

80. Murray Parkes C.M., Parkes J. 'Hospice' versus 'hospital' care: Re-evaluation after 10 years as seen by surviving spouses. *Postgraduate Medical Journal.* 1984; 60: 38–42.

81. Murray Parkes C. M. Terminal care: Evaluation of an advisory domiciliary service at St Christopher's Hospice. *Postgraduate Medical Journal.* 1980; 56: 685–689.

82. Saunders and Winner, Research into terminal care of cancer patients.

83. Saunders C. The challenge of terminal care. In Symington T., Carter R., eds. *The Scientific Foundations of Oncology*. London: Heinemann; 1976: 673–679.

84. Balfour Mount interview with Neil Small, Hospice History Project, 16 October 1995.

85. Balfour Mount interview with David Clark, Hospice History Project, 14 March 2001.

86. Cicely Saunders letter to Robert Twycross, 6 March 1978; Clark, *Letters*, 178–179.

87. Cicely Saunders interview with David Clark, 16 May 2000.

88. Saunders C., Walsh T.D., Smith M. Hospice care in Motor Neurone Disease. In Saunders C., Summers D., Teller N., eds. *Hospice: The Living Idea*. London: Edward Arnold; 1981: 126–147.

89. Saunders, Walsh, and Smith, Hospice care in motor neurone disease, 133.

90. Saunders, Walsh, and Smith, Hospice care in motor neurone disease, 134.

91. Saunders, Walsh, and Smith, Hospice care in motor neurone disease, 128.

92. For example: Holden T. Patiently speaking. *Nursing Times*. 1980; June 12: 1035–1036.

93. Saunders, Walsh, and Smith, Hospice care in motor neurone disease, 1981.

94. Lamerton R. *Care of the Dying*. Harmondsworth: Pelican; 1980.

95. Saunders C. Appropriate treatment, appropriate death. In Saunders C., ed. *The Management of Terminal Malignant Disease*. London: Edward Arnold; 1978: 1–16.

96. Saunders C. Current views on pain relief and terminal care. In Swerdlow M., ed. *The Therapy of Pain*. Lancaster, PA: MTP Press; 1981: 215–241.

97. Clark D. Between hope and acceptance: The medicalisation of dying. *British Medical Journal*. 2002; 324: 905–907.

98. Clark D. The rise and demise of the "Brompton Cocktail." In Meldrum M.L., ed. *Opioids and Pain Relief: A Historical Perspective*. Vol. 25, *Progress in Pain Research and Management*. Seattle: IASP Press; 2003: 85–98.

99. The Brompton Cocktail. *The Lancet*. 1979; 313(8128): 1220–1221 [Editorial].

100. Vere D. In Reynolds L.A., Tansey E.M., eds. *Wellcome Witnesses to Twentieth Century Medicine*. Vol. 21, *Innovation in Pain Management*. London: Wellcome Trust Centre for the History of Medicine at UCL; 2004: 15.

101. David Clark interview with Robert Twycross, Hospice History Project, 4 January 1996.

102. Twycross R.G. Choice of strong analgesic in terminal cancer: Diamorphine or morphine? *Pain*. 1977; 3: 93–104.

103. Twycross R.G. Value of cocaine in opiate-containing elixirs. *British Medical Journal*. 1977; 2: 1348 [Letter].

104. Twycross R.G. The Brompton Cocktail. In Bonica J.J., Ventafridda V., eds. *Advances in Pain Research and Therapy*, Vol. 2. New York: Raven Press; 1979: 291–300.

105. Overy C., Tansey E.M., eds. *Palliative Medicine in the UK c1970–2010*. Vol. 45, *Wellcome Witnesses to Twentieth Century Medicine*. London: Queen Mary, University of London; 2013.

106. Saunders C. The moment of truth: Care of the dying person. In Pearson L., ed. *Death and Dying: Current Issues in the Treatment of the Dying Person*. Cleveland, OH: The Press of Case Western Reserve University; 1969: 49–78.

107. Saunders C. Nature and management of terminal pain. In Shotter E.F., ed. *Matters of Life and Death*. London: Dartman, Longman, and Todd; 1970: 15–26.

108. Baines M. Symptom control in the dying patient. In Saunders C., Summers D.H., Teller N., eds. *Hospice: The Living Idea*. London: Edward Arnold; 1981: 93–101.

109. Saunders C. An individual approach to the relief of pain. *People and Cancer*. London: The British Council; 1970: 34–38.

110. Cicely Saunders letter to Dr Austin H. Kutscher, 1 December 1971; Clark, *Letters*, 151.

111. Cicely Saunders letter to The Rev W. Benjamin Holmes, 9 December 1971; Clark, *Letters*, 151–152.

112. Cicely Saunders letter to Elisabeth Kübler-Ross, 22 August 1972; Clark, *Letters*, 153–154.

113. Cicely Saunders letter to Christer Tovesson, 17 May 1978; Clark, *Letters*, 180.

114. Saunders and Winner, Research into terminal care of cancer patients.

115. Saunders, The challenge of terminal care.

116. Saunders C. The nature and management of terminal pain and the hospice concept. In Bonica J.J., Ventafridda V., eds. *Advances in Pain Research*, Vol. 2. New York: Raven Press; 1979: 635–651.

117. Saunders, Current views on pain relief and terminal care.

118. Twycross, Choice of strong analgesic in terminal cancer.

119. Cicely Saunders interview with David Clark, 6 June 2002.

120. Elizabeth Earnshaw-Smith interview with Neil Small, Hospice History Project, 30 January 1996.

121. Saunders C., Summers D., Teller N., eds. *Hospice: The Living Idea*. London: Edward Arnold, 1981.

122. Thelma Bates interview with Neil Small, Hospice History Project, 19 May 1997.

123. Cicely Saunders letter to Dr W.P.L. Myers, 16 August 1976; Clark, *Letters*, 167.

124. Saunders C. *Beyond All Pain: A Companion for the Suffering and Bereaved*. London: SPCK; 1983.

125. Clark D. An annotated bibliography of the publications of Cicely Saunders— 2: 1968–77. *Palliative Medicine*. 1999; 13: 485–501.

126. Lamerton, *Care of the Dying*, 1980; Lamerton, *Care of the Dying*, 1973.

127. Cicely Saunders letter to Grace Goldin, 5 September 1972; Clark, *Letters*, 154–155.

128. Goldin G. British hospices. *Encyclopaedia Britannica*, Medical Annual. Chicago, IL: Encyclopaedia Britannica Inc.; 1983: 82–83.

129. Cicely Saunders letter to Mother Potier, 22 December 1983; Clark, *Letters*, 243.

130. Cicely Saunders letter to Eric Wilkes, 25 March 1985; Clark, *Letters*, 258–259.

131. Cicely Saunders letter to Sue Ryder, 4 February 1969; Clark, *Letters*, 136–137.

132. Cicely Saunders letter to Dr Brian L. Mishara, 6 December 1972; Clark, *Letters*, 155–156.

133. Clark D. A special relationship: Cicely Saunders, the United States, and the early foundations of the hospice movement. *Illness, Crisis, and Loss*. 2001; 9(1): 15–30.

134. Cicely Saunders letter to Elisabeth Kubler-Ross, 6 March 1975; Clark, *Letters*, 162.

135. Buckingham R.W., Lack S.A., Mount B.M., MacLean L.D., Collins J.T. Living with the dying: Use of the technique of participant observation. *Canadian Medical Association Journal.* 1976; 115(12): 1211–1215.

136. Cicely Saunders interview with David Clark, 19 December 2000.

137. Cicely Saunders letter to Dr H.A. Coperman, 15 April 1977; Clark, *Letters,* 171–172.

138. Cicely Saunders letter to Dr H.A. Coperman, 15 April 1977; Clark, *Letters,* 171–172.

139. Cicely Saunders letter to Henya Elkinund, 25 October 1977; Clark, *Letters,* 175–176.

140. Cicely Saunders letter to Professor Tadeusz Koszwarowski, 29 June 1978; Clark, *Letters,* 181.

141. Cicely Saunders letter to Halina Iwanowska, 13 July 1978; Clark, *Letters,* 182.

142. Cicely Saunders letter to Mrs Y. Dale, 14 May 1970; Clark, *Letters,* 141–142.

143. Cicely Saunders letter to The Right Reverend the Lord Bishop of Southwark, 28 October 1975; Clark, *Letters,* 163.

144. Wilkes E. Where to die. *British Medical Journal.* 1973; 1(844): 32–33.

145. Saunders C. A death in the family: A professional view. *British Medical Journal.* 1973; 1(844): 30–31.

146. Cicely Saunders letter to Professor Kenneth Calman, 6 December 1977; Clark, *Letters,* 177.

147. Cicely Saunders letter to The Mother Superior General, 13 November 1979; Clark, *Letters,* 192–193.

148. Working Group on Terminal Care [The Wilkes Report]. *Report of the Working Group on Terminal Care.* London: Department of Health and Social Services; 1980.

149. Cicely Saunders, pers. comm. with the author, 14 March 2000.

150. World Health Organization. *Cancer Pain Relief.* Geneva: World Health Organization; 1986.

151. World Health Organization. *Cancer Pain Relief and Palliative Care.* WHO Technical Report Series 804. Geneva: World Health Organization; 1990.

152. Cicely Saunders letter to Florence Wald, 14 January 1969; Clark, *Letters,* 136. Cicely Saunders letter to Margaret G. Arnstein, 17 April 1969; Clark, *Letters,* 137. Cicely Saunders letter to Messrs Cotterell and Leonard, 8 July 1969; Clark, *Letters,* 139.

153. Cicely Saunders letter to Dr Claire F. Ryder, 27 June 1969; Clark, *Letters,* 137–138.

154. Cicely Saunders letter to David Frost, 7 November 1974; Clark, *Letters,* 161–162.

155. Cicely Saunders letter to Angela Tilby, 25 August 1976; Clark, *Letters,* 170.

156. King's College London Archives, SAUNDERS, Dame Cicely (1918 – 2005), K/PP149/2/2/20.

157. Cicely Saunders letter to Grace Goldin, 21 January 1980; Clark, *Letters,* 196.

158. Cicely Saunders letter to Professor W.J. Rudowski, 17 March 1981; Clark, *Letters,* 207.

159. Saunders C. Templeton Prize speech, first published in Saunders C. *Selected Writings 1958–2004.* Oxford: Oxford University Press; 1981: 57–62.

160. Cicely Saunders letter to Shirley du Boulay, 17 March 1983; Clark, *Letters,* 236.

161. du Boulay, *Cicely Saunders*.

162. Cicely Saunders letter to Edward England, 30 January 1984; Clark, *Letters*, 245.

163. Doyle D. Review: Du Boulay, S (1984) Cicely Saunders. The founder of the modern hospice movement. London: Hodder and Stoughton. *The Lancet*. 1984; 329(8535): 714.

164. Cicely Saunders letter to Grace Goldin, 28 October 1980; Clark, *Letters*, 205.

165. Cicely Saunders letter to Grace Goldin, 8 January 1981; Clark, *Letters*, 206.

166. Cicely Saunders letter to The Rev Benjamin Holmes, 6 August 1969; Clark, *Letters*, 139.

167. Cicely Saunders letter to Major General the Lord Thurlow, 8 August 1969; Clark, *Letters*, 137.

168. Cicely Saunders letter to Marty Herrman, 3 June 1970; Clark, *Letters*, 143.

169. Cicely Saunders letter to Marty Herrman, 27 November 1970; Clark, *Letters*, 144.

170. Richard Lamerton interview with Michelle Winslow, Hospice History Project, 14 October 2004.

171. Cicely Saunders letter to The Rev W. Benjamin Holmes, 1 December 1970; Clark, *Letters*, 144–145.

172. Cicely Saunders letter to Marty Herrman, 27 November 1970; Clark, *Letters*, 144.

173. Obituary: Ronald Michael Charles Welldon. *The Lancet*. 1970; 296(7683): 1145–1146. Also abbreviated as a biographical note in Welldon R. The 'shadow-of-death' and its implications in four families, each with a hospitalized schizophrenic member. *Family Practitioner*. 1971; 10: 281–302.

174. Cicely Saunders to letter Admiral J.M. Holford, 29 December 1970; Clark, *Letters*, 146.

175. Cicely Saunders letter to Lt General Sir Derek Lang, 15 June 1971; Clark, *Letters*, 148.

176. Cicely Saunders letter to *The Times*, 1 June 1971; Clark, *Letters*, 147.

177. Cicely Saunders interview with Neil Small, Hospice History Project, 7 November 1995.

178. Cicely Saunders interview with Neil Small, Hospice History Project, 7 November 1995.

179. Wye E.A., Mathisen J.H. *A Survey of the Management of Resources at St Christopher's Hospice*. Cranfield: Cranfield School of Management; 1970 [unpublished].

180. Cicely Saunders letter to Thelma Ingles, 25 September 1974; Clark, *Letters*, 160.

181. Saunders C. Care of the dying—1: The problem of euthanasia. *Nursing Times*. 1959; October 9: 960–961.

182. Cicely Saunders letter to Professor Dr A. Sikkel, 31 May 1972; Clark, *Letters*, 152.

183. Saunders, The moment of truth.

184. Saunders C. Caring for the dying. In Lack S., Lamerton R., eds. *The Hour of Our Death*. London: Geoffrey Chapman; 1974: 18–27.

185. Church of England Board of Social Responsibility Working Party. *On Dying Well: An Anglican Contribution to the Debate on Euthanasia*. London: Church Information Office; 1972.

186. Cicely Saunders letter to A.N. Exton-Smith, 2 August 1973; Clark, *Letters*, 158.

187. Saunders, Care of the dying—1.

188. An idea introduced three years earlier, see Saunders, A death in the family.

189. Saunders C. Care of the dying—2: The problem of euthanasia—2. *Nursing Times*. 1976; 72(27): 1049–1052.

190. Cicely Saunders letter to John Fryer, 28 April 1977; Clark, *Letters*, 172.

191. Saunders C. Caring to the end. *Nursing Mirror*. 1980; September 4: n.p.

192. Saunders C. Principles of symptom control in terminal care. *Medical Clinics of North America*. 1982; 66(5): 1169–1183.

193. Cicely Saunders letter to John Fryer, 27 August 1985; Clark, *Letters*, 261–262.

194. Neil Small interview with Sam Klagsbrun, Hospice History Project, 27 February 1996.

6 | Reflection, Illness, Loss, and Death (1985 – 2005)

The creative life that is also the creative suffering of God[1].

Good Times and Bad

In 1985, Cicely stepped down as medical director of St Christopher's hospice. She had been the only occupant of that esteemed position and it had taken some time to prise her out of it. Even then, she acted for a while as if nothing had changed, despite the symbolic and substantive shift to the role of chairman of Council. As her colleagues became more frustrated, things got worse rather than better. New thinking was gaining a hold in the National Health Service and the hospice was more and more having to fight its corner, not only over finance, but also over externally imposed benchmarks for quality, choice, and care standards. Specialty recognition for palliative medicine was also imminent, but this in turn would bring pressures as well as opportunities. Cicely was also beset by growing concerns about her husband's health, with accompanying scares and worries that would gradually escalate. She moved even more into the role of solicitous wife and carer and eased further back from professional commitments, some thought to the neglect of good order in the hospice.

As Chairman

In January 1985, Cicely wrote to two American colleagues explaining that her new role as chairman would allow her to spend more time with her husband. She felt 'the Hospice is well able to develop in its own way now, but I will still be about'[2]. On the one hand, it seemed a plausible scenario, but it was also a potentially dangerous cocktail. In truth, the handover of roles at St Christopher's was not straightforward — and that probably surprised no one. Neither was it Cicely's finest hour. She clung doggedly to her status, her treasured office space, and her degree of influence across 'the house'. The handover took up most of the year. Sensing trouble ahead, she also had Sam Klagsbrun confirmed as hospice visitor. He would have to mediate between her and Tom West when disagreements occurred. If Klagsbrun considered West an appropriate successor to Cicely, one who would allow others to come up through the ranks and express themselves more fully[3], Cicely was not so convinced. She saw West as a very good number two, but 'not at all a good number one'[4]. Later, West couldn't remember when he had taken over as medical director — perhaps a sign that, in Cicely's eyes, it never really happened. But others saw his 'watch' as successful, consolidating, and more consensual in style than that of his predecessor[5]. As he settled into his role, Cicely gradually became more comfortable as chairman. In early 1986, she told Grace Goldin that she was now 'occupied with strengthening and enlightening the Council, not in competition with the Executive'[6]. She became more interested in the workings of hospice governance, even conducting a survey of fifty-five medical directors on their relationship with their boards of trustees. She was also helped in her deliberations by her old friend Gillian Ford, who from 1986 had secured a secondment to work for three years at St Christopher's as director of studies. Together they began to shape some ideas about a form of institute that could be established at St Christopher's and would function as a place of high-level training. They even registered it as a non-profit organisation in New York[7]. Its name was the St Christopher's Hospice International Foundation, and by early 1987 it was receiving donations. Though in any event, it did not develop as intended; it foreshadowed a later foundation that would bear Cicely's own name, that would be established in a university setting separate from St Christopher's and that quite quickly would have a global influence.

The Role of Medical Director

With Cicely unable to travel and needing to stay at home with Marian, the opportunity arose for Tom West to take on more conference appearances and attend international meetings. His sardonic and very English style of delivery pleased external audiences and, when separated by great distances from the hospice, he felt more able to speak his own mind and less constrained to toe the party line[8]. Back at St Christopher's, he developed his ideas about family care, as well as staffing issues and support. He did not last long as medical director, however. By 1990, West, now in his early sixties, was ready to retire. He had been ill, undergone surgery and an extended period of sick leave in 1989, and didn't seem to recover his strength fully thereafter. He gave two years' notice of his intention to leave, having reached a point where he had nothing else to give to the hospice or the wider field and was ready to stop. In particular, the combination of clinical work and hospice administration was proving uncongenial. Neither he nor his wife seemed to be in good health.

He told Cicely: '[W]e are not old but we are ageing'[9]. Though he made his decision without regrets, the lengthy period of his notice was not helpful and only served to prolong another set of uncertainties about succession — and with it further tensions between him and the chairman. If he had seen himself as a bridge between Cicely's era and the one that was to follow, in retrospect he felt he had only succeeded in building its foundations[10]. This was perhaps a self-deprecating assessment. Curiously, the metaphor was one that Cicely also used, in a lecture she was fond of giving, titled 'Hospice as Bridge Builder', that was first delivered (by satellite) to the Montreal Conference of 1990. Unlike West, she was far from ready to settle into an undemanding and sequestered retirement.

Now a new challenge emerged. Finding a replacement for Tom West would be done through an external appointment process. St Christopher's had never selected its medical director in this way before. Two candidates were interviewed and, in June 1992, Cicely wrote to Geoffrey Hanks, Britain's first professor of palliative medicine, to tell him that Dr Robert Dunlop had been appointed[11]. Elected as a fellow of the Royal Australasian College of Physicians in 1986 and with a Ph.D. in Chemistry from Queen's University, Belfast, Dunlop had more recently been working in the palliative-care team at Bartholomew's Hospital in London. Shortly before his appointment to St Christopher's, with his nurse colleague Jo Hockley, he had published a book on the workings and organisation of such teams[12]. He brought substantial clinical experience, scientific knowledge, an awareness of the pharmaceutical industry, an interest in management, and a deep concern for the care of the whole person. He had a big vision for the future of St Christopher's. Cicely wrote to hospice founder and former I.W.G. president Bill Lamers in the United States with all the news. She considered that Dunlop would 'take us on in a stimulating and exciting way' and told Lamers that she would 'stay around as Chairman for the time being over the transition, but perhaps more in the background than you might think'[13]. It wasn't really to be.

Wider Issues

Cicely maintained a high public profile in the interstices of caring for Marian. When in 1992 Dr Nigel Cox, a consultant rheumatologist in Hampshire, England, was found guilty of attempted murder after injecting a seventy-year-old patient with potassium chloride in order to relieve her suffering, Cicely wrote to the Secretary of State for Health, Virginia Bottomley, urging her to encourage wider discussion about difficult decisions at the end of life[14]. She anticipated Lord Walton's ensuing review of medical ethics, that was precipitated by the Cox case, wrote to him early during the deliberations of his House of Lords committee, and was relieved that it recommended no change to the law on assisted dying and euthanasia[15]. Expressing her pleasure at the outcome to Balfour Mount, she nonetheless felt (correctly) that the long campaign from the palliative-care world against euthanasia was still not over[16]. Whilst holding on to this outward-facing role, she also kept up a close interest in the day-to-day issues of the hospice and would write in detail to Sam Klagsbrun long letters containing updates on everything from the state of the budget to a new baby in a staff member's family. She apprised Klagsbrun of recent appointments, marketing plans, National Health Service changes, and internal communications. She also relished his visits and the reports he wrote by way of follow-up. Her orientation was more the over-weaning administrator than the figurehead chairman[17]. She would eventually struggle to maintain these two approaches, and indeed, in time, she could appear Janus–faced, looking simultaneously to the past and to the future; but also like Janus, she would be called upon to preside over the beginning and ending of conflict, even if she was part of its source.

At the same time, Cicely had a global view of things, something she could never have imagined when she started her work in the field in the 1950s. She began collaborating with the American thanatologist Robert Kastenbaum on what became the first overview of international developments in hospice[18]. She published forty-nine works in the decade of the 1990s, moving markedly away from clinical pieces to wider commentaries, historical reflections, several introductions and forewords to the work of others, and five articles on euthanasia. She lobbied the George Soros Foundation to support hospice in Poland and travelled to Eastern Europe to see the situation on the ground in Lithuania and Belarus. She flew to Cyprus, Greece, the United States, and Singapore (1996) for major speaking engagements, to Japan (1997) then to Australia and the Netherlands (1998), followed by an exhausting round of journeys to Germany, Norway, Switzerland, and the United States (1999). As the year 2000 approached, she seemed satisfied with the composition of the hospice trustees and the work of its management team. Despite increasing disability, she was still planning further international visits. Two thousand lights would be lit on the hospice Christmas tree to bring in the millennium. 'What have you that you did not receive' was a text from Corinthians that kept coming back to her[19]. She was not prepared for the storm that would soon envelope St Christopher's and her entire orientation to things.

With Marian

Combined with worries and strains relating to Marian's declining health, the tensions between Cicely and Tom West became a heavy burden and, in response to Sam Klagsbrun's advice, in 1986, she sought outside help. It came from Benita Kyle, a widow, who with her husband Bill had established the Westminster Pastoral Foundation at London's Methodist Central Hall in 1969. Cicely was the wounded healer who found benefit in psychodynamic pastoral counselling sessions, each one beginning with prayer. There was a strong spiritual dimension to the encounters, that suited Cicely well. She continued longer than originally planned and, in the end, it was the newly arrived Rob Dunlop, who told her she no longer needed to go. Nevertheless, she went back for one more session some years later when, as she put it, she had a 'bad attack of Antoni'[20].

In total, Marian had five life-threatening illnesses throughout the course of their marriage. Each time, his recoveries saw him returning to his artwork. It gave routine and focus, and could be accommodated to bouts of tiredness and be accomplished at home or even in a hospital bed. Grace Goldin was particularly fond of the series of small pastel images of the sun he produced. He was keen for her to have one in which the sun emerged brightly over the dark green of an abstract forest — perhaps a hint of the landscapes of his homeland. One drawing was done only four days before he died. In his quirky English, he came out with a steady stream of aphorisms and bon mots, that Cicely was fond of noting in her diary: 'I am happy as I never was', 'You are my complementary colour', and the morning after a little too much of his favourite drink, Dubonnet: 'I have an over-hang'. He continued to maintain a significant output of paintings, drawings, and pastels. After his 1986 spring exhibition, that Cicely arranged for him at the hospice, the works were 'scattered' around St Christopher's, Rugby Ward, and the Study Centre, and were given away to those who wanted them[21]. He was delighted with the occasion. His health and mobility had recently improved and they could even plan some holidays for later in the year, as well as visits to Oxford and Cambridge in June for honorary degree ceremonies. That summer, one of his grand-daughters, Alicja Szyszko-Bohusz, came as a volunteer to St Christopher's and, on her return to Poland, became involved in the work of the Nowa Huta Hospice in Cracow. She was one of several Polish summer visitors at that time who, despite the challenges of visas and passports, managed to come for six weeks in July and August. Fortified by the experience, they returned to Gdansk and elsewhere to contribute to the quickening efforts of the Polish Hospice Movement that was developing there[22]. It was all part of Cicely's Polish – hospice family that meant so much to her.

There was a symbiosis in staying at home with the ailing Marian. She told Balfour Mount that she didn't begrudge the restrictions it imposed[23]. In her late sixties, and after half a century of rushing around, organising, lobbying, and convincing others, or working in the dark days of loss and death with patients and families, the simple domesticity of Lawrie Park Gardens was comforting. If all this made for a quieter life, then that was so much the better[24]. Meanwhile, the health crises and scares with Marian came and went. In early 1987, after extensive investigations, Cicely was reassured that Marian did not have a malignancy but was in fact being troubled by T.B. glands in the neck, that required twice-daily dressings. Marian devoted most of his remaining energy to his pastel works, and some of these were quickly on display in the newly opened

Family Centre at the hospice. Cicely was determined to remind everyone of her continued presence and of the fact that Marian was with her and still shaping the iconography of St Christopher's. Over time, the profusion of Marian's paintings in the hospice would emerge as a site of tension, and a way had to be found to reduce their volume and visibility. But for now, Cicely quietly ensured they were in the ascendant, even as the artist himself was in decline. In late 1987, Cicely wrote to Sister Gilberte at Taizé, with a picture of Marian and a recent drawing, telling her 'how lively he is . . . still painting joyful and splendid pictures'[25]. Friends from afar read such letters and replied, inviting Cicely and Marian to make long-distance visits, but these were always turned down as 'not a viable proposition'[26]. Cicely was, as she put it to Robert Kastenbaum, 'extremely happy as Chairman of St Christopher's and as diligent spouse to an enchanting eighty-seven-year-old'[27]. Marian and Cicely were, by her account, 'blissfully happy'; she was protective of his age and had no grumbles about staying close to home or about the constraints on being away overnight[28]. There was great peace and contentment in these final years of marriage.

Reliance on Others

At the same time, there were practical considerations on the home front. Cicely's own mobility and general health were also in decline, compounded by her long-standing back problems. Here she describes the situation and the help she received from Hanka Jedrosz, who was now widowed and living alone on the floor above:

> While Marian was getting more and more disabled, she was more and more helping and I used to have a helper to wash him in the mornings. I had to start saying, 'I can't bend over to do all this for you'. I did a lot for a long time, but my back really wouldn't [allow it, so] I had a helper in the morning, a care assistant until about three and then she did the evening, and the night was on me. And then he got heavier and Hanka used to come down and wash him at weekends and help him dress. And it was Hanka who made the classic statement one day when we got him on to the commode here, she said, 'Well, he's lost his modesty but he's kept his dignity'. And I had a bell out there and in the last eight or nine months I really couldn't get him on and off the commode in the night and Hanka used to come down and help me and some-times . . . a bad night would be three or four times and a good night maybe once or twice, and so, you know, she was terrific[29].

The demands took their toll on Cicely. She suffered enormously with her stomach — an irritable bowel she called it — that would give her a gripping pain, often in the mornings[30]. Along with her arthritis, it made for slow starts to the day, when her own debilities and the needs of Marian ate into her morning time for reading and spiritual reflection. Marian, despite huge infirmity, but perhaps emboldened by disinhibition, found his own distractions and was able to flirt 'outrageously' with the 'awfully pretty girl' that came in from the private-care agency[31]. He even took an interest in her career ambitions and encouraged her to take an A level in psychology and become a counsellor, which she subsequently did. Cicely looked on it all with tolerant amusement. Marian was maddening; if challenged he would revert to speaking only in Polish, and if under pressure he would casually remove his hearing aid. But there was a love between them which was expressed in the simplest of ways — in home-cooked food, shared meals, and time spent with old friends and family. Christopher, Cicely's brother, admired Marian. Tom West had completely taken to him. Grace Goldin and many of the other American friends of Cicely had all spent time with them as a married couple, enjoying holidays and visits together. Marian's children and grandchildren had become a part of Cicely's life. It was a remarkable gathering up of scattered threads which had not always connected in the earliest days of their relationship.

The Death of Marian

But Marian's life was coming to an end. He had become too challenging for Cicely and Hanka to care for at home, even with extra help. Now he had a bad chest infection. In December 1994, he was admitted to St Christopher's and was looked after in a single room on Rugby Ward, not far from his studio. Twice he nearly died, only to revive again. In the last days he repeatedly told Cicely he was completely happy with his life and that he was ready to go. On 28 January 1995, 'he slipped away peacefully and finally rather unexpectedly'[32]. For Cicely, Rob Dunlop's care for her husband — no easy medical task in the circumstances — was exemplary. She found him holding his patient's hand as she hastened back to the ward, only to learn that Marian had just taken his last breath. It confirmed a point she had so often made in lectures. No one should feel guilt that they are not present at the very end of a loved one's life: '[W]e have to go before they can let go'[33].

They held a requiem mass for Marian at the Church of the Resurrection of Our Lord in Sydenham Kirkdale, not far from their home and from the hospice. The striking modernist architecture and large sculpture of Christ above the entrance door (a less than remote echo of St Christopher's) would no doubt have appealed to Marian and to Cicely. To Cicely's satisfaction, two priests — one Catholic and one Anglican — presided over the occasion, as had happened at their wedding. The hospice chaplain spoke of the love between Cicely and her husband. Marian's friend, Polish violinist and barrister Damian Falkowski, played Vaughan Williams's 'The Lark Ascending'. Marian's large painting of the resurrection was later given by Cicely to the church which had laid him to rest. His ashes were scattered in the garden at St Christopher's, marked by a simple grey stone cross, carved with his Christian name.

After Marian died, the first person Cicely called was her step-daughter Daniela, whose immediate response was to say: '[Y]ou must come and stay with us'. Within weeks, Cicely was on the aeroplane to California. She stayed for nearly a month and came back looking twenty years younger according to her driver, Barry. Marian's death, if anything, strengthened the relationship between the two women. Cicely took a close interest in Daniela's situation and its challenges, including life as a single parent with a daughter going to university. She was also proud of Daniela's achievements, her beautiful house in San Francisco, and her willingness to visit London with her daughter Max and to stay in touch over the years. Through Daniela, she would continue to keep the connection with Marian — really the only man who had ever made Cicely *happy* in an uncomplicated way.

The Developing Field

Within a decade of the opening of St Christopher's Hospice, some were seeking to establish that the principles of hospice care could be practised in many contexts — in specialist inpatient units, but also in home-care and day-care services. Likewise, hospital units and support teams were being formed which engaged with the challenge of bringing the new thinking about dying into the settings of hospital acute medicine. As these services expanded, the focus of intervention also widened, from care of the actively dying to those earlier in their disease progression with symptom problems, and with an increasing focus on care management, quality of life, and a desire to engage with patients' and families' needs and preferences wherever possible. Cicely watched all this with great interest. She had long argued that hospice was not just about terminal care, that it could enhance quality and meaning in life regardless of the time which was left. She could see that this diversification and stretching of the newer concept of palliative care was vital to reaching more people who could benefit, though as she grew older, she seemed less interested in contributing to the many societies and new organisations which began to spring up around the burgeoning field. Yet, she still responded in detail to enquiries from other potential hospice founders and was generous with her time and in passing on information. She was clearly pleased that, through the 1980s, a steady process of hospice expansion was underway in Britain. The 'movement' that she had unconsciously founded was burgeoning, and her part in its formation was by now widely acknowledged.

A Fully Fledged Specialty

As hospice and palliative care developed, there was growing interest in establishing it as a medical specialty which would have its own recognised training pathway for doctors wishing to concentrate their efforts in this area.

Cicely's friend Gillian Ford was instrumental in this. It was she who, from her position in the Department of Health, had written a key briefing paper outlining the value of specialty recognition. As part of the management team at St Christopher's from 1985, Ford started looking at issues such as the training of medical staff around the country who were already involved in palliative care, and presented her results to the newly created Association of Palliative Medicine at one of its early meetings. She surveyed eight hundred G.P.s, asking them what they would identify as their needs in this field. By finding out more about training requirements, realising hospices needed to do things such as appoint senior staff in conformity with the National Health Service, and recognising the value of joint or honorary contracts, she adduced that everything was pointing in the direction of a specialist programme of training for doctors in palliative medicine. At the same time, Derek Doyle, medical director of St Columba's Hospice in Edinburgh and an acknowledged mover and shaker in the field, had been talking to the junior doctors in the Association and asking what *they* needed. The driving force was a requirement for this expanding group of people to be recognised for the clinical work and teaching they were doing, now in many different settings and organisations.

With Gillian Ford's expert manoeuvrings, discussions got underway with a number of key groupings within the Royal Colleges, the most influential of which was the Joint Committee on Higher Medical Training (J.C.H.M.T.). At the time, a growing number of universities and medical schools were calling on those working in hospices to teach students about pain control and physician – patient/physician – family communication, though as yet no formal curriculum on palliative medicine existed. Ford prepared a paper for the J.C.H.M.T. and, at the same time, encouraged the chair of the Specialty Advisory Committee in General Medicine and other senior medical colleagues to visit St Christopher's for an appreciation of the work being done there. The outcome of these deliberations was enormously important for the history of palliative care in the United Kingdom (U.K.) and, arguably, much farther afield too[34]. In 1987, exactly twenty years after the opening of St Christopher's, palliative medicine was established as a sub-specialty of general medicine, initially on a seven-year 'novitiate' which once successfully concluded led to the creation of a specialty in its own right. In that year, all U.K. doctors working full time in hospices were granted specialist registration. Thereafter, entrants into higher medical training for the new specialty were required to be members of the Royal Colleges of Physicians, G.P.s, or psychiatrists; or fellows of the Royal College of Surgeons[35]. Cicely wrote to Josefina Magno at the International Hospice Institute in Washington: 'Good news from here about accreditation. Gillian has managed to get this through our Royal Colleges and be on the inspection team approving hospices for such experience'[36]. Though Cicely had played a minor role in the effort, she was ensuring that St Christopher's remained centrally placed in the unfolding narrative of specialisation, palliative medicine recognition, and the formal growth of the field.

As specialist recognition emerged in this way — indeed, as a pre-requisite for its emergence — there was a need for greater clarity of definition and scope for this new form of activity, as well as more precision about what it could achieve and where its boundaries might begin and end. A major step forward had come through the interest of W.H.O. and its chief of cancer, Swedish oncologist Dr Jan Stjernsward. The W.H.O. definition of palliative care emphasised the active, total care of the patient, focussing on the control of pain and other symptoms as well as providing psychological, social, and spiritual support to improve the quality of and to affirm life, whilst regarding dying as a 'normal process' and seeking neither to hasten nor postpone death[37]. Cicely endorsed the approach and often recommended it to others. If she was not closely involved in the work that was going on through W.H.O., her former clinical research fellow Robert Twycross certainly was and she kept in touch through correspondence and, later when she resumed international travel, at palliative care conferences, with some of the main activists, such as American pain specialist Dr Kathleen Foley and Italian palliative care leader Professor Vittorio Ventafridda. She sensed the W.H.O. orientation was less sympathetic to hospice, favouring a more public health and health systems approach, and was keen to let Stjernsward know that the hospice contribution remained important:

> So long as we maintain our standards and continue with all the volunteers, research and training that is demanded of us, I think we will be a useful resource for perhaps a large number of people who will be working within more traditional medical settings[38].

By 2002, a second definition of palliative care appeared from W.H.O.[39], stating that palliative care is an approach which improves the quality of life of patients and their families facing the problems associated with life-threatening illness, through the prevention and relief of suffering by means of early identification and *impeccable assessment and treatment* of pain and other problems, physical, psychosocial, and spiritual. Palliative care had thus become even more expansive in its goals and had sought to move its influence 'upstream' to earlier stages in the trajectory of illness. At the same time, there was growing interest in *end-of-life care*, viewed more broadly in relation to people with a wide range of conditions and diagnoses. Cicely was noting all this in the last years of her life and remained surprisingly au courant with the unfolding debates. She recognised the different approaches which were developing in Britain and America, in particular the so-called 're-framing' of palliative care, away from the last stages of life, stimulated in part by the concern of patients and families that physicians will abandon them if hospice care is recommended. Palliative care, seen in this way, was no longer something that commences when all else has failed; it becomes an integrated component of mainstream medical practice, to be pursued legitimately alongside other clinical goals. Cicely supported this — indeed, she had argued for it in some of her works, stating in 1995, for example:

> The achievements for which palliative care has aimed have above all been the potential that patients still have in physical ease and activity, in personal relationships and in emotional and spiritual growth. Such treatment may itself not only add to quality but also to length of active life, or even result in referral for more active intervention after all[40].

In due course, this was modified further by others and emerged in an approach to palliative care that increasingly followed the demands and orientations of the patients and those close to them, acknowledging these were changing over time as new treatment possibilities emerged and as cancer therapies in particular began to extend remission and increase survival. It could then be argued that delivering palliative care to achieve better symptom control, improve communication, and produce greater alignment with patient and family wishes had become primary goals. Only when these had been realised was it appropriate to engage with questions of meaning, mortality, and the reality of death. This seemed a departure from Cicely's model of 'total pain' which had been widely adopted by hospices and in which a strong focus was on finding personal and/or religious closure at the end of life, and where a wider social goal of making society better was also being pursued in addition to providing care to patients and families. Indeed, for Cicely and her followers, such work served as a measure of the very worth of our culture. As she put it in a very early article — and continued to maintain over the years: 'A society which shuns the dying must have an incomplete philosophy'[41].

Stepping out of the Spotlight

It may come as no surprise, given her interests, orientation, domestic duties, and advancing age, that Cicely gave opinion and comment mainly from the sidelines as detailed discussions got underway about these matters, and also through the formation of organisations such as Help the Hospices and the Association of Palliative Medicine. Although she was consulted, offered advice, and readily proffered her opinions, she was not in the driving seat. Content to be a passenger, she could watch as others continued the journey, even as a process of 'routinisation'[42] got underway involving the bureaucratic overlay of systems, procedures, guidelines, and rules which might eventually obscure the charismatic origins of hospice as a social movement. Cicely was not unduly romantic about this. In a way, it was others who worried more than her about the putative processes, particularly in relation to spiritual care[43]. Instead, Cicely was the pragmatist. She could see these new organisations and associations, whatever their limitations and self-serving tendencies, would be a necessary step on the road to greater recognition for hospice and palliative care. Meanwhile, she kept her own steady focus on promulgating her ideas through continued writing, lectures, and educational contributions at St Christopher's and farther afield.

Last Years at the Hospice

The late 1990s saw St Christopher's suddenly move into financial difficulties and then a moment of organisational turmoil. Cicely was no stranger to deficit at financial year end, and in her years as medical director and as chairman, had somehow managed to muddle things through, often relying on some windfall or large grant to steady the ship. She called it 'living on faith and an overdraft'[44], but the sums in the past had never been so large as now. The hospice had reached a turnover of £10,000,000 annually, only thirty per cent of which came from contracts with the National Health Service. Problems were looming.

Crisis

In 1998, St Christopher's had a surplus of £500,000. The hospice was becoming larger and more complex. There was talk among the senior staff of ambitious plans to make a big leap forward. The workload had been rapidly increasing and the home-care service had expanded massively. The style of general management, and the requisite skills which went with it, were showing themselves inadequate to the task. In the process, the administrator, Chris Clark, with whom Cicely had been known to have explosive encounters, left his post at the hospice. Then there were some unsuccessful fund-raising appointments. Suddenly, and it seems under the very eyes of the senior management team, surplus was turning into deficit. Unexpected legacies were being used to fund revenue expenditure. With no investment portfolio, St Christopher's was operating from just twelve weeks of running costs in reserve. Then the legacies dried up, with nothing to offset them from the fund-raising people. The half-million surplus of 1998 became an equivalent deficit in 1999. By the summer of that year, the word was out. St Christopher's was in trouble. As medical director and also chief executive, a dual role he had taken on in 1997, when a new senior management team was forged, Dr Rob Dunlop maintained his pressure on the local National Health Service to give extra financial support to the increased service that was being provided by the hospice. But it was clear that he too was struggling under the pressures of the day. Savings would have to be found and they would have to come in part from redundancies. In early 2000, a large meeting of staff and managers took place. The atmosphere was antagonistic toward the chief executive, who seemed unable to respond or win back support. By now the treasurer had resigned, the personnel officer had left, and there was growing anxiety about the future.

Members of the staff were in shock. They had not known of the growing problems. They were not only at risk of losing their jobs, but also they were losing something deeply meaningful in which they had made huge personal investments — a reality which was lost on some of the human resources expertise brought in to manage the process. There were prayer vigils in the chapel, and Cicely focussed her sentiments especially on those whose posts would be made redundant. One nurse of twenty-four years' service came with flowers to say it had been a privilege to work at the hospice. The St Christopher's Prayer Diary, first started by Helen Willans and naming people and groups inside and outside the hospice which should be remembered, was actively revived. Cicely prayed for Dunlop. She had a soft spot for him. He had looked after Marian with skill and empathy, but she could see that, for all his reading in management books, he was not up to the task he faced. Seventy members of staff signed a letter of no confidence in him. It was an extraordinary state of affairs in the most famous hospice in the world. After the previous prevarications of Council, Ian Mills, Chair of the Finance and General Purposes Committee, now moved swiftly. Dunlop was told to clear his desk and take an extended period of absence. He did so, but never came back, quickly finding employment in the private medical sector, after which he largely lost contact with Cicely and with palliative care. Twenty-six redundancies followed, along with an additional ten people who left voluntarily. Barbara Monroe, the social worker who had joined St Christopher's in 1987 and, a decade later, had taken on the role of director of patient and family services, was now appointed acting chief executive.

Throughout it all, Cicely looked to the future and believed that providence would deliver, quoting Psalm 46: 'The Rivers of the flood thereof shall make glad the city of God . . . .'[45] Salvation would come out of adversity. Divine grace like a full and never-failing river would yield refreshment and consolation. Or, as she put in in more secular terms: '*reculer pour mieux sauter*'[46]. It was partly about delaying the inevitable, but also a latent sense that they would emerge stronger and more able. Yet, on the central issues, Cicely (as chairman) seemed to be losing her grip on the situation. On the one hand, deeply imbricated in everything which was going on, she could appear at the same time curiously detached from it. So she observed wryly and rather naively in March 2000, just as the whole series of events was reaching its peak: '[A]t the moment I haven't been blamed. People have been rather sorry for me'[47].

This was soon to change. In late summer and at short notice, she received a message that two members of Council, Sir Adam Ridley and Rodney Bennion, would be coming to see her at home on a Saturday morning. Her secretary, Christine Kearney, saw the unfolding plan. Sir Adam was also seeking a meeting with Sir Edward Ford to encourage him to step down as president of St Christopher's, leaving the way open for Cicely, who would then have to demit office as chairman. In her sitting room, Ridley's opening gambit, that according to Cicely went 'on and on', used the analogy of the family firm where people stay too long. The two men explained that whilst she described herself as a figurehead chairman, she was, in fact, too involved in day-to-day matters — as they put it, sitting in her office and watching constantly to see who was coming and going and what was happening. She listened and then flatly refused to accept their proposal. Later it was said she told her visitors to 'bugger off'. She took some pleasure in recounting this, though claimed it was not true. In her own words: 'What I said was, "No. I'm not going to make up my mind on a Saturday morning, but the person I want to refer to is our visitor, Sam Klagsbrun. That's what a visitor is for, if there are problems. I'm not going to say yes or no, but at the moment I'm saying no, on a Saturday morning out of the blue." Well, pretty well out of the blue'[48]. She quickly spoke to Klagsbrun, who promptly got on an aeroplane and flew to London.

Speaking face to face with Sam Klagsbrun, Cicely acknowledged she must go sooner or later, but absolutely refused to give up her office or to cease coming into St Christopher's each day. It was *plus ça change*, but the visitor supported her. He had a long talk with Mills and then told Cicely that Mills would be the right choice to take over as chairman, for a proposed two-year period. Reconciliation was in the air. Cicely and Mills spoke again on a couple of occasions, at her home and in the hospice. They reached agreement on her proposals and, though he seemed unclear on what he wanted from her in the proposed and neologistic role of 'founder president', she felt she had got the arrangement on her own terms. But Mills also wanted to speak to Cicely's brother Christopher. It seemed a move calculated to undermine her autonomy, seeking the imprimatur of a family member on the arrangement and enlisting Christopher to persuade Cicely to acquiesce. At any rate, Mills achieved his goal. He wrote to Council, explaining Cicely had decided to retire, but would take over her new role from Sir Edward. He, Mills, would be willing to stand as chairman. The new arrangements were fully endorsed at a meeting of Council on 19 October 2000. By now, the head-hunters were seeking applicants for the chief executive post. Five candidates were in the frame, two withdrew before interview and, with Ian Mills in the chair, Barbara Monroe was the choice of the panel. She was fully in post by year end. Meanwhile, public donations came in amounting to £200,000, some of the previous year's deficit was written off, and new income streams were agreed with the National Health Service amounting to £500,000 in revenue monies. The corner had been turned, but Cicely, hurt and angry at first, then resigned and resilient in due course, was left with a sense of mistrust about the key actors and worried about the approach and direction of the new leadership. At a very practical level, she was concerned more for the prospects of her loyal secretary[49]. She need not have been worried; Christine Kearney continued to work at St Christopher's until 2015.

Good Things and Mixed Emotions

With the new arrangements in place by the end of 2000, Cicely, then eighty-two years old, had two tasks in her mind. She wanted to find a settled day-to-day orientation to life at St Christopher's and she also wanted to support the growing plans around a foundation which would share her name. Both would form part of her legacy, but they were not easily compatible. At the same time, she was looking and sometimes sounding frailer. By early evening she was tired, alone at home, and eager for a glass of whisky, perhaps more than one. She ruminated on how to find a modus operandi with the new chief executive of St Christopher's. As she put it in December 2000:

> I think, and Barbara thinks, she can work with me. She thinks she can manoeuvre me and I think I can do my own thing. We can be honest with each other. I think she has truly got St Christopher's to heart, I think she is *extremely* capable.

But there was already a concern within senior circles about where this new Institute (as it was now being called) was heading, and the consequences that would follow for St Christopher's. Cicely could 'foresee a certain amount of hassle and choppy water ahead'. She worried that St Christopher's would drift away from her and become 'A.N. Other Hospice', albeit in a determined effort to meet the profound needs of its local community. She was concerned that the wider international and academic role it could play would be lost, and she believed the new external initiative would rightly address these areas. She concluded in December 2000: 'I have to put my main energies into the Institute. I'm very happy to consider doing that'[50].

By the end of 2001, the Cicely Saunders 'foundation', after slightly intermittent beginnings, was becoming more formalised. John McGrath, chairman of the High Street chemists Boots, was its first formal chairman, taking over from Sir Richard Giordano, who had spearheaded the initiative, and together with Professor Irene Higginson of King's College London and members of the board, had set about creating a strategy, getting approval from the charity commissioners, and raising some initial funds to create an office and appoint administrative staff. Cicely was impressed by McGrath's energy and commitment, as well as his ability to deal with the 'angst' these developments were creating at St Christopher's. At the same time, she feared the hospice might push her out as they had done others of late. As she reflected, these worries 'produced a lot of thinking . . . and clouded the year quite a lot . . . . It's a bit of a muddy pool, isn't it?'[51]

But despite these concerns, there was other great good fortune for Cicely and for St Christopher's. Some two years earlier, Barbara Monroe's husband had seen an advertisement in *The Economist* seeking applications for the Conrad N. Hilton Humanitarian Prize. Initially developed by Rob Dunlop, the bid was signed off by Sir Adam Ridley as a trustee. The Conrad N. Hilton Foundation quickly showed interest and the hospice received a visit from its chief executive, Judy Miller, but the application, although well received, was unsuccessful. However, they were invited to re-apply for the 2001 prize. This time all went well. Miller and her team visited Poland to see the influence of Cicely and St Christopher's that had occurred there. The St Lazarus Hospice in Cracow gave a good account of things, tracing the story back to Cicely's visit of 1978. At a time of feeling embattled at the hospice, that in truth was the beneficiary of the prize, Cicely was pleased to see the $1,000,000,000 award as an endorsement of her own vision, first and foremost, played out though the structures of St Christopher's and its wider influence. The prize-giving was scheduled for September 2001, but had to be postponed because of the terrorist attacks in New York. Rearranged for late November, Cicely travelled with Barbara Monroe, as chief executive, and her secretary, Christine Kearney. They flew on a special ticket called 'Upper Class Virgins', that greatly amused them, and stayed opposite Central Park at the Waldorf Astoria, where the presentation took place and Cicely spoke at a lunch for three hundred people who watched a short film about her work. She was interviewed and photographed for *Time* magazine and several other media outlets. During the next few days she was able to catch up with Florence Wald and Sam Klagsbrun. On the downside, the trip was exhausting. She had to get up at 5 am for her bowels to settle, her back was painful, and by the end she vowed: '[T]this is my last trip'. That said, it was her second visit to America of 2001. Earlier she had visited Brown University and Harvard, where she spoke about medical ethics and palliative care to a full house. The audience had included what she called 'a lovely bunch of oldies from an extremely posh retirement home, old professionals who have a discussion group on ethics, who came and sat at the front'[52]. That year she had also made a quick visit to Germany and taken part in the I.W.G. meeting in the Netherlands. It was to be her final year of international travel — and she was going out on a high note.

In 2002, the new foundation bearing her imprimatur was formally launched. After various deliberations about the name, it was duly called *Cicely Saunders International*, suggesting a modern and outward-facing orientation. Professor Irene Higginson, as a leading international figure in palliative-care research and education, was appointed its scientific director. In due course, and some five years after her death, the foundation would establish the Cicely Saunders Institute, on the Denmark Hill site of King's College Hospital. Meanwhile, early reservations at St Christopher's about the initiative rumbled on, but Cicely felt that, having come out of the crisis of 1999, the house was in better order, and more appropriately managed — evidenced, for example, by major refurbishments of the wards which were then underway.

In the autumn of 2002, a collection of her letters written from 1959 to 1999 was published by Oxford University Press. She considered the volume to be 'a fairly honest story and I'm glad the honest story is going to be published'[53]. It was another element in consolidating the legacy and, to a degree, of setting the record straight. Meanwhile, she was doggedly keeping a close eye on the minutiae and day-to-day details of St Christopher's, no doubt to the enduring frustration of some of those working there. Talking in 2003, she could still list in detail the names of staff and comment on their effectiveness. She was able to draw on insights she got through giving out her special 'coming day cards', that were presented by Cicely face to face to each person on the anniversary of their starting at St Christopher's, and she could still offer opinions on the merits of new appointments. In some ways, she had become a case of what has been called 'founder's syndrome'. The term is used in particular to refer to problematic late-stage behaviours on the part of some creators of non-profit organisations. It has even been thought of as an 'illness'. Its components have been described as displaying grandiosity, ineffective management, the inability to effect smooth transitions to new leadership, and unwavering commitment to the original vision of the organisation[54]. All these elements could be found to some degree in Cicely over the two decades from stepping down as medical director, to her eventual death. She grappled with the dilemmas and could be inconsistent in her reasoning, but no one was really surprised she took the course she did. To have done otherwise would not have been Cicely's way.

Personal Rewards

If the 1984 – 1985 switch from medical director to chairman was painful for Cicely and challenging to her colleagues and the hospice community, it did not serve to interrupt the steady flow of interest in her work from outside and the growing recognition that was bestowed upon her. The academic honours continued to be awarded. In 1986, both Oxford and Cambridge conferred honorary doctorates of laws upon her in a remarkable double-header. Then, in 1989, Her Majesty the Queen awarded her the Order of Merit. Created by King Edward VII in 1902, the 'O.M.' can have only twenty-four members at any one time. Each member, upon investiture, is given a red and blue enamel badge which reads 'For Merit'. A portrait is painted of every recipient, that becomes part of the royal collection. The entire Order meets only every five years. On a member's death, the badge must be returned to the Queen, who receives the next-of-kin personally. It is said to be the highest and most exclusive honour in the British system. Following her award, Cicely joined a club that had included Florence Nightingale, T.S. Eliot, Winston Churchill, Edward Elgar, and Ralph Vaughan Williams. Her fellow members during her time in the Order included Francis Crick, Nelson Mandela, and Margaret Thatcher.

Cicely's major lifetime honours and awards have been fully listed[55]. She won the Aristotle Onassis Prize for Services to Humanity in 1989. There was also the British Medical Association Gold Medal for Services to Medicine and Freedom of the London Borough of Bromley (1987), the Raoul Wallenberg Humanitarian Award (1990), Dame of the Order of St Gregory by his Holiness the Pope (1996), and the Franklin D Roosevelt Four Freedoms Medal for Worship (2000). In April 2003, a *British Medical Journal* survey of doctors found her the third greatest physician of all time. She accumulated a total of twenty-five honorary degrees. It was a dizzying array of acknowledgement which always brought satisfaction, and frequently a sense of fun and excitement as she joined in the accompanying celebrations and ceremonies.

Radio, Television, Interviews

From the mid 1980s, Cicely appeared in a series of radio and television programmes and was the subject of several documentary films. From around the world she was visited by journalists, students, acolytes, and researchers, all of whom were eager to record her story and to relay it to others. One set of interviews conducted in 1997 and 1998 led to an entire book about Cicely, written in German[56]. At the B.B.C. she had developed a good relationship with Shirley du Boulay and her colleagues, as well as Michael Mayne during his time as head of religious broadcasting. She also had fruitful links with religious columnist and broadcaster Clifford Longley, who wrote for the *Times* and later the *Daily Telegraph*, as well as with presenter Mark Tully, who also covered religious subjects in his series 'Something Understood', one of which, broadcast on Remembrance Day 2000, was an interview with Cicely about the possibility of discovering hope in the depths of suffering and grief[57]. In addition to these intellectual media folk, she was likewise at ease in the company of popular television presenters such as Alan Titchmarsh and Esther Rantzen. If she did not become a household name, she certainly appeared on the television screens of many households.

Among all the broadcasts that resulted, one merits particular mention.

Desert Island Discs

The B.B.C. radio programme 'Desert Island Discs' was the brainchild of broadcaster Roy Plomley. Begun in 1942, and continued thereafter with just a small number of presenters who followed its creator, the show amassed more than three thousand episodes in eight decades. It became a classic of B.B.C. radio. During the programme, 'the castaway' chooses eight pieces of music they would take with them to a desert island, one of which one must be singled out as the special choice. In addition, the castaway is allowed the Bible (or another religious text) and the complete works of Shakespeare, plus one book and one luxury of their own choosing. Plomley presented 1,791 editions of the programme stretching over forty-three years, each one meticulously prepared and providing insights into the life and work of the guest, held together through the musical choices and their biographical importance. The archive[58] of 'Desert Island Discs' recordings reveals a stellar list of famous and talented people from across the spectrum of politics, the arts and entertainment, literature, the professions, sport, science, and culture. Cicely was invited onto the programme and the episode was first broadcast on 30 January 1994. Her host was the second of the programme's presenters, former news reader and current affairs anchor-person Sue Lawley.

Cicely's broadcast, much of the story well told and understood from elsewhere, covered her through the days at Roedean ('I hated it'), Oxford, nurse training, her back (which 'finally packed up'), meeting David Tasma, and the subsequent history of the Hospice Movement. She gave a brilliant summary of the 'work' that a patient may have to do in hospice, even when it is not clear how much longer they may have left to live, but when it is a time to review one's life and to be at one's most mature point of reflection. Her favourite piece of music was 'Symphony No. 7 in A Major' by Ludwig van Beethoven. Her luxury was plenty of paper, pens, and pencils so she could write 'bad poetry' when unhappy. Her favourite book was her 'endless fascination' for the Oxford Dictionary of Quotations. As a 'people person', she declared she would be desperate to get off the island at the earliest possible opportunity.

Cicely's initial musical choice was the opening of Chopin's first piano concerto, played by Christian Zimmerman. She wanted to make an early emphasis on her Polish preoccupations. Despite its demanding loud chords and scintillating arpeggios, she described it as a piece she often played whilst writing. Next was music she'd heard at home as a child — Paul Robeson's 'Swing Low Sweet Chariot'. Her choice of the singer, Kathleen Ferrier, took her back to her second period in Oxford and her time in the Bach choir: 'See the saviour's outstretched hands', from the St Matthew Passion. Lacking any obvious warmth for her castaway, Sue Lawley seemed a little snippy with Cicely, even impatient to move her along, perhaps unconvinced by the narrative of Antoni Michniewicz. Schubert's *Auf den Zee*, with its beautiful rippling accompaniment — 'something one almost wants to dance to' — lightened the mood, and then it was on to St Christopher's and the patients who helped to make it happen. Cicely articulated the purpose of modern hospice, explaining to her host that it is not simply a place where people go to die, that it is not all gloom, but indeed a place where profound questions may be asked of the caregiver. Returning to her houseman days in the St Thomas's Hospital choir, Cicely explained that, on a few occasions, they had been conducted by Ralph Vaughan Williams himself — so her choice now was the soaring violin notes of 'The Lark Ascending'. Talking of Marian at the time they married ('we were very old'), she acknowledged that marriage was something she had always wanted. As it turned out, and as we have seen, 'The Lark Ascending' was played at his funeral. Her next choice was for him — the bright and bustling rhythms of Beethoven's seventh symphony. When the inevitable question came on euthanasia, Cicely did not dispute that, for some people, this might be the considered viewpoint, but she argued against it on grounds of the slippery slope and the risk that many would come to see themselves as a burden to others. As to M.N.D. as surely a case when euthanasia might be justified, she replied with the observation: '[W]ithin dependence there is a surprising independence'. Her seventh choice was again back to her singing: 'The Heavens Are Telling the Glory of God', from Haydn's Creation, that a St Christopher's choir had once sung with others in Norwich Cathedral. When asked about her own death, Cicely wanted time to say thank you, to say sorry, and to sort out something of herself to be able to say, '[W]ell, I am me and it's alright'. The journey into death is one into mystery and, for the Christian, it is also one into love. To this end, her final choice was *Lux aeterna* from John Rutter's Requiem, representing a sense of peace at the end of life — one that she had seen so many people reach for themselves over so many years.

Other Profiles

Cicely was the consummate interviewee and never lost her enthusiasm for talking to others about herself, though as she once remarked, she could rarely remember what she had said afterwards[59]. Among the many magazine articles and newspaper features, that had begun in the 1960s and were still much in evidence in the last years of her life, a few of the later ones stand out.

In 2002 she had an unexpected visit from the lawyer and wife of the British Prime Minister, Cherie Booth. *Good Housekeeping* magazine had asked Ms Booth to nominate the woman she would most like to interview. She wanted to choose someone feisty, determined, and British. There seemed no better choice than Dame Cicely. The interview took place in the sitting room at Lawrie Park Gardens, and in the accompanying photographs, Cherie Booth appears fully engaged in the discussion. In the posed image of the two of them, Cicely, newly diagnosed with breast cancer, looks exceedingly well — resplendent in a red jacket and gold jewellery. In the background are her laden bookshelves and vast numbers of her favourite long-playing vinyl recordings. The interview itself covered her entire life in just three pages, touching on all the major milestones and topics. Rather grandiosely, it was titled 'The Woman Who Changed the Face of Death'[60]. Perhaps to Booth's disappointment, Cicely declared 'I'm not a rampaging feminist. The role of women has changed, but it has changed around me and I wasn't particularly conscious that I had anything to do with it'[61]. It was perhaps a fair summing up of Cicely's orientation to matters of gender, and indeed to wider structural issues, other than, of course, to what most preoccupied her — care of the dying.

There was another connection about this time with the higher echelons of the Labour Party. Distinguished and long-serving Labour politician Gordon Brown always found time in his career for side projects, usually of a literary nature. In his later years as chancellor of the exchequer and shortly before he became prime minister, he embarked upon a book about courage. He structured it around eight lives: Edith Cavell, who nursed the wounded of the First World War in Belgium and helped Allied soldiers escape back to Britain; protestant pastor Dietrich Bonhoeffer; businessman and diplomat Raoul Wallenberg; Martin Luther King; Robert Kennedy; Nelson Mandela; Aung San Suu Kyi; and Cicely Saunders. We thus find her in exemplary company, placed by Brown at the highest levels of achievement in modern times. The courage he found in his subject was that of a visionary, who (again in that phrase) 'changed the face of death'. It was also that of one who had the courage to love what she must lose — David and then Antoni. Her courage in turn led her to battle against the medical assumptions of her times. In a chapter of remarkable range and detail, Brown captures much of Cicely's life and achievement and designates her 'one of the greatest humanitarians of our time'[62]. Unrecorded by Brown in the book, his interviewer had asked Cicely: 'What are you afraid of?' The reply was surprising: 'Well, I'm afraid of upsetting other people because I can barge in and catch people off guard . . .'[63]. It was a sensitivity that was lingering with her in these later years and had also cropped up in the Booth interview, when she had commented on her tiresome habit of earlier years, when she could never stop herself from correcting people, even in public. Through the public interview, highly familiar to Cicely, and really a rather routine experience for her, she was also undergoing an incremental process of life review.

Photographs, Portraits, and Sculptures

Cicely was photographed frequently, even from her days at St Joseph's, when she too used her camera to take images of patients. As medical director at St Christopher's, she was the subject of a series of well-crafted images taken by distinguished photographer Derek Bayes. There are also some striking photographs of Cicely by her friend Grace Goldin. Cicely was not photogenic and, though many pictures show her smiling and looking directly at the camera, it is often the stuffiness rather than the warmth that comes across in the posed settings, almost always arranged when she was rather formally dressed. Some more candid, unposed images, particularly in later life capture, her tender side, such as one taken at the Wellcome Witness Seminar on the history of pain, held in London on 12 December 2002. There are remarkably few images, readily seen, of a relaxed Cicely, casually attired and caught in an 'off-duty' mode. An exception is a set of holiday photographs taken with Marian in the English countryside in 1969. There may be others like them, locked away in personal albums or scrapbooks.

Marian painted Cicely several times. He found a sort of quirkiness in her that seems to have been lost on other artists, who tended to emphasise her severity. A full-length portrait of her by Bohusz-Syszko, seen on the cover of this book, shows her seated with legs crossed at the ankles, turned just slightly to one side, but looking with warm attention at the painter. Her plain blue dress is elegant and she is wearing a watch, pearl necklace, and rings. A cardigan or throw on the chair gives a touch of ochre – that sets off the prevailing blues and greens of the background. Her glasses capture the moment. Dark rimmed and oval, they give her a zany air, beautifully matched to her inscrutable expression. Clearly, Marian saw in her some things which were lost on others, but of course he did know her more intimately than anyone else.

Sculpture

At Christmas in 2000, the hospice received a gift of £100,000 from city lawyer and philanthropist Jonathon Stone, with a condition that Cicely have her head sculpted in bronze for display in the entrance to St Christopher's. She had ten sittings with the figurative sculptor Nigel Boonham, of the Royal British Society of Sculptors and the creator of many other major works. But the year had been tainted by misgivings and tensions between Cicely and the hospice, and the artistic result was severe: 'I wouldn't want to cross her!' chuckled Cicely when describing it. On an elongated base, the head is again looking directly at the artist. Her elderly face is beautifully captured. Devoid of glasses and with the hair characteristically swept back from the forehead, there is a nakedness about her that is emphasised by the shallow detailing of the eyes, which appear as if clouded by cataracts. Ambivalently ('I'm not coming walking through reception and seeing my head every day'), she gave way to its display in the hospice entrance next to the lovely kneeling figure that she had herself commissioned in the 1960s[64]. But after her death, the bronze head was removed to the reception area at the Cicely Saunders Institute.

More attractive to her perhaps was *Dame Cicely Saunders*, commissioned for St Thomas's Hospital and placed on display in the Central Hall in 2002. The work of Shenda Amery, this second sculpture is composed of a bronze bust on a fibreglass and column-shaped pedestal, suggesting coloured marble, with gold lettering. It was unveiled on 14 March 2002 by cultural historian and then-director of the National Portrait Gallery Charles Saumarez Smith. In this work, the effect on the viewer is much softer. Cicely is again without spectacles, but now smiling, kindly, her high cheek bones well shown and her hair parted slightly to the left side. We see the almoner, the nurse, and the doctor who had walked the floors of St Thomas's, now content, wise, and full of empathy, and with just a touch of sadness around the eyes.

Final Portrait

A trilogy of works in these years was concluded in 2004 and 2005, with an oil portrait of Cicely. It too depicts her in rather severe manner, but was well received when it appeared. Catherine Goodman trained at the Camberwell School of Arts and Crafts, and the Royal Academy Schools. In 2002 she won first prize in the B.P. Portrait Awards. Cicely's portrait was commissioned from Goodman in 2004 for the National Portrait Gallery. There were some exhausting sittings, twenty-two in total, carried out initially at Cicely's home when her own health was in steep decline, and were concluded at the hospice. Goodman found a rare 'mutual concentration' in their sittings. As Cicely put it: 'You have to concentrate on what is interesting that you have done which, presumably, has an effect on your face'. They talked about Cicely's imminent death and the difference between human and spiritual fear. Goodman found in her none of the former, but a measure of the latter[65]. The work was unveiled, newly completed, in April 2005, only weeks before Cicely died. It drew much attention. On hearing that a friend of the artist had observed a look of 'love and steel' in Goodman's portrait, Cicely is reputed to have said: ' "Love and steel". How kind. Anyone doing hospice work will need plenty of both'[66]. It was a phrase much used by others down the years that followed. Love and steel might not encompass all of Cicely's complexities, but each was certainly part of her life and makeup.

Revisiting the Past: David, Antoni, and Marian

In the aftermath of Marian's death, the past came flooding in. Absolved of caring duties and spending more time alone, Cicely fell to thinking about the three men, all Polish, who had done so much to shape the narrative of her life over nearly half a century. Through many years, Antoni and Marian were, in Cicely's curious syntax, 'both being about'[67]. We can see now that the two men were curiously connected in time and geography. They were born in the same year: 1901. Both had lived on landed estates in the countryside but had also spent extended periods in the city of Wilno. They were educated and had been to university. They had made professional careers. Both had been captured whilst serving in wartime and had been displaced for long periods. Both were Catholic believers. They each arrived in London in the aftermath of the Second World War. Each was patrician and proud. Theoretically, at least, they might have met.

David, by contrast, was born a few years later, in 1907, in Warsaw. A city boy, he lacked formal education, never had a profession, and was, in his own words, 'only a rough old fellow'[68]. Common identity, nationality, and eventually place bound the three together — Polish men, exiled with no hope of return to their homeland, living in the city of London. Cicely's attraction to each of them remains puzzling. In each case she had placed her love on the margins of her cultural experience and background. Her other 'boyfriends' had been her own age or younger, English, urbane, at ease in a social milieu she could navigate and understand. These Polish men, older than her, struggled with the English language, stumbled over their words, and looked to her to articulate their thoughts. They awoke in Cicely a lifelong fascination for their country and drew her into its music, art, and religious life. With her, they generated a complex set of relationships which is perplexing and defies easy explanation, but is also oddly attenuated, even trivialised, in her often glib shorthand use of the term 'my three Poles!'

Antoni Again

Even before Antoni's death, Cicely had begun to dream about him, and this continued intermittently for almost the rest of her life. Some were recorded in handwritten notes. We have seen that her dream about Antoni in 1972 occurred at a time when she was still uncertain about her relationship with Marian. Then, at the age of eighty and on the night of 7 – 8 February 1999, just four years after Marian had died, Cicely had a vivid and last dream about her Polish patient from 1960.

The 1999 dream was very important. Written down the morning after in blue ink on yellow quarto and lined paper, presumably left over from a visit to America, where it is in common use, it comprised just three paragraphs, laid out in a bold hand, without a single correction and with just one missing word. It reads:

> We were in a hospice and he was in bed. I was allowed to show how close we were and to stay. I was able to lie on the bed beside him. We were closely together.
>
> I was involved in a seminar led by Tony Yates[69] and Antoni, well and strong, tall and thin was part of it, one of the contributors. We moved around together; I think we were planning. Then we moved on to go and perform and Antoni picked up a full despatch case; he had a lot of work behind him. We went together in a horse carriage.
>
> Then we were alone together walking through Hadley churchyard. It was quite large and full of trees. It was full of a feeling of security and peacefulness and there was no hurry. All the same I knew we were going to part and go our separate ways. I said, 'I think this [is] where my ashes should be scattered'. I woke up with a great sense of quiet happiness from just walking together hand in hand.

The first paragraph is intense and sexual. Its composition may even have been held in check to protect a sense of modesty. In the dream, the lovers are able to be close in a way which had never been possible in life. There is a sense of consummation in just three sentences. The second paragraph, however, is more opaque, confusing even. Whilst the seminar setting is familiar, the inclusion of a senior male doctor from St Thomas's, known to, but not closely linked with Cicely, is unclear. Although it appears that Cicely and Antoni are both to speak at the seminar, marking them out as equals, and he apparently has a large portfolio of work on which to draw, they seem also to be plotting their exit. When this happens, ambiguously, it is by horse and carriage, suggesting grandeur or an earlier era in time. It may be a link to childhood. From Monkenholt, as a child, Cicely had been taken each day to school by the same mode of transport —a carriage drawn by a horse. Hadley itself is then the setting in which the dream concludes. There, the lovers walk together hand in hand in a funereal but sylvan, calm and unhurried place. Now it is Cicely who has intimations of mortality and averts to a time after her death. But that is not yet to be. Yes the lovers must be parted again, but without sorrow, and on awakening there is a persisting sense of good things.

One day, not long after this occurred, Cicely was having lunch with two colleagues at St Christopher's[70]. They fell to musing on what a brilliant movie her life would make. Her story was taking on a dream-like and filmic quality. When one suggested that Vanessa Redgrave (suitably tall) should play the part of Cicely, she quickly responded: '[A]nd who would be Antoni?' There were awkward glances between her companions and one quickly interjected: 'Well I think we'd draw a veil over that one'. Afterwards, Cicely, still reflecting on her recent dream, was disturbed and thought to herself: '[W]ell, if that's the way it's been talked about, I'd better have the story properly told'. It had been recounted by du Boulay, to whom Cicely had opened up completely. But as Cicely remarked, 'not everybody who's read the biography, *has* read the biography'. She had written of him anonymously on occasions, albeit not concerning the personal relationship between them. It was him to whom she was referring in the oft-repeated narrative:

'Am I dying?'

'Yes', she replied.

'Long?'

'No'.

'Was it hard for you to tell me that?'

'Well yes, it was'.

'Thank you. It's hard to be told but it's hard to tell too. Thank you'.

Although she had also spoken about Antoni on television in 1976 on the B.B.C programme *In the Light of Experience*, she resolved to return to the story and to tell it more fully and personally. Now after her years of happiness with Marian, Antoni had come back and she found herself crying for him. It had all been so unfinished, so brief, so crammed with emotion and powerful sentiment. Yet at the same time, she knew that nothing before or since had brought her closer to God. If she cried, it was not just for Antoni, but for an unprecedented spiritual experience — one that must not be 'mis-reported'[71].

So it was that over a few weeks in June 1999, first at a small conference hosted by the Department of Palliative Medicine at the University of Sheffield, and then again just outside Bergen in Norway in a meeting at a place called Solstrand, she set out in more detail the story of Antoni, St Joseph's, and the summer of 1960, now contextualized and explicated in the light of experience and wider reflection[72]. Forty years on, as she explained to her audience on these occasions, it was not an easy story to listen to, nor to recount. Her experience with Antoni, she thought, might best be expressed in the words of William Blake's four line poem:

> He who binds to himself a joy,
> Does the winged life destroy.
> He who kisses the joy as it flies,
> Lives in eternity's sunrise[73].

She was not seeking to idealise or embellish the story. Her account was shored up by the practical detail and emotional power of the diary and daily prayers she had written down at the time. What occurred in those few weeks in 1960 was the essential foundation of all she subsequently sought to develop, but it was also the fount of a remarkable energy — one of both protest and of gratitude. It was about 'recognizing that an important dimension of being human is the lasting dignity of weakness and of going through the things we did not choose'[74].

As we have seen, Antoni Michniewicz, age sixty, was a widowed Polish electrical engineer who had been admitted to St Joseph's Hospice, Hackney, in February 1960. For some months he was just one of forty-five cancer patients Cicely was looking after, gaining no more or less attention from her than any other, until his daughter, Anna, explained her dying father had fallen in love with his doctor. Cicely was suddenly thrown into a short period of intensified emotion, in which her thoughts, feelings, professional judgements, and personal beliefs collided like atomic particles. She learned about his life in Poland, his wartime experiences, political exile, the death of his wife. Their snatched moments together were in full view of the hospice ward, or concealed by the flimsy curtain around the bed. They kissed just once, on the day that he died. In her talk in Norway, Cicely framed all this in the words of Carlo Caretto: 'Our passing is always a fearful ordeal, like looking at a boundless sea and then the explosion of joy as you watch the sea part — beyond there is nothing but love'[75]. In the years that followed his death, Cicely had to grow into Antoni's maturity, if not Blake's sunrise of eternity. If she was able to attenuate Antoni in her consciousness as her relationship with Marian bumped along and then stabilised, it was many years later that she was finally able to disentangle him from other sorrows and stresses, even those relating to her parents. As she remarked: 'I think Antoni has probably carried quite a load for other things'[76]. But as she also explained, with him: 'I've never been so close to God. So if I cry, it's not just for Antoni; it's for a peak of a spiritual experience'[77].

She had maintained an awkward relationship with Antoni's daughter, Anna. Apart from some photographs, she appears to have had none of his possessions or private documents. Now, in the summer of 1999, she had saluted his presence in her life by publicly declaring her enduring love for him, his ambiguous legacy, and everything she had done thereafter. In her lifetime, Antoni had been fully revealed by Cicely, but always as the source of an authentic suffering which galvanized her theoretical knowledge. Yes, he did become associated with some memorable and repeatable quotations, but they lacked emblematic importance for the Hospice Movement. Her various audiences could therefore be ambivalent about Antoni. Her experience with him perhaps had some generalizable lessons, but to develop such a relationship with a patient and then to struggle for so long to come to terms with it after his death was not a role model to be passed on to others. He could be conveniently labelled 'Cicely's second Pole', but he perhaps still arouses more equivocation than numbers 'one' and 'three'. Ultimately, the story of Antoni, despite his warmth and likeable persona, is perhaps harder for us to somehow accept and endorse, not out of any moral prurience or disapproval, but more from a sense of doubt about whether it should ever have been told.

At Peace with David

Less dramatically, and over many years, David Tasma had entered more prominently into the founding mythology of St Christopher's, captured in countless talks and letters, and immortalised in many publications. Her 'first' Pole now seemed to sit comfortably in her consciousness and in her spirit. He troubled her less than Marian and Antoni. David had left her the window, the hospice had been built around it, and he was permanently associated with its beginning. He was easier to acknowledge in public and was more centrally placed in Cicely's self-conscious narrative of St Christopher's and the wider movement it was to catalyse. She seems not to have dreamed about him, and he caused her no undue and painful reverberations in later life.

Her two Jewish patients-as-lovers, Antoni and David, therefore meant different things for Cicely, as she reflects in this eloquent statement made just a few years before her death:

> Well I think that's what I owe very much to Antoni, because he gave me the authenticity of having really been there, been really close to somebody who was dying, and being very close within bereavement, made me realise the potential that there is in that area, the power of powerlessness is something that you can go on learning about endlessly, so that you move from purely clinical into philosophical and theological insights, and there's no end to discovery

there. David gave me the idea. I was interested in the dying before I started visiting him in 1948. It partly shows why I made such a quick contact with him in the ward. And so he gave me the three basic principles: the openness to challenges of the window; the mind matched with heart, science, and spirit; and the freedom of the spirit is him making his own journey. They're basic principles which have lasted. Antoni gave me the head of steam to do it, because there's a real creativity in bereavement. There's a real desire to do something to make things better for somebody else. After Antoni died . . . there was a kind of ladder out of the very dark hole of grief, in which one upright was 'Oh, my love, how happy you are,' and the other upright was 'Oh God, I am so grateful.' Every time I managed to come back to seeing those I had built another rung on the ladder, and I was a little bit further out. But I still need that ladder sometimes after all these years[78].

More of Antoni

In due course, Cicely renewed her contact with Antoni's daughter, Anna. After periodic outings and exchanges of letters during the 1960s, often with long gaps in between on Anna's part, they had lost touch. Cicely knew the meetings were only for her own benefit and quietly let them drop. Then, when Shirley du Boulay was filming for the B.B.C. programme *In the Light of Experience*, they re-connected, getting Anna's agreement for Cicely to talk about Antoni and show his photograph. Marian and Cicely visited her home from time to time for dinner or tea. Anna was now married with four children. Just after Marian died in January 1995, Cicely was in San Francisco when, via the hospice, Anna's husband contacted her to say that his wife had been diagnosed with cancer of the ovary. Cicely took a close interest in Anna's treatment at the Royal Marsden, that was intense and exhausting. But soon Anna's condition worsened and she was admitted to St Christopher's, where she had a room of her own, and could spend time talking with Cicely and listening to the Mozart Clarinet Concerto, that had been a favourite of her father. There was a coming together between the two women, though Anna was a difficult patient for the ward staff. If it brought back many memories of Antoni and was only months after the death of Marian, Cicely nevertheless was glad of the opportunity to be reunited with Anna, albeit relieved that she was not there at the end, when her lover's daughter, like her father, died in a hospice at the age of sixty. Afterwards, Anna's husband was never heard of again and Cicely soon refrained from sending him a card at Christmas. It was the ending of a line.

But more reminders of Antoni came in 2001, the year Sister Mary Antonia died. She had been in charge of Antoni's ward at St Joseph's and it was under her purview, if not her full awareness, that the relationship between the doctor and the imminently dying patient had unfolded. On one occasion at the time,

Cicely had sensed some disapproval on the part of Mary Antonia, though it was never articulated. Curiously, Cicely wrote to Sister Antonia in May 1990, saying she had recently selected a few of her original notes from St Joseph's and 'finally threw the rest away'[79]. This was at best a half-truth, because many papers from St Joseph's certainly remained after Cicely's death, and they were subsequently archived. In particular, she had most definitely not thrown away her diaries and notes about Antoni. Perhaps there was something that made her want to reassure Antonia that nothing could survive in the record which might show the nursing Sister in a bad light, somehow turning a blind eye to an inappropriate state of affairs occurring on her ward. In her diary from those days, Cicely had, on one occasion, sensed a disapproval from the Catholic Sister and perhaps she felt it lingered with her still. Quietly, if disingenuously, Cicely had sought to give reassurance.

Then, in August 1997, Cicely wrote to Antonia:

> At this time of year I often think of Antoni Michniewicz, and that time in your ward remains as vivid as ever. You were very good to us in quiet support, and although you said you did not realise what was really going on, that in itself was a comfort. It is nice to know there is someone else who knows how special he was[80].

Perhaps it is no coincidence that Cicely's beloved patient and her dear nursing Sister had names in common, with just one letter of difference between them. They inhabited, for a brief time, the same emotional space, with Cicely as its fulcrum. The shared meaning of their names is 'priceless', 'praiseworthy', and 'beautiful'. With Antoni's daughter dead, the Irish nun had been the only other person left alive who had known Antoni at the time of his death. By 2001, Mary Antonia was gone too. Cicely had the comfort of knowing she was 'safely gathered'[81] and was perhaps with Antoni in heaven.

Moreover, Cicely had always believed that it was Antoni who led her to Marian. In March 1965, she had written one and a half foolscap pages of thoughts about Antoni[82]. She no longer felt the pain of their separation or the grief of watching his weakness and weariness. Now she felt they were not even apart, 'for he is so completely woven into all that I do and think'. It was her sorrow after his death that drove Cicely out that day in 1963, when she had discovered the exhibition in the Drian Gallery and Marian's painting of the crucifixion, 'and that is a joy both ways; it makes me so sure that he is still looking after me, and Marian is such a joy in himself and needed for St Christopher's'[83].

Marian's Continued Influence

Alongside all this, Cicely knew that it was Marian who had changed her for the better[84]. At one level she became 'much more bland . . . smoothed over', less likely to jump in on an issue or a person, more tolerant. He also put right the uncomfortable memories of when her friends were marrying, having children, and she was not. She no longer had to feel unwanted. More remarkably still, he was 'so sexually aware . . . even at his age he certainly was in all sorts of subtle ways too. He really could make somebody feel good'. When Cicely observed that 'he made all his pupils feel their paintings were worth something', she was undoubtedly referring to herself as well. After all, the cruel teasing that Cicely had received from her father was, as she put it so many years later, 'paid back by Marian'[85].

Eighteen months after his death, Cicely made a visit to Marian's place of origin. He was born in 1901 in the disputed territory of Byelorussia, that became the independent republic of Belarus in 1991. Like Antoni Michniewicz, Marian grew up there on a large estate (that Cicely always maintained belonged to his family), but the Russian advance of 1914 saw him driven off the land and moving with his grandmother to Wilno. He never returned to his birthplace or to anywhere else in Poland. In the spring of 1996, Cicely was visited by the Belarussian ambassador who wished to celebrate Marian with a permanent exhibition of his work, in his home village of Trokienniki. He invited Cicely to visit and look at the proposed location.

After discussing the sensitivities with the Polish ambassador, and mindful of the sensibilities of Marian's family in Poland, Cicely agreed to make the visit. In July, accompanied by her late husband's friend, barrister Damian Falkowski, and his wife, she made the journey, staying in Lithuania, just outside Vilnius. From there they took a day trip over the border into Belarus, travelling on through forest and farmland to Marian's village. There, in Trokienniki, the welcoming party included Dr Gorchakova, a children's palliative-care activist from Minsk and also Professor Maldis, Minister for Heritage. They were served with bread and salt, and presented with gifts. A group of six women sang to them and then they were given a lavish meal in the house which had been proposed as the home for Marian's paintings. Later, in a nearby church, a Polish priest celebrated a requiem mass for Marian and his parents, and Cicely's parents also. Deeply moved in the church where she was sure Marian must have been baptized, she left a white stone for him in the graveyard and was given two granite stones to bring back to London. One she kept at home by his photograph; the other she placed where his ashes had been scattered in the hospice garden. She found 'the Poles and Belarussians living well together' and agreed to donate drawings and prints to the collection in Trokienniki and an oil painting to the Minsk Academy[86]. It had been a remarkable journey and one never made by her with Marian. At last she had connected with the place from which he sprang. It was an element of closure for both of them, achieved when she was seventy-eight, and more than a year after he had died.

At the same time, Marian lingered on as a source of concern, if indirectly. By 2000, issues about his paintings were emerging more openly. This was a rare thing. In the past, ambivalence about them was largely unstated, except for one notable occasion in the late 1960s, when Richard Lamerton had openly scorned them. In the middle of a St Christopher's staff meeting he suggested, 'They're like scrambled eggs thrown at the canvas. They're hideous. They're badly damaging the atmosphere here and they're bad for the patients because they're disturbing to the mind. They're a disturbance'. At this, Cicely went black in the face and the next morning appeared in Lamerton's office, visibly angry. She explained that she had changed her will and the pictures were going to stay, even after her death. Lamerton told her: 'When I'm medical director here and you're dead, if that's what your will says, I will have a room made in the basement and we'll put them all down there, and if anybody wants to go mad, he can go down there any time he wants. Why should we all have to put up with these hideous things just because Dr Saunders's boyfriend painted them?' At this point, according to Lamerton (and allowing for his theatrical storytelling), she drew herself up to her full height, as 'icicles formed on all the windows' and said: 'Because it's true!'[87]

Likewise, there was truth in the ambivalence that surrounded the paintings. It finally surfaced again, when Cicely was much more vulnerable in later life, and as she was making the transition to founder president. In 1999, Cicely asked Michael Mayne, a Council member and former dean of Westminster, to convene an occasional group at St Christopher's to explore questions of spirituality as they related to the hospice. It comprised other Council members, some senior staff, and various associates — of varying shades of religious belief as well as those of no belief at all. During the discussions, Marian's paintings emerged as a focus for wider issues. They represented something about what the hospice stood for. They were a strong component it its iconography and were a constant presence for patients, families, staff, volunteers, and visitors. Not everyone felt this was a good thing. Some even began to speak about it more publicly, outside the hospice[88]. Cicely stated she would be very distressed if they were ever taken down. She had many examples where family members still showed interest in and enthusiasm for the pictures. Rob Dunlop told her they would never be removed whilst he was there. A large painting of the resurrection, once declined by the Vatican when proffered as a gift, and never Cicely's favourite, was a particular object of contention. As we have seen, Cicely neatly body-swerved that one by offering it to the local church, that was pleased to accept it after Marian's death. By 2003 she had sent the *Blue Crucifixion* and the painting called *Christ and People*, that had hung in the chapel, to the hospice in Cracow[89]. She planned to do the same with another resurrection painting. But it was a rear-guard action. Soon, other paintings were coming off the walls in the public spaces. It was suggested they be brought together in the former Draper's Wing as an exhibition — an idea Cicely thought ridiculous because she felt the paintings were there to nourish the soul of patients, visitors, and staff, not as works to be displayed, as in a gallery. After various discussions, Cicely changed her will again, to state that if they were not wanted at St Christopher's after her death, they should be offered to (what would eventually be) the Cicely Saunders Institute. Paradoxically, Marian may well have been affirmed, even amused, by all this. It was precisely the situation an artist might relish. The debates, tensions, and dissensions that were going on revealed the enduring power of his art — sparking emotion, firing controversy, and even shaping events and decisions.

Belief and the 'Cantus Firmus'

Religion, faith, and religious observance were a constant part of Cicely's day-to-day life beginning in the late 1940s. She prayed, she read, she attended formal worship, she conversed with others on spiritual matters, and she wrote at length on these subjects as they related to hospice and palliative care. It was a combined discipline which formed what her friend Michael Mayne, taking a musical analogy, described as the 'cantus firmus'. He was referring to 'the firm ground, the absolute rather than the relative, learning to hold firm to the heart of the matter and light to the rest'[90]. There is a sense here not only of the absolute, but also of a constant repetition, the *continuo*, which can be at the centre of a human life. Bonhoeffer had inspired this thought, writing to a friend that the 'cantus firmus' is that to which the other melodies of life form a counter-point. For Cicely, the bundle of her religious practice was exactly such ground. All other things — her work, her three Poles, her family, her pleasures — were secondary. When any one of these failed, after her conversion, she could always rely on her own *obligato*, not just as a way of believing, but also as a way of creating these primary beliefs through her daily routines. It was something echoed in Cicely's conviction, drawn from the poetry of Anne Ridler, that to learn to live is 'an exacting joy'[91].

Although she had started with it from soon after her conversion, in December 1953 her friend Stephen Smalley, later the dean of Chester, had given her a copy of *Daily Light*, sometimes known, according to Cicely, borrowing a phrase from Baptist theologian Glen Stassen, as a volume of 'kangaroo exegesis'[92]. We have seen that Cicely embraced it somewhat mechanistically, as others might a horoscope, to confirm or refute particular courses of action at a given time. She was still using the tattered and personally annotated copy given to her by Smalley, right up to the end of her life.

Paradoxically, the happy and absorbing years with Marian had also served to take away from some aspects of this spiritually organised life. Her daily attention to reading and prayer in the morning was eroded by the duties of wife and carer. Shirley du Boulay considered her 'prayer life' to have been attenuated at this time. After Marian died however, she had time for herself again, and this unleashed a powerful period of spiritual reflection that continued up to the very end. There were several aspects to this, ranging from matters of deeply personal belief and insight, through private and public religious observance, to further questioning about the place of religion and spirituality within the broad ethos of palliative care and, in particular, within the life of St Christopher's as an institution.

Religion, St Christopher's, Palliative Care

The hospice had been founded on Christian principles, but the decision had been taken that it was first and foremost a medical organisation. Over the years, the relationship between these had been much debated. Cicely's personal path had also broadened. This meant St Christopher's had found ways to shape and adapt itself to changing circumstances, but never (in Cicely's lifetime) losing its Christian ethos. But as her life drew to its end, and as her moral authority and practical influence came into question or was diminished in the hospice, so too did questions surface about its Christian orientation. As we have seen, the issue of Marian's paintings (most of which were, in fact, *not* religious in subject matter) became a flashpoint. They had come to represent a particular definition of the place, and this now came under wider scrutiny. The main objection was rooted in a concern for those of other faiths. But it may be that the works also represented too much about Cicely and her boundary-blurring ways — a set of pictures she had encouraged from the man who eventually became her husband, and which now spoke more of the past than the future. Incremental changes started to come into effect. In the chapel, a blind was installed in front of Marian's 1967 triptych (Figure 6.1); but, as Cicely noted in 1999, two visiting Imams declined the offer to use the blind when praying there, saying: 'No, you must keep your integrity and then we can keep ours'[93]. Indeed. Cicely felt, like the then-chaplain — Len Lunn — that it was the 'secular fundamentalists' who were more threatened by such images. She tried to emphasise the importance of St Christopher's 'keeping its own values', but also 'constantly learning', and by such means finding a way to meet with others of different beliefs and orientations[94]. These points related to two wider issues which concerned her in later years: one, the so-called secularisation of hospices and, two, the social exclusion of people of other faiths. There were also some linked issues which troubled Cicely at this time — the closure of the Draper's Wing being prominent among them — which she felt marked a significant change in the nature of community at the hospice, and where 'community' had been so closely tied to religious life and fellowship. She clung tenaciously to these matters of concern, as we have seen, inviting Council member Michael Mayne to explore them through a specially convened group which could look again, and in addition to the 'Foundation Group', at religious and spiritual issues in the hospice. But she was now losing traction, and after

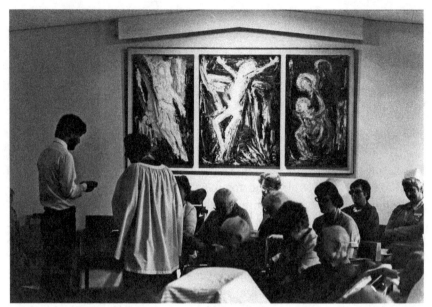

FIGURE 6.1 Cicely, the triptych, and the chapel. *Source: kept by Cicely Saunders.*

her death, the issue would later gather further momentum in ways she would not have approved.

An Evolving Faith

Cicely's religious worldview in late life fully embraced doubt, uncertainty, and the falling short of faith. It perhaps equipped her well for the personal and professional trials she encountered during her final years. She saw herself as still exploring, still reading diligently, marking things in her current Bible, following *Daily Light*, and the *Daily Psalms*, spending thirty-five to forty minutes in this way every morning at home from exactly 6:55 am, before then devoting ten minutes to prayer in the hospice chapel. Reading was key for her ('I'm not somebody who sits and goes off into a contemplative thing. And I don't sit and do Ignatian meditation. I've had a look at things like that and it's no good, I can't do it, so I don't try.'[95]). Here, in December 1999, she describes her morning devotions:

> I always start with saying a prayer, one which has been going on for months now is the prayer at the beginning of communion: 'Oh, My God, to whom all hearts are open, sense the thoughts of my heart . . . .' I find that very helpful. And then I concentrate on *Daily Light* and perhaps pick out a verse and think about that and make it into a prayer maybe. And then I read the Psalm for the day and maybe use a bit of that. And then I'm reading. I've gone back to the

Gospels at the moment. I had patches when I didn't read the Bible much and I read other spiritual books . . . it's a constant discovery. A lot of feeling of the Communion of Saints and remembering all the people — not just David, Antoni, and Marian — but a whole crowd of people who have been in the Draper's Wing and Jack Wallace and Carleton and all the others; from time to time, I sort of salute them and think of them in my prayers[96].

About 1960, the sister of Madge Drake, Eileen, had introduced Cicely to the English mystic Julian of Norwich. Julian's work *Revelations of Divine Love*, formed at the end of the fourteenth century, is thought to be the first book in the English language to be written by a woman[97]. We know it gave Cicely comfort in the immediate aftermath of Antoni's death. She had read the various translations as they appeared over the years and found deep solace in the rhythms of Julian's sorrowful, but eventually uplifting, prose. In late life, Cicely deepened her reading of Julian and could talk about her spontaneously and in rich detail:

When she was about thirty, when we think she was probably married and had lost children in the Plague . . . she was desperately ill, and the priest brought the crucifix to hold in front of her and she saw it bleeding and she describes it coming as thick and fast as water off the eaves. And she has a series of sixteen what she calls 'showings'. In one of them, she sees something in her hand as small as a hazelnut and said softly, 'What is this?'

And God said, 'It is all that there is'.

She wondered how it could last, and God said, 'It lasts because I made it and because I keep it and because I love it'.

And then she gets better and she becomes a hermit, or an 'anchoress', and has a little cell built on the side of St Julian's Church in Norwich. And after twenty years she writes a short version, and then after twenty years she writes the long version.

'Why did he show it to you?'

'For love'.

'What did he show to you?'

'Love. There will be never anything else to see but love'.

And God says to her, 'I will do a great deed which nobody will know until it happens and then all shall be well'.

She's gentle but very strong, and she has this feeling that somehow every-thing will be alright.

And she never sees any wrath in God, and God says to her, 'But all the wrath is in you. It's in people. It's not in Me. I'm nothing but Love and I cannot live with any wrath'[98].

In 2001, Cicely wrote the foreword to Michael Mayne's book *Learning to Dance*, a work exploring big themes in the encounters between contemporary life, the cosmos, art, faith, relationships, grace, and the promise of heaven. Its subject matter exactly reflected Cicely's own journeying, and the time of its publication found her in reflective mood in a year when her widespread travels were coming to an end and in which Sister Antonia's death had broken the last living bond with Antoni. She considered Mayne's book to be enchanted and enchanting. She was delighted at his various references to Julian and found that both authors, separated by half a millennium, could confront the issue of how 'all can be well' even when such pain, trouble, and distress come to God's creatures. Cicely was reassured that Mayne, in the manner of Julian, and ultimately rather like herself, was *content to live with the questions*[99].

Illness and Death

Cicely's living arrangements at 50 Lawrie Park Gardens continued to serve her well over the years. When Mr and Mrs Jedrosz retired in the middle of the 1980s, Cicely bought out their share of the house at its then increased value, thereby helping them financially. They stayed on, however, and things were otherwise unchanged. The action says something about Cicely's loyalty to them, and in time it was repaid handsomely as Hanka did so much to help Marian and then Cicely herself as her own condition deteriorated. But Vladeck became ill with Parkinson's disease and dementia and died in October 1988 in Hithergreen Hospital in Lewisham, southeast London. The two widows kept their own space on the upper and lower floors of the house, so the place never felt empty. Hanka did some shopping for Cicely and they would have a chat together every evening before bedtime. In 1998, Cicely had a knee replacement, followed by a second one the next year. To her surprise, she found she could not tolerate the opioid analgesics she was prescribed afterwards — a rich irony for one who spent most of her professional life promoting their use[100]. By 2000, Hanka was bandaging Cicely's legs every night to keep them from swelling. Despite their individual problems, the situation suited them and, for a few more years, it seemed to provide each with a measure of companionship and security, not least as Hanka was now herself much disabled by varicose ulcers and circulation problems.

In 2001, Cicely had done a considerable amount of travelling[101]. In particular, as we have seen, she had been in the United States for the Conrad N. Hilton prize-giving and had spoken at Brown University and Harvard. It had proved arduous, the packing hurt her back, and whilst she was away she had stomach problems. Barbara Monroe and Christine Kearney travelled with her and noted afterwards that she had needed much more help than on previous trips. Even her infamous and previously tried and tested methods of avoiding jet lag (a combination of alcohol, melatonin, and sleeping pills) were not working as well as before. Her account of the last visit and her general situation at that time is not pleasant:

> That was just a trip which was fairly exhausting and my back was hideous when I got there. And then my guts don't like getting up in the morning in strange places much; they grip me. I'm sure that's purely an irritable bowel, you know — psychosomatic. It did it a lot while I was looking after Marian and then, after he died, it stopped. But it's quite difficult to walk across a room with it, you know, to get yourself the whisky and the diazepam which you take while you sit and read your holy books and hope that it's going to go off. So I'd get up about five o'clock in the morning so that it has its hour or two to get settled down before you start doing anything. But it really did make me think[102].

Despite all this, she felt the American visit had gone extremely well, but it was time to stop. She was now turning down invitations from the United States. The I.W.G. meeting in the Netherlands that year and her contribution to the 'transformation group' had also been a success, but she would not attend its next meeting in Norway. Always the optimist, Cicely felt she could end her travels on a successful run.

One morning in January 2002, whilst taking a shower, Cicely noticed that her left breast was looking bigger than usual. She 'kept an eye on it' [103], examined it once or twice in the following weeks, and eventually found a lump. Her reaction was not the 'terrible great sinking of heart' which might have been expected, but rather a sense of relief: '[A]h, it's come at last'. She had long reckoned on it, even hoped for it. Big of build, a dominant person who never had children and had been on hormone replacement therapy 'for ages', she considered herself a likely candidate for breast cancer. Moreover, she understood the disease, had seen it close up on countless occasions, and knew it would afford many opportunities — to tidy things up, to make preparations, to say goodbyes. She had always said she didn't want to die of something like a stroke, but rather to go from cancer, 'which gives you time'. Her G.P. confirmed Cicely's suspicions and congratulated her on a skilled self-examination. The doctor could see that Cicely was going to be very pragmatic and would not have to be worried about. Cicely came out of the surgery and told her driver Barry, then in the evening she telephoned her god-daughter, Rosemary 'Bud' Burch, the daughter of Rosetta. Bud was the clinical nurse specialist running the breast clinic at St Thomas's. With her help, an appointment was fixed for Cicely to attend the Edward VII Hospital within a few days as a private patient, though without charge. When he saw Cicely, consultant Tony Young was slightly doubtful about the diagnosis made on the basis of an examination only. He ordered a mammogram and took a biopsy, but immediately confirmed Cicely's suspicions. They decided to delay admission for about a fortnight to allow Cicely to attend the unveiling of Shenda Amery's bronze bust. Despite the seriousness of the situation, things would be done without disruption to plans and without undue haste.

The mastectomy operation — or 'bunfight', as she termed it — took place on 19 March 2002. Cicely's self-described ample bosom made the procedure quite challenging. It also included, partly as a diagnostic procedure, the auxiliary clearance of lymph nodes. Standard management procedure at the time, it did indeed confirm palpable lymph nodes. She was totally impressed with the anaesthetist, who had been nervous of her, especially when told she would be nauseated by an opioid for pain relief. 'He did brilliantly because I came round in recovery in very good nick. I was operated on about two o'clock in the afternoon and by seven o'clock in the evening I was eating ham sandwiches'. She slept soundly between 11 pm and 4 am, woke with good arm movement, was given a 'most wonderful blanket bath', and (to her considerable amusement) was told by a nurse that she had a 'P.M.A.' — positive mental attitude. She then spent a few days over the weekend in the private ward upstairs, where she was visited by the chaplain and took communion on the Sunday. She had flowers and cards in abundance, and 'just the right number of visitors'. By Tuesday, she was back at home. Hanka too was in hospital at this time, but Barry brought in shopping and Christine Kearney visited every day. There would be no chemotherapy or radiotherapy. Cicely was established on a six-month course of tamoxifen and felt 'it couldn't be a more simple story'. Bud came in most days and, on some occasions, she drained fluid from under the lymph node scar tissue. One day, when Bud arrived with a temporary prosthesis, they collapsed in gales of laughter at the 'soft falsie'. It looked 'exactly like a chicken breast in a supermarket'. By the time Cicely had been to the premises of Rigby and Peller, corsetiers to the Queen, she felt totally happy with her appearance. Experts in such matters, they provided the exact kind of support that was needed, not least to hold up her rather heavy Order of Merit medal on special occasions. Though she looked a little fat in the mirror, it was certainly not enough to make her 'go on a diet or stop drinking'. She and Bud made giggly shopping trips together to a favourite place in Esher — 'always great fun' — and spent lots of money on new outfits. It was a chance to re-kindle something of Cicely's 'girly' side which had previously found an outlet only with her closest friends, like Rosetta Burch and Gillian Ford.

Returned from hospital, Hanka was, in due time, back upstairs, though much less able to help Cicely. They shared a washing machine, but when the laundry became too much for both of them, Cicely enlisted help from her cleaner, who also took ironing home. If it came back smelling of cigarettes, it only served to conjure up pleasant memories of Gordon, her father, who had been an assiduous smoker. Soon, Cicely's strength returned and, in around six weeks, she resumed her daily sessions in St Christopher's. The only modification to her routine was a slightly later start. Previously going in at 8:30 am for prayers in the chapel, at 8.45 she now listened to B.B.C. Radio 4 until 9:45, followed by the World Service daily religious programme. She then called Barry to drive her to St Christopher's. Despite these latest complications, she was resolute in her daily routine.

Hanka died on 12 October 2003. The local Polish priest had come on Saturday evening to deliver a house mass. Cicely had let him into the house and called up to Hanka that he had arrived, but there was no answer. He went upstairs and sat in Hanka's living room but felt uneasy as it was all too quiet. The priest too called out to her as he knocked on the doors to the different rooms and eventually found her in bed, her book open but no longer being read, and a cold cup of tea by her side. It was very strange without Hanka in the house. They had lived under the same roof since 1969. Cicely was relieved that after many years of bitterness and agnosticism about God, Hanka had come back to the Roman Catholic Church just three weeks before she died. A requiem mass was held for her, with personal tributes from several people and Cicely judged it 'a very, very good send-off'[104]. Another chapter had closed and another link with Marian had been severed. Cicely needed to find continuity and, inevitably, she looked to St Christopher's, despite the many changes that were taking place there.

The St Christopher's Foundation Group continued to meet in the hospice and the prayer group met at her house. She managed to get to the communion service in the chapel every Sunday at 10:30, often joined by Gillian Ford before her move from London to Lewes, as well as by a handful of patients and elderly volunteers. The numbers were usually in single figures, rarely more than twenty. There was also a service of blessing and laying-on of hands in the hospice chapel every second week, and on Monday, Wednesday, and Friday at 12:30 pm, Cicely was a regular attender for the chapel volunteers' short prayer meeting. This was important to her; it meant she was still able to 'pray for the hospice in the hospice'. The daily prayers in the chapel had been a part of her routine from the early days, and then lapsed for ten years while she was looking after Marian. When he died, she had enjoyed a return to them, but now they too were becoming harder to sustain. In her eighty-fourth year, she mused: 'I can't go on doing it forever. There must be a moment when I decide that I really must behave a little more like my age'.

One of the highlights of 2003 was a lecture at Westminster Hall in June. Her theme was 'Consider Him' in which, as on many previous occasions, she returned to the areas of personal faith, the inspiration for therapeutic work, the lessons taught by individual patients, and the need for community and fellowship in the care of the dying. It was a splendid affirmation of her life and philosophy. Approaching the end of her own existence, she could speak of the 'healing of wholeness and of many little resurrections'. She observed that 'the way care is given can reach the most hidden places . . . but you do have to face all the little deaths of living in this free and dangerous world'[105].

But by that summer, additional health problems were surfacing[106]. For some years publicist and lobbyist Geoffrey Tucker and his wife Naomi had been in the habit of taking Cicely and a group of friends to lunch at the Savoy Grill, around the time of her birthday. He had done so much for British Gas behind the scenes and had then been drawn into the work of the National Council for Hospice and Palliative Care, which was how he met Cicely. Tucker died in 2002, but his widow insisted they keep up the tradition the following year. When they duly assembled, as a group of ten, for lunch in the restaurant, there was a misunderstanding about the lift. Cicely found herself walking up a flight of steps, when suddenly her hip became extremely painful. The subsequent x-ray revealed a suspected secondary. A bone scan at St Thomas's confirmed a 'hot spot'. An M.R.I. scan revealed nothing else. At the end of July, Cicely was given one 'shot' of radiotherapy and another followed in due course. She was not alarmed by any of this, remarking, 'I only want another couple of years'. Meanwhile, her carers sought to control her side effects and settle her stomach, whilst she planned further social engagements, such as an event at Buckingham Palace in October for 'pioneers', and bought more clothes.

But towards the end of the year, other problems loomed[107]. The swelling in her legs got worse and she became breathless, weepy, and worried. She was glad to be welcomed into St Thomas's by Bud, where she was admitted to a 'staff bed' on the twelfth floor, to a room with en suite facilities and a wonderful view across to Big Ben and the Houses of Parliament. It was sixty-three years to the month since she had begun her nurse training there. The hospital did not forget its own, and of course she was now a great name in the world of medicine and palliative care. A registrar at the hospital recalled the scene:

> Looking after Dame Cicely was something akin to looking after the Queen. I knew who she was but was under strict instructions by the consultant that she was to have the utmost attention. This wasn't difficult as she was a very engaging patient. Dame Cicely was on the 'special' ward for 'special' patients, that was at the top of the hospital with single rooms, for a talc pleurodesis for the malignant effusion she had developed. It must have been a painful procedure but she seemed quite un-phased by the admission and happily chatted to me, mainly about the view. She had three bottles of whisky on a shelf in her room and I mentioned that was quite a collection to have in hospital and to congratulate her on getting them past the nursing staff, to which she replied with a glint in her eye that they were for her 'visitors'[108].

After twelve days of successful treatment, Cicely went to St Christopher's, where it looked like she would spend Christmas 2003; but, responding to antibiotics, she quickly improved further and was back at 50 Lawrie Park Gardens before the festive season got underway. She was showing her 'usual resilience'. On the one hand, happy with the quick turnaround in her symptoms, she was also ambivalent: 'Quite frankly, David, I thought I'd probably got a pleural effusion and thought "That's marvellous, God, because that means I might be getting ahead and getting off to Paradise, which would suit me down to the ground" '[109]. But that wasn't to be just yet.

Her two shots of radiotherapy had not been successful. The cancer spread from the hip into the pelvis. By the spring of 2004, it was becoming very difficult for Cicely to walk straight[110]. The orthopaedic surgeon said she would be walking round in circles soon. Joking apart, when he saw the x-ray his face darkened. She was presenting quite a clinical challenge and it was going to require quite a radical operation. She spoke welcomingly about the possibility of 'dying on the table'[111], but was at the same time still eager to see how things would progress at St Christopher's and in the hospice world beyond. She wished to call it a day, but also wanted to continue. The operation was carried out in May, in Guy's Hospital, London, and again she had the support of Bud, who smoothed the arrangements as much as she could. That autumn, Cicely described the procedure: 'I heard they were about two hours at it and they'd dug a lot of secondary out and put in a sort of plate and three screws, like my little finger, and sort of cement and so on. The oncologist brought me the x-ray to see, which did look as if they'd been pretty busy'[112]. She was in Guys Hospital for twelve days. She deemed the medical care 'excellent', the nursing 'quite good', the physiotherapy 'not so good'. Her brother Christopher visited her on a couple occasions, there were masses of flowers, and she began to improve quite quickly. To convalesce, she went to St Christopher's. There, in the following weeks, from the patient perspective, she did a similar personal audit of the care being practised. At the hospice, the physiotherapy was 'very good' and the nursing 'wonderful'. If not everyone was 'absolutely terrific', some were 'outstanding'. As her strength came back, she began to watch more carefully what was going on around her, even eavesdropping on conversations with other patients.

As my room was opposite the day room, where families would be going when a patient was admitted and were sitting around and so on, what impressed me was to watch them gradually being settled and comforted and children playing in a sort of different way during the course of the morning when they stayed two or three hours after grandmother was admitted. Quite a few of them came across and said 'Hello' and they saw my name on the open door. And they kept saying, 'Everybody here is so kind,' and I talked to one family and one of the sons who's a night-time taxi driver came across and was talking to me and said, 'What made you do this?' and I gave him a bit of sort of history of the question of pain and all, and isolation of patients and so on. But after he'd gone, I thought that I'd left out that I really did this as a vocation. Well, as it happened, the next day his sister came in and I said, 'You know, I really left something out when I was talking to your brother', and I just briefly mentioned it. But the day after that he came to say goodbye because he knew I was going out almost immediately and our chairman was sitting with me, and so I said to him, you know, 'And I was talking to you about how it started and it was really important, this is something that God wanted done, and so if you find yourself saying, "Why should God have let my mother have had cancer and where is he in this?", where he is, is he got the Hospice Movement started and he got St Christopher's there to welcome her'. And I was quite glad to have a chance of saying that in front of the chairman[113].

Cicely didn't have much pain and got moving quite quickly. But her bowels ('par for the course') continued to give 'endless problems'. Returning home, she was hugely reassured that her carer, Dell, was there to help her. Described by Cicely as 'a dynamic sixty-five-year-old Jamaican who's been a very senior nurse and midwife too, ran a home for the elderly for about fifteen years, and has a great sense of humour', she and Cicely had been together since late 2003. Cicely adored her and benefitted hugely from the daily help. Dell came from eight to nine in the morning and from six to eight in the evening. Along with Wendy, the cleaner, she ensured Cicely was safe and secure. With St Christopher's around the corner, Barry on hand to drive her when needed, practical care at home, and the ever-watchful eye of Christine Kearney, Cicely was getting through some major medical challenges but, more and more, turning her attention to her own demise.

Before 2004 ended, she was going back into her office in the hospice, sitting at her desk, and meeting people on a couple of occasions each week. She gave up the ritual of Coming Day, though she made an exception in one case for a twenty-fifth anniversary. She missed going in to welcome the families of patients who had died a year earlier. On these occasions, her themes had always been about memories, about not feeling guilty if they weren't there at the last moment, and the importance of recalling a whole life — not just the last part of it, which might have been difficult. She missed the life of St Christopher's but was less sad about it than she had expected. If she worried about how spiritual care at the hospice had gone after the retirement of Len Lunn as chaplain, she had faith that it would go on developing, if not in the way she had originally envisaged. She could 'trust God to keep an eye on it'[114].

As had now become her pattern at Christmas, after attending the morning service in St Christopher's she spent the rest of the day in 2004 with Bud and her family[115]. In the new year she wrote the foreword for an edited collection about palliative care in Ireland. Christine Kearney came to her home every day with the post. Dell was there morning and evening. Then one morning Cicely had severe pain in her hip, she could no longer bear weight on her right leg, and was placed on a larger dose of oxycodone. The situation was 'tiresome', but it did not prevent her attending the Foundation Group at the hospice or from holding the prayer group at home or from writing a piece of one thousand words on Elizabeth Kübler-Ross in which she likened the two of them to the blades in a pair of scissors: one focussed on changing public attitudes, the other on the recognition that pain could be overcome. But in her talks with Bud every weekend, it was clear things were becoming more and more difficult. They got the flat above ready for a live-in carer. She then had a fall and had to call for emergency services. Dell attentively laid out her lunch on leaving each morning and did everything she could to help Cicely, who was now only able to move around her rooms with the aid of a rather incongruous tea trolley for support. She never grumbled to Dell, but her carer could see that, at times, she was 'grey with pain'. Cicely was taken on by the St Christopher's home-care service and her G.P. called to see her. But when another x-ray was done which showed the cancer now far advanced round the pelvis (a procedure during which she painfully pulled a muscle in her shoulder), it was decided she must go back into the hospice. A week's respite for Dell to take a holiday had already been booked for Easter at the end of March, but now things were brought forward. On the afternoon of Friday, 25 February 2005, paradoxically the anniversary of David Tasma's death, with snow on the ground and no ambulance available, Cicely was pushed in a wheelchair from her home in Lawrie Park Gardens to St Christopher's in Lawrie Park Road. She was accompanied by the hospice medical director, Nigel Sykes, who carried her suitcase and belongings. With the hospice physiotherapist taking care of the wheelchair, the three made an unlikely procession.

Cicely considered that Dell had given her an extra eighteen months at home, but she was now established in a single room on Nuffield Ward (Figure 6.2). Despite this, her anxieties rose. The Draper's Wing, which would have been highly suited to her situation, had gone. In these modern days of 'acute'

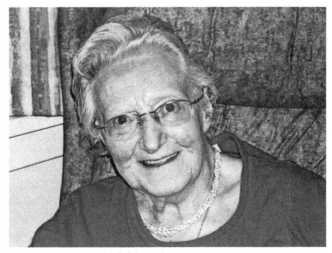

FIGURE 6.2 Last months at St Christopher's. *Source: David Clark.*

palliative care, with hospice length of stay influenced by commissioners, it might not be possible to remain there for an uncertain, possibly extended duration. The thought of being 'shunted off to a nursing home', hinted at on some occasions, appalled her. Matron stepped in to give reassurance; the whole matter had been agreed with the Primary Care Trust and Cicely was staying where she was. She admitted she had begun to feel lonely at home. This was 'home from home'. Nowhere else could have been more familiar. There was light, movement, interest, a constant stream of visitors, and a twenty-four-hour sense of being safe. She was 'very much in the hub of things' and soon had an established daily routine:

> I do get extremely tired by the evening. I'm in bed by seven and dozing, but I wake up early and have a cup of tea at about six and do my morning reading because if I don't get it done then and the prayers said, it doesn't happen later in the day, and it's nice to do that then. And I get my hot-water bottle refurbished a couple of times in the night when I get out for the commode, and I suppose I've got to come to terms with the degree of disability. I have breakfast about half past eight and then somebody helps me with a wash and dress, so I'm sort of up and in my chair by about half past ten, and lunch at half past twelve and visitors popping in and out. What I'm quite frankly hoping is that the cancer's going to turn up somewhere else. With this, one may go on for months and years even, and that, I think, would be a bit tiresome. I really don't want to go on indefinitely, but we don't have a choice unless the euthanasia people would think so and I can't be saying that after all I've said about them in the past[116].

But in the same breath she continued to talk of tasks and projects which were keeping her going. Christine Kearney saw her every day to go through the post and keep up with her correspondence. She began to think of her room at the end of Nuffield Ward as a mini Draper's Wing. She liked the new hospice chaplain and being able to go to chapel. When the good weather came, Mary Baines and others were able to push her down the roads to home in her wheelchair, where she could do some sorting out.

In the next few months, the visitors came in droves. There were many goodbyes, that she bore with great fortitude. Nevertheless, she felt it was all taking too long, and told Christine Kearney she was not 'dying well'. On 3 June she even received an honorary degree from the University of Bath, at a ceremony in the conservatory on Nuffield Ward. That month, as the full English summer came into bloom, she was still discussing Lord Joffe's euthanasia bill with Baroness Finlay. She asked Gillian Ford if she had really done enough in her life. She was able to see the cover of the new book of her selected writings, due out later in the year, and even hoped she might be sending it to friends at Christmas[117]. Her eighty-seventh birthday came and went with modest celebration. When Tom West called her, they went through the hospice farewell mantra: 'sorry, thank you, goodbye'. She told another visitor: 'I have been a nurse, I have been a social worker, and I have been a doctor, but the hardest thing of all is learning to be a patient'. Towards the end of the month there was a crisis point, when Cicely contracted a chest infection. Visibly shaking, Nigel Sykes discussed with her the option of using anti-biotics or letting nature taking its course. She looked at him with her characteristically steely eye — and opted for the anti-biotics. Next morning, she was much improved and sitting up in bed eating porridge.

It ushered in the final period of farewells, and she used the brief time purposefully. Then everything came crashing back and her condition worsened. She told Christine Kearney she would be gone within a week. As Cicely's life began to expire, death on a mass scale came to London in a series of terrorist explosions that took place on the public transport system during 7 July, killing fifty-two people and injuring more than seven hundred others. As London and its people tried to make sense of what had happened, Cicely's condition was deteriorating. This time, there would be no treatment. Her lungs, full of fluid and presumably tumour, were causing severe breathlessness. Though emotionally and spiritually ready for death, it took time to loosen her physical grip on life. For three days she could no longer be roused. Rosemary Burch was there at night and Christine Kearney was her constant companion in the daytime. The hospice chaplain, Andrew Goodhead, also spent extended periods of time sitting at the bedside.

On 14 July 2005, senior colleagues and trustees gathered for St Christopher's annual general meeting, something Cicely had always enjoyed and prepared for meticulously. It would be the first one to be held without her, though her dying presence pervaded the meeting. At the noon hour, a bell sounded in the hospice to commence two minutes' silence for those who had died in the bombings of the previous week. As the city of London in which she had spent most of her life came to a grieving standstill, so Cicely gave one big sigh, and her life came to an end. The 'exacting joy' was over.

Notes

1. Cicely Saunders interview with David Clark, 19 February 2003.

2. Cicely Saunders letter to Margaret and Mary Scott, 8 January 1985; Clark D. *Cicely Saunders: Founder of the Hospice Movement: Selected Letters 1959–1999.* Oxford: Oxford University Press; 2002: 256–257 (hereafter *Letters*).

3. Sam Klagsbrun interview with Neil Small, Hospice History Project, 27 February 1996.

4. Cicely Saunders interview with David Clark, 16 May 2000.

5. du Boulay S., with Rankin M. *Cicely Saunders: The Founder of the Modern Hospice Movement.* London: SPCK; 2007 edn.

6. Cicely Saunders letter to Grace Goldin, 30 April 1986; Clark, *Letters*, 281–282.

7. Cicely Saunders letter to Marty Herrman, 27 January 1987; Clark, *Letters*, 290.

8. Tom West interview with Neil Small, Hospice History Project, 28 January 1997.

9. Cicely Saunders letter to Sam Klagsbrun, 20 March 1992; King's College London Archives, SAUNDERS, Dame Cicely (1918 – 2005), Correspondence and related papers, 1948 – 2005, K/PP149/3/1-5.

10. Tom West interview with Neil Small, Hospice History Project, 28 January 1997.

11. Cicely Saunders letter to Professor Geoffrey Hanks, 8 June 1992; Clark, *Letters*, 340–341.

12. Dunlop R., Hockley J., eds. *Terminal Care Support Teams: The Hospital–Hospice Interface*. Oxford: Oxford University Press; 1990.

13. Cicely Saunders letter to Dr William Lamers, 4 August 1992; Clark, *Letters*, 341.

14. Cicely Saunders letter to The Right Honourable Virginia Bottomley, M.P., 18 November 1992; Clark, *Letters*, 34–3.

15. *Report of the House of Lords Select Committee on Medical Ethics*. HL Paper 21. London: Her Majesty's Stationery Office; 1994.

16. Cicely Saunders letter to Professor Balfour Mount, 11 March 1994; Clark, *Letters*, 350.

17. Cicely Saunders letter to Sam Klagsbrun, 14 January 1994; Clark, *Letters*, 348–349.

18. Saunders C., Kastenbaum R., eds. *Hospice Care on the International Scene*. New York: Springer; 1997.

19. Cicely Saunders Christmas letter to friends and colleagues, December 1999; Clark, *Letters*, 378–379.

20. Cicely Saunders interview with David Clark, 25 September 2003.

21. Cicely Saunders letter to Grace Goldin, 30 January 1986; Clark, *Letters*, 274–275.

22. Cicely Saunders letter to Dr Halina Bortnowska, 5 August 1986; Clark, *Letters*, 285.

23. Cicely Saunders letter to Professor Balfour Mount, 27 August 1986; Clark, *Letters*, 287.

24. Cicely Saunders letter to Marty Herrman, 27 January 1987; Clark, *Letters*,: 290.

25. Cicely Saunders letter to Soeur Gilberte, 19 November 1987; Clark, *Letters*, 301–302.

26. Cicely Saunders letter to Dr Josefino Magno, 11 January 1988; Clark, *Letters*, 302–303.

27. Cicely Saunders letter to Dr Robert Kastenbaum, 17 June 1988; Clark, *Letters*, 307.

28. Cicely Saunders letter to Sandol Stoddard, 17 October 1988; Clark, *Letters*, 309.

29. Cicely Saunders interview with David Clark, 16 May 2000.

30. Cicely Saunders interview with David Clark, 12 December 2001.

31. Cicely Saunders interview with David Clark, 22 December 2003.

32. Quoted from du Boulay with Rankin (*Cicely Saunders*, 208) and attributed to Cicely.

33. Cicely Saunders interview with David Clark, 14 March 2000.

34. Hillier R. Palliative medicine, a new specialty. *British Medical Journal*. 1988; 297: 874–875.

35. Doyle D. Palliative medicine: The first 18 years of a new sub-specialty of General Medicine. *Journal of the Royal College of Physicians of Edinburgh*. 2005; 35: 199–205.

36. Cicely Saunders letter to Dr Josefina Magno, 11 January 1988; Clark, *Letters*, 303.

37. World Health Organization. *Cancer Pain Relief and Palliative Care*. W.H.O. Technical Report Series 804. Geneva: World Health Organization; 1990.

38. Cicely Saunders letter to Dr Jan Stjernsward, 7 February 1991; Clark, *Letters*, 329.

39. Sepúlveda C., Marlin A., Yoshida T., Ullrich A. Palliative care: The World Health Organization's global perspective. *Journal of Pain and Symptom Management*. 2002; 24(2): 91–96.

40. Saunders C. A response to Logue's 'Where hospice fails — The limits of palliative care'. *Omega*. 1995/1996; 32(1): 1–5.

41. Saunders C. And from sudden death . . . . *Nursing Times*. 1962; August 17: 1045–1046.

42. James N., Field D. The routinization of hospice: Charisma and bureaucratisation. *Social Science and Medicine*. 1992; 34(12): 1363–1375.

43. Bradshaw A. The spiritual dimension of hospice: The secularisation of an ideal. *Social Science and Medicine*. 1996; 43(3): 409–419.

44. Cicely Saunders interview with David Clark, 14 March 2000.

45. Cicely Saunders interview with David Clark, 14 March 2000.

46. Cicely Saunders interview with David Clark, 14 March 2000.

47. Cicely Saunders interview with David Clark, 14 March 2000.

48. Cicely Saunders interview with David Clark, 20 September 2000.

49. Cicely Saunders interview with David Clark, 20 September 2000.

50. Cicely Saunders interview with David Clark, 19 December 2000.

51. Cicely Saunders interview with David Clark, 12 December 2001.

52. Cicely Saunders interview with David Clark, 12 December 2001.

53. Cicely Saunders interview with David Clark, 6 June 2002.

54. Schmidt E. Rediagnosing "Founder's Syndrome": Moving beyond stereotypes to improve nonprofit performance. *Non Profit Quarterly*. 2013; July 1, https://nonprofitquarterly.org/2013/07/01/rediagnosing-founder-s-syndrome-moving-beyond-stereotypes-to-improve-nonprofit-performance/, accessed 22 April 2017.

55. du Boulay with Rankin, *Cicely Saunders*.

56. Hoerl C. *Cicely Saunders: Brücke in eine andere Welt*. Freiburg: Herder Spektrum; 1999.

57. Something Understood, http://genome.ch.bbc.co.uk/3b14279d142347dda7f0ea1 aafb0ff3f, accessed 10 August 2017.

58. B.B.C., 'Desert Island Discs', http://www.bbc.co.uk/programmes/b006qnmr, accessed 26 February 2017.

59. Cicely Saunders interview with David Clark, 25 September 2003.

60. Booth C. The woman who changed the face of death. *Good Housekeeping*. 2002; October: 64–66.

61. Booth, The woman who changed the face of death, 66.

62. Brown G. *Courage: Eight Portraits*. London: Bloomsbury; 2007: 204.

63. Cicely Saunders interview with David Clark, 25 September 2003.

64. Cicely Saunders interview with David Clark, 12 December 2001.

65. Dickson EJ. Painting Dame Cicely. *The Times*. 2005; May 7: 22.

66. Robert Twycross tribute at memorial service for Cicely Saunders, Westminster Abbey, 8 March 2006, http://www.pallcare.ru/en/?p=1229768584&id=1238830227, accessed 15 April 2017.

67. Cicely Saunders interview with David Clark, 19 December 2000.

68. du Boulay S. *Cicely Saunders: The Founder of the Modern Hospice Movement*, 2nd ed. London: Hodder and Stoughton; 1994: 54.

69. Mathews J.A. Consultant rheumatologist at St Thomas's Hospital (1966–1990), died 13 September 2004, http://www.bmj.com/content/suppl/2005/01/20/330.7484.200-f.DC1, accessed 4 February 2017.

70. Cicely Saunders interview with David Clark, 23 August 1999.

71. Cicely Saunders interview with David Clark, 23 August 1999.

72. Saunders C. Kjaerlighet. *Omsorg*. 2000; 1: 5–10.

73. Eternity, by William Blake (1757 – 1827).

74. Saunders, Kjaerlighet. Also: Talk for Norwegian Conference, June 1999, manuscript in possession of the author.

75. Caretto C. *Letters from the Desert*. London: Darton Longman & Todd; 1990.

76. Cicely Saunders interview with David Clark, 25 September 2003.

77. Cicely Saunders interview with David Clark, 23 August 1999.

78. Cicely Saunders interview with David Clark, 2 May 2003.

79. Cicely Saunders letter to Sister Antonia, 8 May 1990; Clark, *Letters*, 320.

80. Cicely Saunders letter to Sister Antonia, 11 August 1997; Clark, *Letters*, 369.

81. Cicely Saunders interview with David Clark, 12 December 2001.

82. Cicely Saunders manuscript of 31 March 1965, in possession of the author.

83. Cicely Saunders manuscript of 31 March 1965 in possession of the author.

84. Cicely Saunders interview with David Clark, 25 September 2003.

85. Cicely Saunders interview with David Clark, 25 September 2003.

86. Cicely Saunders Christmas letter to friends and colleagues, December 1996; Clark, *Letters*, 366–368.

87. Richard Lamerton interview with Neil Small, Hospice History Project, 30 January 1997.

88. Cicely Saunders interview with David Clark, 15 December 1999.

89. Cicely Saunders interview with David Clark, 22 December 2003.

90. Mayne M. *The Enduring Melody*. London: Dartman, Longman and Todd; 2006: 3.

91. Ridler A. Christmas and the common birth. In *Collected Poems*. Manchester: Carcanet; 2016: 16.

92. Cicely Saunders interview with David Clark, 15 December 1999.

93. Cicely Saunders interview with David Clark, 15 December 1999.

94. Cicely Saunders interview with David Clark, 15 December 1999.

95. Cicely Saunders interview with David Clark, 15 December 1999.

96. Cicely Saunders interview with David Clark, 15 December 1999.

97. Julian of Norwich. *Revelations of Divine Love*, trans. Elizabeth Spearing. London: Penguin Classics; 1998.

98. Cicely Saunders interview with David Clark, 20 September 2000.

99. Saunders C. Foreword. In Mayne M. *Learning to Dance*. London: Dartman, Longman and Todd; 2001: 1–2.

100. Cicely Saunders Christmas letter to friends and colleagues, 1998; Clark, *Letters*, 375–376.

101. Cicely Saunders interview with David Clark, 12 December 2001.

102. Cicely Saunders interview with David Clark, 12 December 2001.

103. Cicely Saunders interview with David Clark, 6 June 2002; also the sources of quotes following in this section.

104. Cicely Saunders interview with David Clark, 22 December 2003.

105. Saunders C. Consider Him. In Saunders C. *Watch with Me*. Sheffield: Mortal Press; 2003: 48, 39–50.

106. Cicely Saunders interview with David Clark, 25 September 2003.

107. Cicely Saunders interview with David Clark, 22 December 2003.

108. Pers. comm. to the author.

109. Cicely Saunders interview with David Clark, 22 December 2003.

110. Cicely Saunders interview with David Clark, 5 October 2004.

111. Telephone conversation with the author.

112. Cicely Saunders interview with David Clark, 5 October 2004.

113. Cicely Saunders interview with David Clark, 5 October 2004.

114. Cicely Saunders interview with David Clark, 5 October 2004.

115. Cicely Saunders interview with David Clark, 9 March 2005.

116. Cicely Saunders interview with David Clark, 9 March 2005.

117. Saunders C. *Selected Writings 1958–2004*. Oxford: Oxford University Press; 2006.

Epilogue: Making Sense of Cicely Saunders

C ICELY SAUNDERS MARRIED LATE in life and had no children. Her closest personal relationships were complicated. Her steely look and assured manner masked years of vulnerability, poor self-image, and struggles with her femininity. She got into situations where the boundaries between her personal and professional life were seriously blurred. Her commitment to a lifetime of service to others was forged in the crucible of twentieth-century war, and she became the unlikely pioneer of an improbable movement. Stripping away the hagiography and the sheer mass of plaudits, there is no doubt she shaped a new field of medicine which was gaining significant ground by the time of her death, and one which made further progress in the decade following. A whole generation of palliative-care professionals was trained at St Christopher's, the hospice she founded, and many of them spread their knowledge and expertise in other places. The hospice ideal transferred and translated around the world — and eventually led to universal support through the encouragement of the W.H.O. This epilogue contains a brief assessment of her legacy — and the complex and demanding life that shaped it.

Reverberations

When Cicely died, the obituaries and tributes came flooding in. They appeared in the major broadsheet newspapers, periodicals, academic journals, and newsletters, and on websites. They came from contributors in many countries. In the main, they followed well-trodden ground. Most of them did not stint on hyperbole. As the *Times* put it, Cicely was the '[v]isionary founder of the modern hospice movement who set the highest standards in care for the dying'[1]. *The Telegraph* observed: 'Though she was widely revered as a sort of secular saint, it was only through being tough and authoritative, and often downright difficult, that she succeeded in forcing the medical profession to acknowledge what medicine can do for the dying'[2].

Cicely had been assiduous in creating and re-creating her own biographical narrative. Now its major landmarks, twists, turns, and accompanying aphorisms were well documented in the accounts of those who saluted her. The obituary writers crammed a life into a few hundred words, often with enviable clarity and insight. If Cicely was one of scores about whom they had written, their respect and admiration were nevertheless palpable. Others wrote as those who had known her, had seen her influence in their own lives, and had become caught up in the *habitus* of hospice and palliative care. In this context, Balfour Mount deserves particular mention[3].

Writing in the world's first-ever specialist publication in the field, the Canadian–based *Journal of Palliative Care*, Mount drew together a series of personal observations and snapshots. Starting with the well-told story of how he had first come to know and work with Cicely at St Christopher's, he referred to her as a 'hurricane', and spoke of her 'bulldog leadership' and 'penchant for candid expression of her opinions'. One of many that came to mind was an occasion in March 1981, at a symposium on human value organised by Richard Lamerton and held in the presence of His Royal Highness (H.R.H) Prince Philip. The opening speakers were South American liberation theologian Dom Helder Camara, followed by American civil rights activist and politician Jesse Jackson. They each 'stunned and humbled' the audience. Yet during the interval, over coffee, H.R.H. declared them to have been 'wide of the mark'. Lamerton and Mount were at first uncharacteristically lost for words, before blankly nodding agreement. Cicely was not one to concur. 'Nonsense!' she declared forcefully. 'They were absolutely marvellous'. Relief exuded from the tongue-tied colleagues and H.R.H. was apparently highly amused as well.

There must be a thousand such stories of Cicely's direct-ness, but Mount also highlights some of her other capacities — an enquiring mind (at age seventy-six, Cicely told Mount that 'one must stay curious; stay on the learning curve') and a capacity for growth until the very end. On the latter, he quotes a remark she made to me in 2002, and which I used in the introduction to *Watch with Me*: 'I don't believe so many things today as I did before, but my beliefs now are certainly held more deeply'[4]. Ultimately, for Mount, as for others, her death was also a renewed call to action. The work she had started was still unfinished. Much remained to be done. It was time to 'get on with it'. As her long-time friend concluded, 'Cicely's legacy is now in our hands'[5].

That legacy was fully articulated at her memorial service in Westminster Abbey on 7 March 2006, a warm, rainy spring day which saw a packed congregation set the seal on all she had been and all she had accomplished. They came from many countries and constituencies — kith and kin, colleagues, friends, devotees, admirers, and representatives of wider institutions. The mood was calm, expectant, but also troubled, with a curious mixture of oscillating sorrow and joy. There were two extended tributes[6]. Robert Twycross was eloquent in teasing out Cicely's personal and professional qualities, and he portrayed her unequivocally as the 'wounded physician' who had thereby been enabled more readily to empathise with and support the patients and families who came under her care. Sam Klagsbrun saw her as a leader of biblical proportions, whose strength came from the power of her personal example and of her teachings. As their words faded into the nooks and crannies of the Abbey, they were followed by the notes of Vaughan Williams's 'The Lark Ascending', once again played by Damian Falkowski, along with Robert Quinney at the organ. The congregation made a collective re-dedication to follow Cicely's example. The final hymn was 'Ye Holy Angels Bright, Who Wait at God's Right Hand'. Cicely had run her earthly race and could now behold the face of her Saviour.

For those left behind, there was much still to do. Cicely had broken through the carapace of indifference to the dying which had been allowed to develop in the modernising ethos of the British National Health Service and the wider culture of medicine. She had done this by stepping off the tracks and creating a charitable alternative to state provision, but nevertheless one which, over time, had increasingly to work with the structures and procedures of the public health system. Although home care had been a key feature at St Christopher's from the early years, hers was still largely an institutional model. The teaching, the research, the public face and presence, the diverse forms of care and support at St Christopher's were very much focussed on the hospice building itself. It fell to her successors to turn the hospice inside out and re-balance its orientation to the local community. More widely, the Hospice Movement would have to re-appraise its role now that palliative care had moved from the margins of medicine and health care into a much more central position of concern and recognition[7]. Within a decade of her death, there was in England a national strategy for end-of-life care, a palliative medicine professor in charge of it, and a growing desire to 'roll out' the principles of hospice into mainstream settings where they could benefit larger numbers of patients and families. As this unfolded, it was hard for some not to see a diminution in Cicely's influence and approach. New rhetorics were emerging — of choice, quality improvement, personalised care, and shared decision making. Cicely would have had no problem with any of these, but would have wanted to know *to what end?* The response of *better measurable outcomes* may not have fully satisfied her. Hospice, as Claude Levi Strauss might have put it, should be 'good to think' as well as 'good to do'. It should be about meaning just as much as action. Deep engagement with patients and families, the attention to personhood, the possibilities and contradictions of belief, the mysteries of doubt and uncertainty might all prove difficult to maintain within a changing external environment. This slightly uneasy combination of priorities was in evidence a decade after her death when, in the summer of 2015, many of her friends and colleagues gathered at St Christopher's for an afternoon titled 'Remembering Cicely'. Everyone present was holding on to her memory in some way, but among the touching personal recollections, there were also contributions which pointed to the unfolding legacy of Cicely's work — the international spread of hospice and palliative care and, in particular, the milestone resolution, passed one year earlier by the World Health Assembly, calling on all governments to integrate plans for palliative care into their national health strategies[8].

Despite these achievements, within a decade of her death some concerns were also being raised about her *diminishing* influence and the threat this posed to the 'essence' of palliative care. There was a sense that some aspects of Cicely's early vision and direction were being lost, thereby stimulating countervailing arguments about maintaining and nourishing her under-pinning ideas and Christian beliefs, and their relevance to contemporary palliative care, some of which configured around a sustained interest in her *Watch with Me* collection[9].

Capacities and Contradictions

Cicely had a work rate, energy, and a measure of resilience that astonished those who knew her. Her detailed letters show how, over many decades, she laboured to achieve her multiple goals. She had to create organisational strategies to test out and deliver her ideas. She needed clinical acumen and experience to forge a more meaningful philosophy of care in the shadow of modern medicine. She had to raise money, garner support from others, commission a building, develop its programmes of work, and engage with the countless enthusiasts who were drawn to it.

Robert Twycross observed in Westminster Abbey that Cicely was fond of saying: 'I did not found hospice; hospice found me'[10]. The notion has a hermeneutical feel about it. We can over-inflate our agency in the creation of things. Sometimes those things seek us out and compel us accordingly. As musician and writer Robin Williamson puts it: 'I sing to send songs back to themselves'[11]. The origin of things can be outside us, yet feel deeply a part of us. In Cicely's case, we can probably infer that God had sent hospice to find her — just like Mrs G.'s God, who sent people to tell her stories. For Cicely, as for her American colleagues, from whom she probably acquired the notion, hospice was an adjective as well as a noun. The noun refers to the formal organizational structures in which hospice care is delivered — the setting or building, the mode of delivery. The adjective describes the conceptual framework of care — the premise that when the quantity of life is limited, then the quality of life must be optimal. There are connections between the two and, clearly for Cicely, there was something about the inter-twining setting and philosophy that was very powerful indeed. Recalling the historical roots of hospice but acknowledging the modern variant, she observed: 'Hospice has come a long way in a short time . . . but the match today between "mind and heart" has opened up new possibilities of humanising life as well as death'[12].

One specific combination of capacity and contradiction in Cicely was her propensity to bring herself into the narrative. Encompassed in assured and upper-middle-class tones and values, Cicely lived in a self-referential world. Her ability to empathise with patients and families, to capture the apparent essence of their concerns, was often articulated in ways that brought recognition to her as somehow the conduit for the expression of their discontents. In later years she picked up on the idea of hospice as a 'voice for the voiceless', but so often it was her own voice that predominated in this. She was fond of referring to public speaking as 'a drug of addiction', but it was a habit she could not kick. She was always happy with an audience, whether it was one person visiting in her office or a gathering of thousands at an international meeting.

Another contradiction within Cicely was her tendency sometimes to trample over established boundaries, protocols, and norms. Despite her impeccable manners and poise, she could ride roughshod over conventions of practice, formal organisation, or rule keeping. This seems perplexing in one who was a nurse, a social worker, and a doctor, and was therefore no stranger to matters of professional ethics. Perhaps in a later era it could have been her downfall. Somehow, she turned the stories of David and Antoni into the founding myths of the Hospice Movement, when it might have gone the other way. Without the indulgence, or perhaps the studied myopia, of some of those around her at the time, these events could indeed have been her downfall. It is an astonishing thought that the early hospice ideal might have foundered on professional admonishment or disgrace. Instead, boundary blurring, if not outright rule breaking, was built into the story of its evolution.

Cicely wrote more than fifty pieces in which religious and spiritual matters featured centrally. A similar number touched on these issues more tangentially. Interestingly, they were spread evenly across her entire publishing career. As Ruth Ashfield[13] has identified, these works highlight a number of dimensions, including Cicely's personal journey, questions of pain and suffering, witnessing to pain, and the biblical themes of fall, sin, suffering, and death. Cicely's faith was interwoven in all of this. It sustained decades of personal enquiry and searching that deepened as she grew older. Even in the times when Marian was at his most dependent, and notwithstanding du Boulay's comments about her prayer life at that time, Cicely was still reading Julian of Norwich in the bath, eager to replenish her spiritual capacity and deepen her understanding. She never lost her capacity for reading, for serious reflection, and for seeking out an intellectual world that could illuminate her questions and shed light on her faith. This was also harnessed to a sense of daily discipline in prayer and worship. Ultimately, she did not need to found a closed community to establish her own rule and order. Her daily pattern bolstered and nurtured her, not least in some of the sorrows and stresses of her last decade.

She remained implacably opposed to the practice of euthanasia. In her early writing, she begins by addressing euthanasia from a Christian perspective and went on to focus on how it denies any positive achievement in dying. In her later works, she discussed the questions of dependence, freedom, and the fact that the dying person exists in relation to others and in community. She became more and more convinced of the dangers of euthanasia leading to an obligation to die among older people. She was convinced of a slippery slope which would extend the criteria for euthanasia and accelerate its take-up, and she buttressed against this through the conviction that where palliative care is available, then the cry for life to be ended disappears. Her warnings have been born out in some contexts but not in others, and in one remarkable example in Flanders, euthanasia and palliative care have made common cause. If she preferred to debate with the protagonists of euthanasia about inherent rights and wrongs, much of the subsequent discussion has been about consequences rather than principles.

Future Scholarship and Influence

We are fortunate that Cicely retained a vast quantity of her correspondence, papers, and memorabilia. During the early 1960s, she casually remarked she would need an archivist one day to sort everything out. That process first got underway thirty years later; then, after her death, a huge quantum of material was consolidated at King's College London, in two tranches in 2006 from St Christopher's Hospice and the Saunders family, and then in 2009 from the papers held by me which had formed the initial tranche of cataloguing. At King's the collection is arranged into ten sub-series according to principal subject or type, and within each the ordering is chronological. Cicely's books are housed as a special collection within the King's College library and can also be accessed through the archive.

Over the years, Cicely held on to things, conscious of the legacy she was creating. Whilst she sought to appear casual about this — to be otherwise would have seemed self-serving — she was nevertheless deeply aware of the value and interest of these materials. They comprised files and correspondence, reports, offprints of articles, drafts of her own publications, notes and transcriptions of conversations with patients, and digests of her own vast reading. There were personal appointment diaries (made by Letts) that were maintained for almost sixty years. As we have seen, there were also the prayer diaries of the 1960s. Holidays and foreign visits were captured in travelogues, with photographs, brochures, and details of places of interest. She kept concert programmes, music scores, postcards from friends and family, and bundles of foreign stamps, some which she forgot to pass on to their intended recipients. She hoarded with a casual air, never sorting, tidying, or listing what she had, but always aware of its steady accumulation and, in many cases, future significance. There were thousands of slides for teaching and lecturing, typescripts of the talks that accompanied them (these often heavily annotated). From her American visits, she seems always to have returned with quantities of yellow quarto paper which she was fond of using for drafts and notes. She was an inveterate maker of lists. Sometimes, a tiny torn strip of paper would be retained — itemising things to do, odds and ends or clothing to be taken on holiday, people who should be sent postcards, or reminders of tasks to be undertaken. She had a prodigious collection of books, long-playing records, family photograph albums, and cuttings from newspapers and magazines. There were prizes, medals, and trophies which accompanied her major awards and many tours and lectures she undertook at home and abroad. And, of course, there were Marian's paintings, sketches, cartoons, and pastel works.

If all of this made up the ramshackle *bricolage* of her intense and varied life, it was still, after a fashion, 'curated'. When I first spoke to Cicely about archiving some of it, she proffered a false modesty as to its interest to others. But, this soon gave way to an active engagement in what might happen to it all after her death. It was as if she had been waiting for some formal acknowledgement of the question, whilst in the meantime, her papers accumulated in old cardboard boxes in the basement of St Christopher's, crammed on shelves under heating pipes, and were, on one occasion, damaged by flooding. During the late 1990s, she and I visited the beautifully constructed history of medicine archives at the headquarters of the Wellcome Trust, under the Euston Road in London. Her back went into spasm as we toured the meticulously ordered collection, but she was fascinated by the commitment to preservation and documentation that could be seen there. Eventually, as discussions about Cicely Saunders International got underway, it was clear to her that King's College London should house her archives, and work on this began soon after her death, though the full catalogue and collection were not opened for access until late 2015. As Yasmin Gunaratnum has observed, it is an archive that constitutes more than a collection of historical records in a physical space: '[I]t includes dreams, promises and windows'[14]. Seen in this way, an archive can be opened, but it also opens those who encounter it. The archive can create a fever in those who enter, thrilled by the journey of discovery, but also a susceptibility — as we move through and between the different objects and materials it comprises, we are in turn shaped by them.

Her publications merit particular attention. A bibliometric Ph.D. thesis of 2006 was dedicated to them[15]. It identified 340 works, of which 313 were 'formally published'. They included works translated into eight languages and published in eighteen countries other than the United Kingdom. The bibliography contains 110 journal articles, fifty-eight book chapters, thirty-seven prefaces, twenty-one published letters, eighteen authored or co-authored books or booklets, thirteen edited or co-edited books, ten editorials, twenty-seven published conference contributions, and a selection of other items including second or subsequent editions and re-prints. Although I possess most of these works, they need to be collated and preserved. The archive is an authentic guide to the context and time of their production, but there should be a catalogued library of her works which can be accessed easily by scholars and interested readers, preferably online.

For me, it is the letters and publications of Cicely Saunders that make up the 'solid ground' of her documentary legacy. Allowing for their textuality and situated character, recognising that the former have gaps, omissions, and perhaps deliberate deletions, nevertheless they provide a journey through her life and times that can be chronicled and detailed for a period of almost fifty years. Despite all of my own efforts in more than twenty years of study, I do not have the full measure of them. Far from it. Rather, I contend they yet hold much potential for research, interpretation, and verification in future years. Added to these are the shakier sources of oral testimony, interviews with Cicely and about Cicely, commentaries by journalists and other writers, documentary films, images, interpretative works of art — and much more.

As I conclude this work, the second full-length biography of Cicely Saunders to be attempted, I am left with a feeling of things not covered, areas unexplored, and paths not taken. Already I have begun to wonder what a third biographer will make of Cicely's life. I am also conscious that there is enormous scope for additional more detailed and focussed studies of aspects of her experience, work, philosophy, beliefs, and influences. I hope we will see more 'Saunders studies' emerge from scholars of varied disciplines. The potential is enormous and the value high. To paraphrase the famous remark of Norman Barrett, her mentor and inspiration: *There is so much more to be learned about Cicely.*

Notes

1. Cicely Saunders. *The Times*, July 15, 2005.

2. Dame Cicely Saunders, OM. *The Telegraph*, July 15, 2005, http://www.tele-graph.co.uk/news/obituaries/1494039/Dame-Cicely-Saunders-OM.html, accessed 12 January 2018.

3. Mount B. Snapshots of Cicely: Reflections at the end of an era. *Journal of Palliative Care*. 2005; 21(3): 133–135.

4. Clark D. Foreword. In Saunders C. *Watch with Me*. Sheffield: Mortal Press; 2003: xii.

5. Mount, Snapshots of Cicely.

6. For tributes to Cicely Saunders, http://www.stchristophers.org.uk/about/damecicelysaunders/tributes, accessed 2 September 2017.

7. Clark D. From margins to centre: A review of the history of palliative care in cancer. *The Lancet Oncology*. 2007; 8(5): 430–438.

8. World Health Organization. Strengthening of palliative care as a component of integrated treatment within the continuum of care. Document EB134.R7, http://apps.who.int/gb/ebwha/pdf_files/EB134/B134_R7-en.pdf, accessed 12 January, 2018.

9. See, for example, Larkin P. *Compassion: The Essence of Palliative and End-of-Life Care*. Oxford: Oxford University Press; 2016.

10. See Twycross tribute, http://www.stchristophers.org.uk/about/damecicelysaunders/tributes, accessed 2 September 2017.

11. Williamson R. I pray to God in God's absence. *The Island of the Strong Door*. Cardiff: Pig's Whisker Music; 1999.

12. Saunders C. Origins: International perspectives then and now. *The Hospice Journal*. 1999; 14(3/4): 1–7

13. Personal communication with the author, February 2013.

14. Gunaratnum Y. *Death and the Migrant*. London: Bloomsbury Academic; 2013: 27.

15. Whan P.J. The palliative care knowledge system: A case study of Cicely Saunders' pioneering role. Unpublished PhD dissertation. University of Queensland, 2006.

INDEX

References to figures are indicated with an italicized *f.*

Academy of Fine Art in Krakow, 138
Advances in Pain Research and Therapy
  (Bonica and Ventafridda), 224
Afrikaaner Bond political party, 19
Agam, Yaacov, 137
A.I.D.S., 234
Aldwinckle, Stella, 41
Allbrook, David, 54*f*, 55
The Allegory of Love (Lewis), 41
Allen, Mildred, 170
Allen, Sir Donald, 158, 160
All Nations Bible College, 48
Allport, Gordon, 170–71, 172, 173
All Souls, 53, 62, 71, 88, 89, 119,
  148, 157
almoner. *See* evangelical almoner
The Almoner (journal), 51
American Cancer Society, 170
American Journal of Nursing
  (journal), 144
American Psychiatric Association, 199
Amery, Shenda, 282, 298
Amin, Avnita, 159, 161
Amulree, Lord, 160, 251
Anderson, W. Ferguson, 238
Andrews, Lucilla, 35
Annals of the Royal College of Surgeons
  (journal), 136

Archway Hospital, 56, 59, 60
Aristotle Onassis Prize for Service to
  Humanity, 278
Ars Moriendi, 240
Ashfield, Ruth, 315
Association of Palliative Medicine,
  269, 271
awards, 242–44, 277–78

Bailey, Margaret, 133
Baines, Mary, 190, 193, 196, 198, 225,
  226, 232, 304
Banderanaike, S.W.R.D., 169
A Bar of Shadow (van de Post), 125
Barrett, Howard, 64
Barrett, Norman, 94, 318
  advice for getting into medicine, 76–77
  Cicely Saunders and, 71–81
  influence on Cicely, 71–81
  motivating and sowing seeds, 75–76
Barton, A. E., 188
Bates, Thelma, 231–32, 240
Bayes, Derek, 281
Becket, St. Thomas, 77
Beecher, Henry, 128
Beethoven, Ludwig van, 279
Bell, Gertrude, 30
Bellamy, John, 137

du Boulay, Shirley, 1, 5, 20, 34, 60, 87, 96, 97, 139, 211, 278, 292, 315
   biographer, 244–45
Duff, Ray, 195
Dundee, John W., 136
Dunlop, Robert, 263, 265, 267, 272, 273, 276, 291
Durrell, Gerald, 20
Dyke, Margaret, 54*f*

Earnshaw Smith, Elizabeth, 230
The Economist (magazine), 276
education
   Cicely at Roedean, 11–16, 12*f*, 140
   St. Christopher's Hospice, 197–200
Edwards, Muriel, 157
Edwards, Philip, 201
Edward VII (King), 24, 277
Edward VII Hospital, 297
Elgar, Edward, 277
Eliot, George, 53
Eliot, T. S., 277
Ella Lyman Cabot Trust, 171, 173
Ellie, Edward, 24
Elliot, Charlotte, 49
Emergency Bed Service, 108
emotional planning, 239
euthanasia, 111–12, 316
   case against, 130–31
   opposition to, 249–51
Euthanasia Education Council, 251
Euthanasia Society, 111
evangelical almoner
   conversion, 48–50
   new friendships, 52–55
   qualifying as, 55–56
   service of, 50–51
evangelical circles, 87–90
Evans, Anthony and Sidney, 195
Exton Smith, Arthur Norman, 111, 129–30, 131, 249

faith, ups and downs of building in, 164–69
Falkowski, Damian, 267, 290, 313
Faull, Christina, 136

Feifel, Herman, 172
Fellows, Sydney, 219
Ferrier, Kathleen, 279
first Oxford interlude, 29–33
   entering into war, 31–32
   making a decision, 32–33
   see also second Oxford interlude
First World War, 34, 45, 51, 138
Flagiole, Maria, 205
Foley, Kathleen, 227, 270
Foote, Meg, 48, 49, 89
Ford, Gillian, 103, 119, 190, 200, 202, 209, 229, 241, 269, 298, 304
Ford, John, 19
Ford, Sarah Christian, 19
Ford, Sir Edward, 273–74
Ford, Susan, 19, 20
Frankl, Viktor, 176, 232
Franklin D Roosevelt Four Freedoms Medal for Worship, 278
Franks, Oliver Sherwell, 14
Fraser, Antonia, 27*n*.20
The Friedenheim, 64, 74
Frost, David, 241–42
Fryer, John, 240, 251, 252
Fryer, John E., 199
Fundamentalism and Evangelicalism (Stott), 88

Galton, Barbara (Mrs G), 115, 189, 314
   case of, 84–87
   death of, 121
   inspiration of, 112–13
Galton, Helen, 190
Galton, Jack, 189
Gardner, Lilian, 22, 47, 202–3
Garnier, Jeanne, 233
Gault, Fernand, 85
Gavey, C. J., 213
George, Lloyd, 8
George Soros Foundation, 264
George VI (King), 71
Geriatrics (journal), 144
Gibbs, Peggy, 51
Gilbran, Kahil, 125
Gillie, Annis, 124

St. Mary's Hospital Gazette (journal), 65

St. Thomas's Hospital, 33, 34–35, 51, 55, 68n.88, 77–78, 174, 212, 279, 282, 285

St. Thomas's Hospital Gazette (journal), 5

Sancte e Sapienter, 77

Sandle, Michael, 137

Saunders, Barbara, 232

Saunders, Christopher Gordon Strode, 11, 124, 203, 301
  family dynamics, 20–22, 46
  holiday time, 23, 23f

Saunders, Cicely Mary Strode
  awards, 242–44, 277–78
  beginnings of, 7–8
  capacities and contradictions, 314–16
  challenges, 245–53
  changing roles, 251–53
  correspondence, 2
  death of, 3
  death of father, 121–23
  death of Marian, 267–68
  death of mother, 202–4
  death of Ron Welldon, 246–47, 246–54
  declining health of Marian, 264–68
  emerging to womanhood, 24–26
  emotional landscape of family, 8–11
  as evangelical almoner, 48–56
  evolving faith of, 294–96
  family dynamics of, 20–22
  father Philip Gordon Saunders, 16–18
  first Oxford interlude, 29–33
  friends, family and marriage, 201–12
  future scholarship and influence, 316–18
  at Hadley Hurst, 15–16, 25–26, 46
  holiday in Scotland, 23–24
  honours and plaudits, 241–44, 277–78
  illness and death of, 296–305
  influence of Norman Barrett, 71–81
  interactions with David Tasma, 56–62
  legacy of, 311–18
  life with Saunders, 20–24
  marriage to Marian Bohusz-Szyszko, 209–12, 252
  material living, 22–23, 23f

media engagements, 241–42

meeting biographer Shirley du Boulay, 244–45

meeting Marian Bohusz-Szyszko, 138–40

mother Mary Christian Knight, 18–20

nurse training in wartime, 33–40

opposition to euthanasia, 249–51

origin of name, 8

patients and their worlds, 81–87

personal rewards, 277–78

photograph, 236f, 303f

photograph in Roedean uniform, 12f

photograph of parents, 9f

photographs, 281–82

photograph with Balfour Mount, 235f

photograph with friends, 54f, 80f

photograph with mother, 10f

photograph with patient, 108f

'Polish kibbutz' of, 206–9

portrait, 283

reflections, 5–6

reverberations after death of, 311–14

revisiting Antoni's case, 284–87

at Roedean, 12f, 13–15

schooldays of, 11–16

sculpture, 282

second Oxford interlude, 40–48

separation of parents, 45–48, 126–27

see also doctor, becoming a

Saunders, Elizabeth, 16

Saunders, John Frederick Stacy, 9, 124, 203, 207
  family dynamics, 20–21, 46

Saunders, John Henry, 16

Saunders, Philip Gordon, 16–18, 102
  Dauntsey's Agricultural School, 17–18
  death of, 121–23
  family life, 8–11, 20–24
  John D. Wood and Co., 18
  photograph in later years, 81f
  photograph with wife, 9f
  separation from wife, 45–48
  support for daughter's medical studies, 76–77
  visit to Grandchamp, 121–23

Sayers, Dorothy L., 30, 43–44
Scheffer, Richard, 237
'The Scheme' (manifesto),
    147–48, 156–57
Schrödinger, Erwin, 79
science and art, of hospice, 214–17
Scotland, Saunders family in, 23–24
Scott, John, 218
Scott of the Antarctic (film), 53
second Oxford interlude, 40–48
    Dorothy L. Sayers, 43–44
    searching, 44–45
    Socratic Club and C. S. Lewis, 41–43
    see also first Oxford interlude
Second World War, 22, 35, 45, 51, 82, 88,
    138, 191, 206, 283
Selected Letters (Clark), 4
Selected Writings (Saunders), 2, 5
Sembal Trust, 162, 164, 167
Settlement Movement, 50–51
Shaw, George Bernard, 25
Sheppard, David, 197
Simpson, Sir John, 12
Sir Halley Stewart Clinical Research
    Fellow, 229
Sir Halley Stewart Trust, 102, 166
Sister of Charity
    Sister Zita Marie Cotter, 195, 202, 246
    See also Catholic Sisters
Small, Neil, 1, 4
Smalley, Stephen, 81, 292
Smith, Charles Saumarez, 282
Smith, Justin (Peter), 158, 161, 165, 168
Smith, Stevie, 79
social work, at hospice, 229–30
Society of Home Students, 29, 31, 33
Socratic Club, C.S. Lewis and, 41–43
Solomon, F. O., 17
Somerville College, Oxford, 14
Specialty Advisory Committee in General
    Medicine, 269
Speech Day, 14, 17
Stassen, Glen, 292
Steel, Joan, 121, 165
Stefan Batory University, 138
Stewart, Harold, 102, 163

Stjernsward, Jan, 240, 241, 270
St Mary's Hospital Medical School, 102
Stoke Mandeville Hospital, 86
Storr, Anthony, 124
Stott, John, 87, 88–90, 148, 156
Strauss, Anselm, 132, 144, 174
Strauss, Claude Levi, 313
Streptococcus, 111
Strode, Sir John, 19–20
Student Christian Movement, 34, 49
Summers, Dorothy, 198, 199–200, 231
Suu Kyi, Aung San, 281
Sweetser, Carleton, 172, 202, 211, 232
Swerdlow, Mark, 222, 228
Sykes, Nigel, 303, 305
Szyszko-Bohusz, Alicja, 265

Tasma, Ela Majer (David), 56–62, 68*n*.95,
    84, 115, 189, 231, 315
    Cicely revisiting the past, 287–88
    Cicely writing about, 118, 122, 146
    death of, 62–63
    funeral of, 61
    photograph of, 57*f*
The Telegraph (newspaper), 311
Temple, William, 44
Templeton Prize for Progress in
    Religion, 243
terminal care, 133–35
Thackeray, William Makepeace, 10
Thatcher, Margaret, 188, 277
The Therapy of Pain (Swerdlow), 228
Thompson, E. P., 50
Thurlow, Lord, 162, 165, 166, 245, 247
Tilby, Angela, 242
Time (magazine), 276
The Times (newspaper), 18, 64, 247,
    278, 311
Titchmarsh, Alan, 278
Tokirska, Harnia, 104
Tolkien, J.R.R., 41, 79
Tonsley, Cecil, 38–39
total pain, 125–28
    concept of, 221, 225
    exploration of, 225–27
transverse myelitis, 85

Trollope, Anthony, 10
Trotman, Dawson, 89
tuberculosis (T.B.), 72, 91, 265
  Brompton Cocktail for advanced,
    73–74, 109
Tucker, Geoffrey, 300
Tully, Mark, 278
Twycross, Robert, 193, 218, 222–25, 240,
    247, 270, 312, 314
Tyrrell, George, 125

Union Society, 251
United States, connections in
    hospice, 169–75
University of Glasgow, 14
University of Oxford. *See* Oxford,
    University of

van der Post, Laurens, 125
Vanier, Jean, 213
Vaughan Williams, Ralph, 53, 267,
    277, 279
Ventafridda, Vittorio, 224, 227, 228, 270
Venter, Henrik, 237
Vere, Duncan, 223, 224, 247
Veterans Administration, 172
vindauga (eye of the wind), 59
voluntary aid detachments (V.A.D.s), 33,
    35, 36, 40, 66*n*.17
Voluntary Hospital Movement, 91

Wald, Florence, 174, 195, 197, 202,
    245, 276
Walker, Ronald, 124
Wallace, Jack, 79, 148–50, 156, 158, 160,
    162, 165, 248
Wallace, Lucie, 149
Wallenberg, Raoul, 278, 281
Wallenstein, Stanley, 128
Wallis, Alfred, 22
war of 1914–1918, 8
Warren, Shirley, 21
Warsaw Uprising, 40
wartime, nursing training in, 33–40
Watch with Me (Saunders), 2, 312, 314

Water and Wine (Tyrrell), 125
Wates Foundation, 198
Watson, James, 82
Watts, George, 12
Weisman, Avery, 234
Weist, Verena, 189
Wellcome Trust, 1, 317
Wellcome Trust Investigator Award, 3
Welldon, Ron, 193, 223, 229
    death of, 246–47
Wells, H. G., 21
Wessel, Morris, 195
West, Betty, 119, 152
West, Tom, 78–80, 96–97, 98*n*.15, 119,
    190, 199, 200, 208, 209, 218, 225,
    236, 240, 251–52, 267, 305
    as medical director, 262–63
Westminster Pastoral Foundation, 264
Whittington Hospital, 59, 111
Wilkes, Eric, 131, 238, 239
Willans, Helen, 188, 190, 230, 273
Williamson, Robin, 314
Wilson, Harold, 167
Winner, Albertine, 157, 161, 195, 197,
    215, 218, 247, 251–52
Wolfson Foundation, 166–67, 198
The Women at Oxford (Brittain), 31
Wood, Barbara, 21
Wood, J. D., 21
Worcester, Alfred, 75, 94–95
World Health Assembly, 314
World Health Organization (W.H.O.),
    189, 240–41, 270, 311
World Wars. *See* First World War; Second
    World War
Worshipful Society of Apoethecaries, 243
Wren, Christopher, 15
Wright Mills, C., 4
writing
    American connections in, 145
    craft of, 140–41
    Nursing Times series of 1959, 141–43
    successes, 143–44
Wyon, Olive, 147, 150–52,
    153, 248